The Periodontic Syllabus

Fourth Edition

The Periodontic Syllabus FOURTH EDITION

Edited By

Peter F. Fedi, Jr., DDS, MS

Professor Emeritus
University of Missouri-Kansas City
Formerly:
Rinehart Professor of Dentistry
Director of Predoctoral Periodontics
Chairman of Advanced Education Program
University of Missouri-Kansas City School of Dentistry
Kansas City, Missouri

Arthur R. Vernino, DDS

Professor Emeritus
University of Oklahoma
Oklahoma City, Oklahoma
Courtesy Clinical Professor
University of Florida
Gainesville, Florida

Jonathan L. Gray, DDS

Associate Professor
Director of Graduate Periodontics
University of Florida, College of Dentistry
Gainesville, Florida

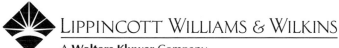

LIPPINCOTT WILLIAMS & WILKINS
A **Wolters Kluwer** Company
Philadelphia · Baltimore · New York · London
Buenos Aires · Hong Kong · Sydney · Tokyo

Editor: Larry McGrew
Managing Editor: Angela Heubeck
Marketing Manager: Debby Hartman
Production Editor: Lisa JC Franko
Design Coordinator: Mario Fernandez

Copyright © 2000 Lippincott Williams & Wilkins

351 West Camden Street
Baltimore, Maryland 21201-2436 USA

530 Walnut Street
Philadelphia, Pennsylvania 19106-3621 USA

Printed in the United States.

First Edition, 1985
Second Edition, 1989
Third Edition, 1995

Library of Congress Cataloging-in-Publication Data
The periodontic syllabus / [edited] by Peter F. Fedi, Jr., Arthur R.
  Vernino, and Jonathan L. Gray. — 4th ed.
      p.   cm.
    Includes bibliographical references and index.
    ISBN 0-683-30668-5
    1. Periodontics.   I. Fedi, Peter F.   II. Vernino, Arthur R.
  III. Gray, Jonathan L.
    [DNLM: 1. Periodontal Diseases.   WU 240 P4473 1999]
  RK 361.P462   1999
  617.6'32—dc21
  DNLM/DLC
  for Library of Congress   99-32590
                                                   CIP

The publishers have made every effort to trace the copyright holders for borrowed material. If they have inadvertently overlooked any, they will be pleased to make the necessary arrangements at the first opportunity.

To purchase additional copies of this book, call our customer service department at **(800) 638-3030** or fax orders to **(301) 824-7390.** For other book services, including chapter reprints and large quantity sales, ask for the Special Sales department.

For all other calls originating outside of the United States, please call **(301) 714-2324.**

Visit Lippincott Williams & Wilkins on the Internet: **http://www.lww.com.** Lippincott Williams & Wilkins customer service representatives are available from 8:30 am to 6:00 pm, EST, Monday through Friday, for telephone access.

02 03
3 4 5 6 7 8 9 10

Preface

The fourth edition of *The Periodontic Syllabus* reminds the editors and contributors that the ever-expanding information base in periodontics makes it difficult to "keep up to date." The practice of periodontics is dynamic and continually changing to reflect the evolving approaches to therapy. It is no wonder that the practicing dentist and dental hygienist find it difficult to keep current.

The fourth edition, just as its predecessors, attempts to focus attention on the biologic approach to treatment modalities. We strive to continue the "cookbook" approach for easy access to different methods for treating diseases of the periodontium and replacing missing components of the dental arches. *The Syllabus* is not a complete and detailed textbook, but it should complement the textbooks on the subject. Our objective is dedicated to present a concise and current syllabus.

We originally targeted the dental student and the general practitioner as primary users. Because more and more periodontal therapy is provided in the general practice, the dental hygienist's role has become increasingly important in the treatment of periodontal diseases. Consequently, a greater emphasis has been placed on including material that would be useful to the dental hygienist and the dental hygiene student.

We have received many requests to re-include the chapter on occlusion as it related to periodontal pathogenesis and treatment. This chapter, "The Role of Occlusion in Periodontal Health and Disease," addresses the status of occlusion and periodontal disease. In addition, the chapter on dental implants (Chapter 20) has been expanded. We may have covered too much material for a syllabus, but we did want to convey the need for cooperative treatment of patients requiring implants.

We welcome suggestions and critiques. Such critiques allow us to provide you, the user of *The Syllabus,* what you want and need. We expanded the reading lists for each chapter in the hope that the continuing student who desires more information on each subject will find these lists helpful.

We want to dedicate this edition to all of our contributors, past and present, without whom these four editions could not have been written.

Contributors

Jane Amme, RDH
Clinical Associate Professor
Department of Periodontics
University of Oklahoma College
  of Dentistry
Oklahoma City, Oklahoma

Sherry Burns, RDH, MS
Clinical Associate Professor
Department of Periodontics
University of Missiouri-Kansas City School
  of Dentistry
Kansas City, Missouri

Donald Callan, DDS, MS
Private Practice, Periodontics
  and Implant Dentistry
Little Rock, Arkansas

Peter F. Fedi, Jr., DDS, MS
Professor Emeritus
University of Missouri-Kansas City
Formerly:
Rinehart Professor of Dentistry
Director of Predoctoral Periodontics
Chairman of Advanced Education Programs
University of Missouri-Kansas City School
  of Dentistry
Kansas City, Missouri

Lorraine Forgas, RDH, MSHE
Assistant Professor, Department
  of Periodontics
University of Missouri-Kansas City School
  of Dentistry
Kansas City, Missouri

Marlin Gher, DDS, MSc
Private Practice, Periodontics
Chula Vista, California

Jonathan L. Gray, DDS
Associate Professor
Director of Graduate Periodontics
University of Florida, College
  of Dentistry
Gainesville, Florida

William J. Killoy, DDS, MS
Professor and Chairman, Department
  of Periodontics
Director of Clinical and Applied
  Research
University of Missouri-Kansas City School of
  Dentistry
Kansas City, Missouri, 64108

Joseph J. Lawrence, DDS, MS
Retired, Professor and Chairman,
  Department of Periodontics
Louisiana State University School
  of Dentistry
New Orleans, Louisiana

John Rapley, DDS, MS
Director of Advanced Education
  in Periodontics
Department of Periodontics
University of Missouri-Kansas City School of
  Dentistry
Kansas City, Missouri

Terry Rees, DDS, MS
Professor and Chair of Periodontics
Baylor College of Dentistry
Dallas, Texas

Arthur R. Vernino, DDS
Professor Emeritus
University of Oklahoma
Oklahoma City, Oklahoma
Courtesy Clinical Professor, University of
  Florida
Gainesville, Florida

Raymond A. Yukna, DMD, MS
Professor, Department
  of Periodontics
Coordinator of Postdoctoral
  Periodontics
Louisiana State University School
  of Dentistry
New Orleans, Louisiana

Contents

Preface.   v

Contributor List   vii

1   The Periodontium.   1

2   Etiology of Periodontal Disease.   14

3   Systemic Contributing Factors   22

4   Plaque-Related Periodontal Diseases: Pathogenesis   31

5   Host Defenses and Periodontal Disease.   41

6   Diagnosis, Prognosis, and Treatment Planning.   51

7   The Role of Occlusion in Periodontal Health and Disease   70

8   Plaque Control   75

9   Scaling and Root Preparation   86

10 Wound Healing.   96

11 Principles of Periodontal Surgery   107

12 Nonsurgical Antimicrobial Therapy: The Role of Antimicrobial
    Agents in the Treatment of Chronic Adult Periodontitis.   124

13 Management of Soft Tissue: Gingivoplasty, Gingivectomy,
    and Gingival Flaps.   136

14 Management of Soft Tissue: Flaps for Pocket Management   145

15 Management of Soft Tissue: Mucogingival Procedures   152

16 Management of Osseous Defects: Osseous Resective Surgery   160

17 Management of Osseous Defects: Bone Replacement Grafts.   168

18 Management of Osseous Defects: Furcation Involvement 174

19 Management of Osseous Defects: Additional Techniques
and Summary 181

20 Dental Implants 185

21 Implant Maintenance 201

22 Periodontal Emergencies 205

23 Periodontal Maintenance Therapy (Recall) 218

24 Mucocutaneous Diseases of the Periodontium 225

25 Instrument Sharpening 239

Index 251

The Periodontium

Peter F. Fedi, Jr.

The periodontium is composed of the gingiva, junctional epithelium, periodontal ligament, cementum, and alveolar process.

GINGIVA

Terminology

The gingiva is composed of keratinizing epithelium and connective tissue. The following terminology is used when describing the gingiva (Fig. 1-1):

1. *Marginal (free) gingiva.* The portion of the gingiva surrounding the neck of the tooth, not directly attached to the tooth, and forming the soft tissue wall of the gingival sulcus. It extends from the gingival margin to the gingival groove.
2. *Gingival groove.* The shallow line or depression on the surface of the gingiva dividing the free gingiva from the attached gingiva. The gingival groove often, but not always, corresponds to the location of the bottom of the gingival sulcus. The gingival groove is not always present.
3. *Keratinized gingiva.* The band of keratinized gingiva extending from the gingival margin to the mucogingival junction (Fig. 1-2). The width of the keratinized gingiva varies from less than 1 mm to 9 mm. Teeth that are prominent in the arch, such as the

mandibular canines and premolars, frequently have a narrow zone of keratinized gingiva. Coronally located frenum and muscle attachments are likewise associated with a narrow width of keratinized gingiva. Often, patients who maintain healthy keratinized gingiva have less than 1 mm of attached gingiva. However, no band of attached gingiva is present, and extension of the lip or cheek results in a pull on the free gingival margin, an increased susceptibility to tissue breakdown may result. An adequate width of attached gingiva may then be defined as the amount of keratinized tissue necessary to assist in maintaining the gingival margin in a stable position and in a state of health.

4. *Attached gingiva.* The portion of the gingiva extending apically from the area of the free gingival groove to the mucogingival junction. In the absence of inflammation, the attached gingiva is clearly defined, except in the hard palate where there is no clinical demarcation between the attached gingiva and the remaining masticatory mucosa. The attached gingiva is normally covered by keratinized or parakeratinized epithelium that has marked rete ridges extending into the connective tissue. There is no submucosa, and the attached gingiva is bound tightly down to the underlying tooth and

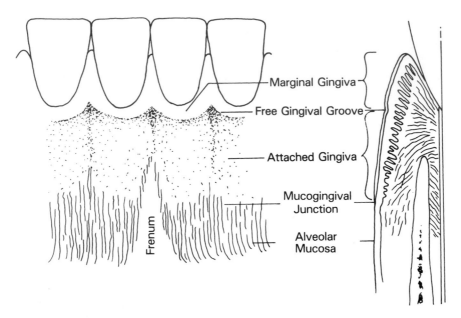

Fig. 1-1

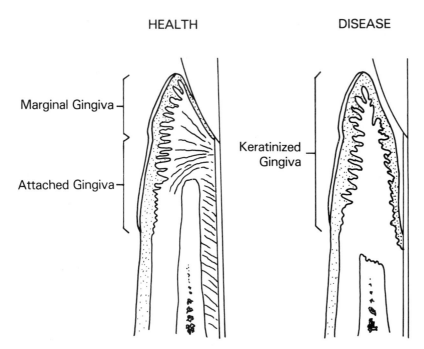

Fig. 1-2

bone. It is apparent that this part of the gingiva is designed to withstand the rigors of mastication, tooth brushing, and other functional stresses.

5. *Mucogingival junction.* The scalloped line dividing the keratinized gingiva from thc alveolar mucosa (Fig. 1-1).

6. *Interdental groove.* The vertical groove, parallel to the long axes of adjacent teeth, found in the interdental area of the attached gingiva.

7. *Interdental papilla.* The portion of the gingiva that fills the interproximal space between adjacent teeth. The interdental papilla is concave, faciolingually. This saddle-like depression has been referred to as the col (Fig. 1-3).

8. *Gingival sulcus (crevice).* The space bounded by the tooth and the free gingiva and having the junctional epithelium as its base.

Epithelium

Gingival epithelium is of the stratified squamous type. It is parakeratinized or keratinized—except for the portion lining the gingival sulcus.

Lamina Propria

This term is used to describe the connective tissue component of the gingiva. Just as other tissues of the body, it consists of cells (fibroblasts, mesenchymal cells, mast cells, and macrophages), formed elements (collagenous fibers), ground

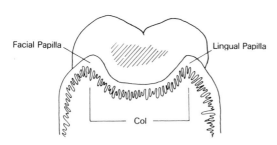

Facial Papilla — Lingual Papilla

Col

Fig. I-3

substance (a polysaccharide-protein complex), and a neurovascular network. Primarily, the collagenous connective tissue fibers are oriented into course bundles, which are grouped according to location and direction, and are sometimes referred to as the gingival fiber apparatus.

Gingival Fiber Apparatus

1. *Gingival group.* These fibers extend from the cementum in three groups (termed a, b, and c) and represent the bulk of the lamina propria facially and lingually (Fig. 1-4).

2. *Circular group.* This group encompasses the teeth from the margin of the gingiva to the alveolar crest (Fig. 1-5).

3. *Transseptal group.* These fibers extend interdentally from the cementum of one tooth to that of the adjacent tooth. Some authors classify this fiber group with the principal fibers of the periodontal ligament rather than with the gingival fiber apparatus (Fig. 1-6). The basic function of the gingival fiber apparatus is to maintain the free gingiva and junctional epithelium in close approximation to the tooth.

Alveolar Mucosa

The epithelium of the alveolar mucosa is thin and nonkeratinized, and it lacks distinct rete ridges. The connective tissue consists of a thin lamina propria and a vascular submucosal layer. The predominant connective tissue fibers are elastic; therefore, unlike the attached gingiva, the alveolar mucosa is bound loosely to the underlying periosteum of the alveolar process. Clinically, the mucogingival junction separates the gingiva and alveolar mucosa. On the facial aspects of the maxillary and mandibular arches, the alveolar mucosa extends to the vestibular fornix. On the lingual aspect of the mandibular arch, the arrangement is similar, but no demarcation in the maxillary

GINGIVAL GROUP

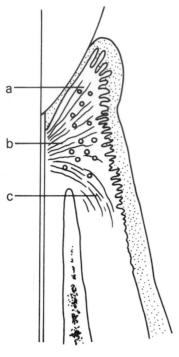

Fig. 1-4

arch exists. In the maxillary arch, the gingiva blends with the palatal mucosa, which is dense and firmly attached to the underlying periosteum. It should be emphasized that the alveolar mucosa is not designed to withstand the forces of mastication; therefore, it cannot serve as gingival tissue.

Clinically Healthy Gingiva

Several terms used in describing the gingival tissues are important. A concept of what is clinically healthy will enable one to recognize what is abnormal during an examination of the gingiva. The following terms are used most often to describe normal gingiva:

1. *Color.* Normal gingiva is described as coral pink, but shading varies widely among individuals. The presence of melanin-containing cells (melanocytes) is normal for people of African and Asian descent.
2. *Size.* Any increase in size of the gingiva is a sign of periodontal disease.

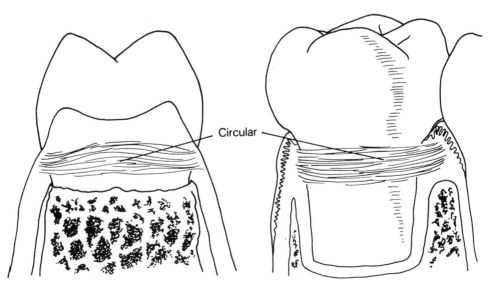

Circular

Fig. 1-5

TRANSSEPTAL GROUP

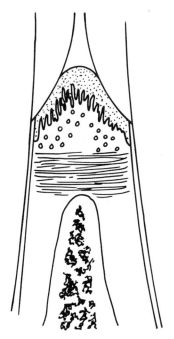

Fig. 1-6

3. *Contour.* This term refers primarily to the festooned appearance of the gingiva.
4. *Consistency.* The gingiva is firm, resilient, and tightly bound to the underlying bone.
5. *Surface texture.* A stippled appearance is normal in the attached gingiva; loss of stippling may be a sign of periodontal disease. Stippling is caused by projections of the papillary layer of the lamina propria, which elevate the epithelium into rounded prominences that alternate with indentations of the epithelium.
6. *Tendency to bleed upon palpation or gentle probing.* Clinically healthy gingiva will not bleed when a periodontal probe is gently inserted into the sulcus or when the marginal gingiva is palpated with the finger. The gingival sulcus is lined with a nonkeratinizing, stratified squamous epithelium. The bottom of the sulcus is formed by the coronal attachment of the junctional epithelium (Fig. 1-7). The sulcus epithelium has been likened to a semipermeable membrane through which bacteria and injurious bacterial products pass into the gingiva. Gingival crevicular fluid seeps out into the sulcus.

Junctional Epithelium

This term refers to a collar-like band of nonkeratinizing basal and stratum spinosum-type cells that varies in thickness from 15 to 20 cells coronally to 1 to 2 cells apically. The cells of the junctional epithelium have relatively wider intercellular spaces and fewer desmosomes compared to the gingival epithelium. Its location on the tooth depends on the stage of tooth eruption, but in the adult it is normally considered to be at or near the cementoenamel junction. Migration of the junctional epithelium apical to this junction is no longer considered by many

DENTOGINGIVAL JUNCTION

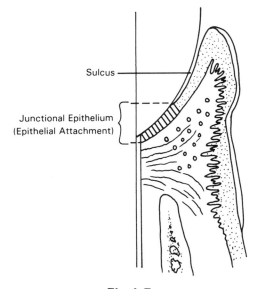

Sulcus

Junctional Epithelium
(Epithelial Attachment)

Fig. 1-7

dentists to be a physiologic process of aging, but rather a pathologic process.

The attachment of the sulcular epithelium to the tooth is comparable to the epithelial-connective tissue attachment found in skin or other body surfaces. There is a basal lamina (basement membrane) that consists of two layers: the lamina densa (adjacent to the tooth surface) and the lamina lucida, to which hemidesmosomes (attachment plaques) are attached. A sticky coating (proline and/or hydroxyproline and mucopolysaccharide) that is secreted by the epithelial cells also binds the junctional epithelium to enamel or cementum.

Dentogingival Junction

The gingival fiber apparatus serves the important function of bracing the gingiva and epithelial attachment against the surface of the tooth. The junctional epithelium and the gingival fibers act as a functional unit, the dentogingival junction (Fig. 1-7).

Blood, Lymphatic, and Nerve Supply of the Gingiva

Gingival tissue has a rich vascular supply formed by a plexus of arterioles, capillaries, and small veins that extend from the sulcular epithelium to the outer surface of the gingiva. The blood supply of the gingiva is derived mainly from supraperiosteal branches of the internal maxillary arteries. Vessels from both the alveolar bone and the periodontal ligament merge with the supraperiosteal vessels to form the gingival plexus (Fig. 1-8).

The lymphatic drainage of the gingiva begins in the connective tissue and progresses into a network that lies external to the periosteum of the alveolar process. Lymphatic vessels drain to regional lymph nodes, particularly the submaxillary group. In addition, lymphatics beneath the epithelium extend into the periodontal ligament and accompany the blood vessels. Innervation of the gingiva comes from labial, buccal, and palatal nerves and from fibers in the periodontal ligament.

Attachment Apparatus

The attachment apparatus comprises alveolar bone, periodontal ligament, and cementum. The root is attached to bone by numerous bundles of collagenous fibers (principal fibers) that are embedded in cementum and bone (Fig. 1-9). These embedded fibers are named according to their location and direction of attachment (alveolar crest, horizontal, oblique, and apical). Interradicular fibers are observed on multirooted teeth.

PERIODONTAL LIGAMENT

The periodontal ligament comprises the white, collagenous connective tissue fibers that surround the root of the tooth and attach to the alveolar process. There are relatively few elastic fibers in the periodontal ligament. The apparent elasticity is a result of the wavy configuration of the principal fibers, which permits slight movement when the tooth is placed under stress.

Functions

The functions of the periodontal ligament are as follows:

1. It maintains the biologic activity of cementum and bone.
2. It supplies nutrients and removes waste products via blood and lymph vessels.
3. It maintains the relation of a tooth to hard and soft tissues.
4. It is capable of transmitting tactile pressure and pain sensations by the trigeminal pathway. The sense of localization is imparted through proprioceptive nerve endings.

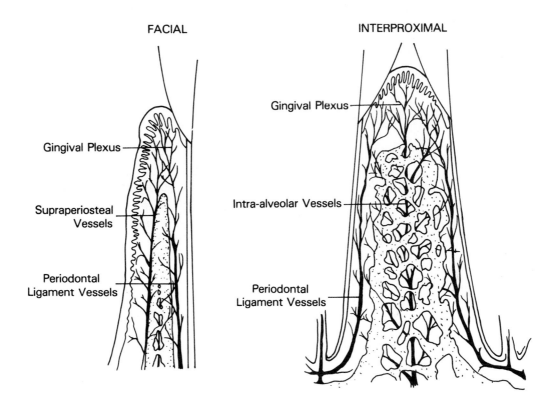

Fig. 1-8

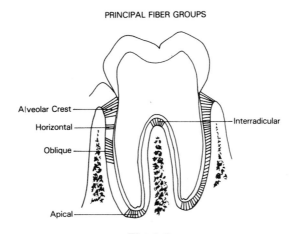

Fig. 1-9

Width

Width of the periodontal ligament space varies with age, location of the tooth, and degree of stress to which the tooth was subjected. The mesial side is thinner than the distal side, owing to the physiologic mesial drift of teeth. A tooth that is not in function has a thin periodontal ligament, with loss of direction of the principal fibers. A tooth under normal use has a thicker periodontal ligament and a normal configuration of the principal fibers. A tooth in functional occlusion has a periodontal ligament space of approximately 0.25 mm, plus or minus 0.10 mm. A tooth subjected to abnormal stress has a considerably thicker periodontal ligament space.

Blood Supply of the Periodontal Ligament

This is derived from three sources:

1. Blood vessels entering the periodontal ligament from the apical area.
2. Interalveolar (interdental) arteries passing into the periodontal ligament from the interdental alveolar process.
3. Anastomosing vessels from the gingiva.

Nerve Supply

Nerves are both myelinated and naked. They vary from knoblike swellings to free endings between fibers. The nerve bundles follow the course of the blood vessels. Their primary purpose is to transmit proprioceptive sensations via the trigeminal pathways, which give a sense of localization when a tooth is touched.

CEMENTUM

Cementum is the calcified structure that covers the anatomic roots of teeth. It consists of a calcified matrix containing collagenous fibers. The inorganic content is approximately 45 to 50%.

Cementum and Cementoid

When first formed, cementum is uncalcified and is known as cementoid. As new layers are formed, the previously formed matrix is calcified and becomes mature cementum. Microscopically, cementum can be divided into two types, cellular and acellular; functionally, however, there is no difference. The cellular cementum consists of lacunae that contain cells called cementocytes. The cells communicate with one another by means of canaliculi. The distribution of cellular and acellular cementum on the roots of teeth varies. Typically, cementum covering the coronal portion of a root is acellular, whereas that covering the apical region is cellular. Cellular cementum is also more prevalent in the bifurcation and trifurcation areas and around the apices of teeth, and is the type of cementum initially formed during wound healing.

Functions

The various functions of cementum are as follows:

1. To anchor the tooth to the bony sockets by means of the principal fibers of the periodontal ligament.
2. To compensate, by continuing growth, for the loss of tooth structure through wear.
3. To facilitate physiologic mesial drift of teeth.
4. To permit a continual rearrangement of the periodontal ligament fibers.

Cementum is deposited throughout the life of a tooth. The presence of cementoid is considered a barrier to the apical migration of the junctional epithelium and to resorption of the root surface.

Cementoenamel Junction

The relationships of the cementum to the enamel at the cementoenamel junction have clinical significance. There are three types of relationships, as demonstrated in Figure 1-10. In 60 to 65% of patients, the cementum overlaps the enamel, and in 30%, there is a butt joint. In 5 to 10% of patients, however, the enamel and cementum do not meet; thus, the dentin is exposed. Patients with exposed dentin may exhibit extreme thermal and tactile sensitivity if recession occurs. This defect also enhances the accumulation of plaque and calculus. Calculus that forms in this defect defies removal, even when visible.

Cervical Projection of Enamel

Enamel projections often extend varying distances (grades 1, 2, and 3) from the cementoenamel junction to the midfurcal area (Fig. 1-11). Their role in the spread of disease into the furcation area is unknown. Cervical projections of enamel, however, are covered by junctional epithelium rather than cementum and connective tissue fibers. An epithelial attachment is potentially weaker than a connective tissue attachment and could

represent a possible pathway for early involvement of a furcation.

Palatogingival Groove

Another defect often associated with advanced periodontal destruction is the palatogingival groove (Fig. 1-12). This groove is most frequently observed on the maxillary central and lateral incisors, and it often extends from the cingulum to the apex. The palatogingival groove presents a difficult, if not impossible, management problem for the patient and clinician.

ALVEOLAR PROCESS

The alveolar process is that portion of the maxilla and mandible that forms and supports the sockets (alveoli) of the teeth.

Divisions

On the basis of function and adaptation, the alveolar process can be divided into two parts:

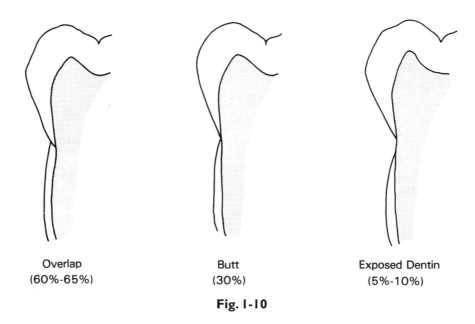

Overlap (60%-65%)   Butt (30%)   Exposed Dentin (5%-10%)

Fig. 1-10

ENAMEL PROJECTIONS

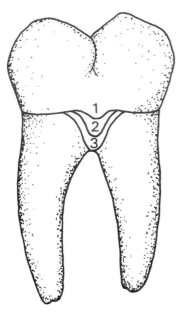

Fig. 1-11

1. *Alveolar bone proper.* A thin layer of bone that surrounds the root and gives attachment to the periodontal ligament. This bone is also known as the lamina dura or cribriform plate.
2. *Supporting alveolar bone.* The portion of the alveolar process that surrounds the alveolar bone proper and gives support to the sockets. It consists of:
   a. Compact or cortical bone found on the vestibular and oral aspects of the alveolar process.
   b. Cancellous bone (spongy bone) that lies between the alveolar bone proper and the cortical bone. Cancellous bone contains marrow that, in the adult, is mostly of the yellow or fatty type. Foci of red marrow can be found in the maxillary tuberosity and, on occasion, in the maxillary and mandibular molar and premolar areas.

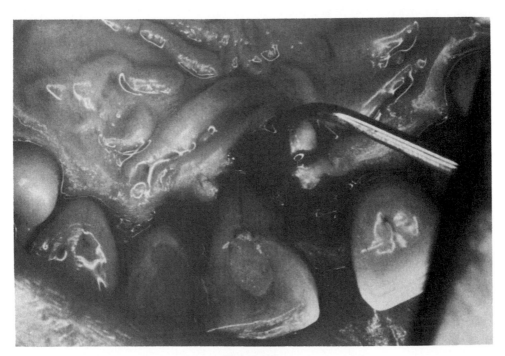

Fig. 1-12

Blood Supply

The vascular supply of bone is derived from intra-alveolar arteries, vessels that penetrate the cortical plates (Fig. 1-8). In circumstances under which cortical bone and alveolar bone proper are fused, as on the facial aspect of the anterior teeth, the blood supply is derived chiefly from supraperiosteal vessels.

Bundle Bone

Portions of the alveolar bone proper frequently contain "bundles" of calcified collagenous fibers from the periodontal ligament (Sharpey's fibers). This bone is termed bundle bone. It is not a special type of bone peculiar to tooth sockets. Bundle bone is present throughout the body wherever tendons, ligament, or muscles attach to bone.

Contours

The contour of the alveolar process conforms to the prominence of the roots and the position of the teeth. The height and thickness of the facial and lingual plates are affected by tooth position, root form and size, and occlusal forces. Teeth that are prominent or in labioversion often bulge through the process, resulting in either an alveolar dehiscence or an alveolar fenestration.

Teeth that are extruded, intruded, or inclined have an angular interdental crest (Fig. 1-13). Studies have shown that, in health, the alveolar crest maintains a constant distance from the cementoenamel junction. For example, when a tooth extrudes, bone formation occurs at the alveolar crest, and the distance between the crest and the cementoenamel junction is maintained. This observation becomes an important factor in the radiographic interpretation of infrabony defects.

When the contour of the cementoenamel junction is broad and flat buccolingually (molars and some premolars), the contour of the alveolar process is broad and flat buccolingually (Fig. 1-14). Conversely, the buccolingual contours in the anterior region are narrow and pointed, owing to the configuration of the cementoenamel junction. It has been reported that the cervical margin of the alveolar bone is often thickened in response to increased functional demands; this is called lipping, or peripheral buttressing bone formation.

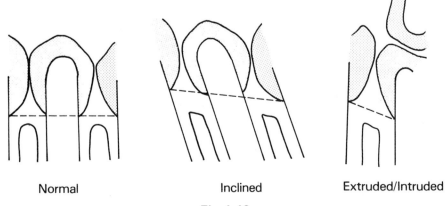

Normal   Inclined   Extruded/Intruded

Fig. 1-13

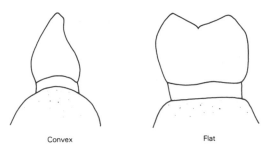

Convex   Flat

Fig. 1-14

ALVEOLAR DEFECTS

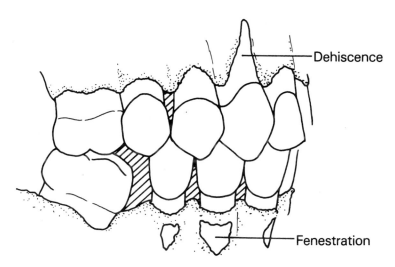

Dehiscence

Fenestration

Fig. 1-15

Lability

Alveolar bone, the least stable of the periodontal tissues, is extremely sensitive to both internal and external stimuli. The contour and internal structure of alveolar bone depend on the stresses placed on it. For instance, in hypofunction, bone is resorbed and density decreases, creating fewer and thinner trabeculae and larger medullar spaces. This state is sometimes termed disuse atrophy. Conversely, in hyperfunction, bone trabeculae are aligned in the path of tensile and compressive stresses, and density increases. When alveolar support has been weakened by periodontal disease, bone forma-

tion often occurs centrally or peripherally in an attempt to support the tooth against the occlusal forces (buttressing bone formation). When the attachment apparatus can no longer adapt to occlusal forces, the injury that occurs is termed trauma from occlusion.

Dehiscence and Fenestration

Two defects of the alveolar cortical plate, dehiscence and fenestration, have clinical and therapeutic significance. Dehiscence denotes the cleftlike absence of the alveolar cortical plate, resulting in a denuded root surface. Alveolar fenestration is a circumscribed defect in the cortical plate, exposing a facial or a lingual root surface (Fig. 1-15).

Only a very thin layer or combined cortical plate-alveolar bone proper exists over the root surfaces of teeth in labioversion, or over those with large roots. In such cases, there is only minimal, if any, interalveolar blood supply; blood supply to the bone is derived chiefly from supraperiosteal vessels. The raising of a mucoperiosteal flap and the severing of the supraperiosteal vessels may result in the loss of cortical plate, exaggeration of a dehiscence, or a fenestration becoming a dehiscence. When such defects are suspected, every effort should be made to leave connective tissue to cover the radicular surface. To this end, a mucosal flap (partial-thickness flap) which preserves the supraperiosteal blood supply is used.

A similar problem arises if bone contouring is performed over the root surfaces. According to the results of studies on wound healing, bone should rarely be removed from radicular surfaces, particularly from the cervical one-third. After osseous surgery on radicular surfaces, bone resorption continues during healing and may result in extensive osseous dehiscences.

CHAPTER

2

Etiology of Periodontal Disease

Arthur R. Vernino

Periodontal disease may be defined as any pathologic process that affects the periodontium. The vast majority of inflammatory diseases of the periodontium result from bacterial infection. Although other factors may affect this region, the dominating causative agents of periodontal disease are microorganisms that colonize the tooth surface (bacterial plaque and their products). Figure 2-1 represents the interaction of etiologic factors that cause periodontal disease. Numerous systemic disorders adversely affect the periodontium (see Chapter 3), but no systemic disorder is known to be the initiating cause of periodontitis in the absence of bacterial plaque. In addition, there are other local factors that act in conjunction with bacterial plaque to produce chronic disease of the periodontium. Two factors that may initiate periodontal disease in the absence of bacterial plaque are malignancies and primary occlusal traumatism. The role of each factor in the initiation and progression of periodontal disease is discussed in this chapter.

TOOTH-ACCUMULATED MATERIALS (TAM)

To discuss bacterial plaque and its relationship to periodontal disease, it is nec-essary to define the various materials that accumulate on the tooth surface (TAM).

1. *Bacterial plaque.* There are many types of bacterial plaques, but the ones that are closely allied to periodontal disease can be divided into two major types. The first type consists of a mat of densely packed, colonized, and colonizing microorganisms, that grow on and attach to the tooth. This type may be supragingival or subgingival. The second type is a subgingival plaque that is "free floating" or loosely attached between the soft tissue and the tooth. The attached bacterial plaque is not removed with a forceful water spray, but is readily removed by other mechanical means. The loosely attached plaque consists primarily of anaerobic bacteria.

2. *Acquired pellicle.* The thin (0.1 to 0.8 micron) primarily protein film that forms on erupted teeth and can be removed by abrasives (e.g., polishing materials). It quickly reforms after being removed. The source of pellicle is apparently from constituents of saliva. It can form whether or not bacteria are present. Acquired pellicle will stain light pink by erythrosin, a red dye commonly used to stain bacterial plaque.

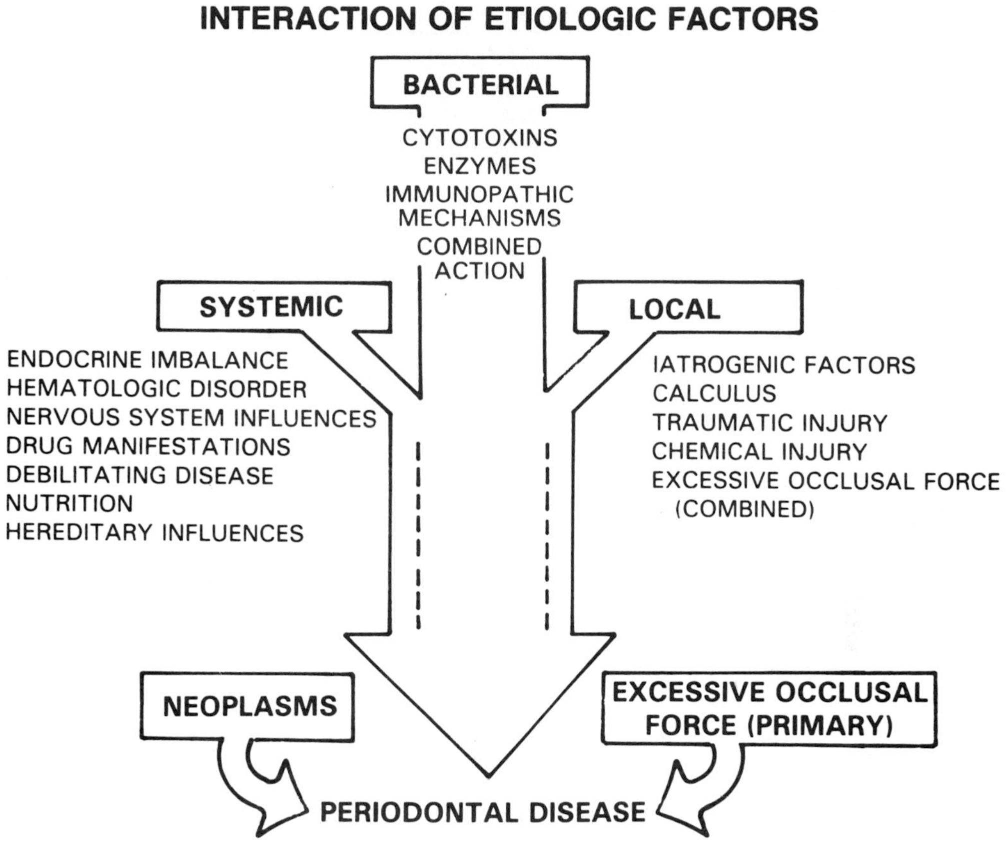

INTERACTION OF ETIOLOGIC FACTORS

BACTERIAL

CYTOTOXINS
ENZYMES
IMMUNOPATHIC
MECHANISMS
COMBINED
ACTION

SYSTEMIC

ENDOCRINE IMBALANCE
HEMATOLOGIC DISORDER
NERVOUS SYSTEM INFLUENCES
DRUG MANIFESTATIONS
DEBILITATING DISEASE
NUTRITION
HEREDITARY INFLUENCES

LOCAL

IATROGENIC FACTORS
CALCULUS
TRAUMATIC INJURY
CHEMICAL INJURY
EXCESSIVE OCCLUSAL FORCE
 (COMBINED)

NEOPLASMS

EXCESSIVE OCCLUSAL
FORCE (PRIMARY)

PERIODONTAL DISEASE

Fig. 2-1

Pellicle is not removed by forceful rinsing, and its role in periodontal disease is unknown.

3. *Calculus.* Calcified plaque that is usually covered by a soft layer of bacterial plaque.
4. *Food debris.* Food that is retained in the mouth. Debris, unless impacted between the teeth or within periodontal pockets, is usually removed by action of the oral musculature and saliva, or as a result of rinsing or brushing.
5. *Materia alba (literally, white matter).* A soft mixture of salivary proteins, some bacteria, many desquamated epithelial cells, and occasional disintegrating leukocytes. This mixture adheres loosely to the surface of the teeth, to plaque, and to gingiva, and can usually

be flushed off with a forceful water spray. The toxic potential of materia alba and its role in the formation of bacterial plaque are not known. Table 2-1 summarizes some of the differences between plaque, materia alba, and debris.

BACTERIAL FACTORS IN PERIODONTAL DISEASE

Morphology of Bacterial Plaque

Studies with light and electron microscopy have yielded evidence to indicate there are distinct morphologic differences between supragingival and subgingival plaque. The morphology of supragingival plaque is similar in patients with

Table 2-1   Some Differences between Plaque, Materia Alba, and Debris

Characteristic	Plaque	Material Alba	Debris
Adherence	Close	Loose	None
Effect of rinsing	None	Dislodged by forceful rinsing	Dislodged readily
Structure	Definite	Amorphous	None

gingivitis and those with periodontitis. The bacterial cells appear to be densely packed on the tooth surface and the deposits may be thick (0.5 mm or more). The composition of the microbial deposits includes coccoid and relatively numerous filamentous forms of bacteria. Some of the filamentous bacteria are covered with coccal organisms, which appear as "corncob" formations. Flagellated forms and spirochetes are observed apically and on the outer surface of the supragingival plaque.

Subgingival plaque in periodontitis patients is composed of an inner and an outer layer. The inner layer of tightly adherent bacteria is continuous with, but is thinner and less organized than, supragingival plaque. Outside this tightly adherent layer, and adjacent to the soft tissue of the pocket, is a loosely adherent layer of microorganisms. This layer consists of numerous spirochetes, gram-negative bacteria, and bacteria grouped into "bottle brush" or "test-tube brush" formations.

Microorganisms of Plaque

The type of microorganisms found in plaque vary among individuals and sites within the mouth, and with age of the plaque itself. Young plaque (1 to 2 days) consists primarily of gram-positive and some gram-negative cocci and rods. These organisms normally grow on an amorphous mucopolysaccharide pellicle, less than 1 micron thick, which is attached to the enamel, cementum, or dentin.

From 2 to 4 days of growth, undisturbed plaque changes in the numbers and in the types of organisms present. The number of gram-negative cocci and rods increases and fusiform bacilli and filamentous organisms become established.

From 4 to 9 days, this ecologically complex population of microorganisms is further complicated by the presence of increasing numbers of motile bacteria, namely, spirilla and spirochetes.

It was shown recently that there are apparent qualitative differences in the microbial flora associated with periodontal health and disease. Dark-field microscopy has revealed that spirochetes and motile organisms are often associated with disease whereas coccoid forms are usually associated with health. Studies in which plaque bacteria have been cultured show that certain gram-negative bacteria may be associated with specific types of periodontal disease. For example, Porphyromonas (Bacteriodes) gingivalis shows a strong association with adult periodontitis; Prevotella (Bacteroides) intermedius has been associated with pregnancy gingivitis. Haemophilus (Actinobacillus) Actinomycetemcomitans and strains of Capnocytophaga are associated with juvenile periodontitis. Prevotella intermedius and Spirochetes are found in large numbers in Necrotizing Ulcerative GingivoPeriodontitis.

Other Constituents of Plaque

Although colonized organisms are the primary constituents of plaque, additional components can be identified by phase-contrast microscopy.

1. *Epithelial cells*. These are found in almost all samples of bacterial plaque in vary-

ing stages of anatomic integrity. They may range from recently desquamated cells with discrete nuclei and clearly defined cell walls to what may be described as "ghosts" of cells swarming with bacteria.

2. *White Blood cells.* Leukocytes, usually polymorphonuclear neutrophils (PMNs), may be found in varying stages of vitality in the several stages of inflammation. It is of interest that vital white cells may be found adjacent to clinically healthy gingiva. Microorganisms are often present within the cytoplasm of the granulocytes. In areas of obvious exudation and purulence, it is often difficult to find any apparently vital cells among the numerous granulocytes present.

3. *Erythrocytes.* These are readily seen in samples taken from tooth surfaces adjacent to ulcerated gingiva.

4. *Protozoa.* Certain genera of protozoa, notably Entamoeba and Trichomonas, can often be seen in plaque taken from surfaces adjacent to acute gingivitis and from within periodontal pockets.

5. *Food particles.* Occasionally, microscopic shreds of food are seen. Those most readily recognized are muscle fibers, distinguishable by their striations.

6. *Miscellaneous components.* Nonspecific elements, such as crystalline-appearing particles (which may be fine fragments of cementum, beginning calcification, or unidentified foodstuffs) and what appear to be cell fragments, may also be found in plaque.

Mechanisms of Bacterial Action

1. *Invasion.* Bacterial invasion is not necessary for gingival inflammation to occur. All that is required is that enough bacteria (and possibly specific pathogenic bacteria) be fixed to the tooth, near the gingiva, for a sufficient length of time to challenge the tissue with their toxic products. No specific organism or group of organisms has been positively or exclusively identified as the cause of periodontal breakdown, but there appears to be a strong association of certain microorganisms with periodontal disease states. There is evidence that bacterial invasion of the connective tissue does occur.

2. *Cytotoxic agent.* Endotoxins, which are lipopolysaccharide constituents of the cell wall of gram-negative bacteria, can be a direct cause of tissue necrosis, as well as an initiator of inflammation by triggering an immunologic response and activation of the complement system. Also, endotoxins from certain oral organisms stimulate bone resorption in tissue culture.

3. *Enzymes.*
   a. Collagenase depolymerizes collagen fibers and fibrils, the major formed elements in the gingiva and periodontal ligament. It is of interest that leukocytes are also known to produce collagenase and are present in large numbers in the lesions of the early stages of gingivitis.
   b. Hyaluronidase hydrolyzes hyaluronic acid, an important tissue-cementing polysaccharide, and can act as a "spreading" factor to increase tissue permeability. This enzyme is produced by microorganisms and by the host.
   c. Chondroitinase hydrolyzes chondroitin sulfate, another tissue-cementing polysaccharide.
   d. Proteases, a family of enzymes, contribute to breakdown of noncollagenous proteins and increase capillary permeability.

4. *Immunopathologic mechanisms.* Studies have demonstrated that several plaque antigens induce inflammation in animals by stimulating the immunologic response. Both the humoral and the cell-mediated

types of immune response have been observed in patients with periodontitis. The role of the immunologic response in periodontal disease is not completely understood; however, the potential to cause tissue destruction is apparent. The role of the immune response in gingivitis and periodontitis is discussed further in Chapter 5.

5. *Combined action.* It is possible that more than one mechanism may be involved in the initiation and progression of inflammatory periodontal disease. For example, it is conceivable that bacterial enzymes and/or cytotoxic substances exert a direct effect on the sulcular and subsulcular tissue, as well as initiate an indirect immunopathologic response.

The exact mechanism of action of bacterial plaque is unclear; however, there remains little doubt that bacteria are the primary etiologic agents for inflammatory periodontal disease.

RISK FACTORS AND RISK INDICATORS

Modern medical terminology refers to ARisk Factors@ and ARisk Indicators@. Risk factors have a reasonably certain causal relationship with a disease process. Risk indicators are less well substantiated. That does not mean that risk indicators may not be categorized as risk factors in the future, but current research does not support that relationship.

Risk Factors for Periodontitis

Bacterial Plaque

This topic is discussed elsewhere in this text.

Smoking and Periodontitis

Smoking is a major risk factor for periodontitis, and may alter its pathogenesis.

One study showed an increased odds ratio of 2.0 to 5.0 using attachment loss as the measurement tool. Smokers appear to have different flora, and do not respond as well to treatment as nonsmokers. When all other factors are eliminated, smoking is as destructive as bacterial plaque.

Systemic Modifiers

This topic is discussed elsewhere in this text.

Genetic Factors

Familial patterns have been documented for LJP for decades. Studies of twins have had mixed results. Human leukocyte antigens (HLA) have been associated with various forms of periodontal disease. For example, HLA-A9 increases in the presence of severe adult periodontitis. Recent research has shown that patients who are positive for the IL-1 genome are at greater risk for periodontal destruction. This topic requires more study. Nevertheless, commercial tests for genetic susceptibility for periodontitis are available. There is a great deal of promise in these new tools, but it remains to be seen how they will be applied in clinical practice. It is conceivable that the pathogenesis of periodontitis may differ in these patients and that alternate treatment modalities may be required.

History of Previous Periodontitis

Patients who have been treated for periodontal disease are at much greater risk for periodontal destruction in the future.

Risk Indicators for Periodontitis

Risk factors for periodontitis include male gender, African-Americans, socioeconomic status and age. These may be associated with a greater incidence of periodontitis.

SYSTEMIC FACTORS AND PERIODONTAL DISEASE

Systemic factors related to periodontal disease are discussed in Chapter 3. However, it should be mentioned that any condition that might reduce the resistance of the periodontium to toxic insult should be expected to contribute to the initiation of inflammation and to influence the rapidity and severity of the disease process.

LOCAL CONTRIBUTING FACTORS AND PERIODONTAL DISEASE

1. *Anatomic factors.*
   These include:
   a. Root morphology (size and shape).
   b. Position of tooth in arch.
   c. Root proximity.
2. *Iatrogenic factors.* There are a number of procedures, techniques, and materials used in dentistry that indirectly, and on occasion directly, contribute to the initiation and/or progress of periodontal disease.
   a. *Operative procedures.* Most injuries to the gingiva that occur during restorative dentistry procedures are of a minor nature and heal readily without loss of form or function of the periodontium. Some precautions, however, should be observed. For example, if a large portion of papilla is destroyed by careless use of a wedge during matrix stabilization, it is likely that the papilla will not regenerate to normal contour. Also, retraction cord, impression tubes, diamond stones, and temporary restorations may result in irreversible damage to the periodontium if either of the following conditions exists.
      (1) Minimal amount of attached gingiva at the operative site. The gingiva can easily become macerated and detached, with ultimate loss of all attached gingiva. Operative procedures performed under such circumstances may result in tissue loss if there is a frenum attachment at the mucogingival junction.
      (2) The gingiva is stripped from a tooth and an overextended temporary restoration is placed, or cementing material is forced between the tooth and the detached tissue and is left in place. In either situation, epithelium will attempt to cover the detached tissue; when the temporary restoration (or cement) is finally removed, a deepened, epithelial-lined pocket will exist. The longer the materials remain interposed between tooth and soft tissue the greater the certainty of permanent loss of the gingival attachment.
   b. *Restorative materials and restorations.* Except for plastics, in which excess free monomer is present, no restorative material used in dentistry today has been shown to be, in itself, capable of producing inflammation. Restorations may play a role similar to that of rough calculus if they have overhanging margins or rough surfaces. Overhanging margins and surface irregularities provide sites for plaque formation and retention. The presence of overhanging margins and rough surfaces makes plaque removal difficult and provides protected areas for microorganisms to multiply and exert their toxic effect.
   c. *Removable partial dentures.* If a prosthesis is so designed as to impinge on the soft tissue or to exert torque on the teeth, direct damage to the periodontium can occur. In the presence of bacterial plaque, these insults can result in rapid, severe destruction of periodontal structures.

d. *Fixed partial dentures.* In addition to the necessity for marginal excellence on abutments, the design must also be such that the patient can clean all surfaces of the restoration. This requirement demands that open interproximal embrasures and generally convex surfaces should be design elements to enhance cleanliness of the prosthesis. These principles are especially critical in pontic design. Failure to instruct patients in the methodology of cleaning fixed partial dentures is the first step toward eventual breakdown of the periodontium.

e. *Exodontics.* When extractions are performed so that the attachment apparatus of an adjacent tooth is damaged at or near the dentogingival junction, the damage is frequently irreversible. For example, the soft tissue and bone supporting an adjacent tooth can be destroyed if they are injudiciously used as a fulcrum for a surgical elevator. Poor flap design, as well as poor approximation and fixation of wound edges, can result in tissue contours that are conducive to plaque and food retention. Failure to remove calculus from adjacent tooth surfaces at an extraction site may negate an excellent opportunity for pocket elimination and regeneration of the attachment apparatus around the remaining teeth. This oversight indirectly enhances the progression of periodontal disease.

f. *Orthodontics.* Fixed appliances (bands and wires) present excellent harbors for bacterial growth and can thus contribute significantly to inflammation. Temporary extracoronal splints, whether composed of welded orthodontics bands, wire, or wire and acrylic resin, may also be included in this category. On final analysis, it is evident that poor dentistry of all types may create sites for the accumulation of plaque, intensify its production, and prevent its mechanical removal.

3. *Calculus formation.* Calculus is calcified dental plaque. It should **not** be considered a direct cause of inflammation. Calculus is important in the progression of disease, however, serving as a "coral reef" within which microorganisms can multiply and release their toxic products. The rough surface of calculus makes it difficult, if not impossible, for the patient to remove associated bacterial plaque. There is ample evidence that complete removal of calculus is necessary for resolution of periodontal pockets.

4. *Traumatic factors.* Trauma to the periodontium can result in the loss of the attachment apparatus and can contribute to the initiation and progression of periodontal disease.

a. *Toothbrush abrasion.* This can completely destroy a narrow band of attached gingiva and result in extensive recession. In fact, toothbrush abrasion is one of the two most common factors associated with recession, the other being tooth position. Such abrasion also results in extensive grooving of the root surfaces, which causes cleaning problems for the patient and management problems for the dentist.

b. *Factitious disease.* Occasionally, patients are encountered who persistently gouge or "scratch" their gingiva with their fingernails (factitious disease). This action usually results in extensive exposure of the root surface and localized inflammation. This rare entity is a difficult diagnostic problem. Whenever isolated areas of recession are noted and a thorough evaluation fails to identify the etiology of the condition, factitious disease should be considered.

c. *Food impaction.* This is one of the more common local factors that contribute to the initiation and progression of inflammatory periodontal disease. Open contacts, uneven marginal ridges, irregular positions of teeth, and nonphysiologic contours of teeth and restorations can result in the impaction of food on the gingiva and into the gingival sulcus. Some investigators believe that food impaction is an important factor in vertical bone loss. It is not clearly understood what produces the initial breakdown in an area of food impaction or food retention. It is speculated that the forceful wedging of food beneath the gingival tissues can produce inflammation from physical trauma, in addition to tearing of the epithelial attachment. It is just as likely, however, that the initial injury is a result of food degradation and chemical irritation. It is also possible that food impaction and retention afford an excellent breeding ground for bacteria that initiate the disease process.

5. *Chemical injury.* Indiscriminate use of topically applied aspirin tablets, strong mouthwashes, and various escharotic drugs may result in ulceration of the gingival tissue. In addition, dentists may inadvertently permit strong bleaches or salts of heavy metals, such as silver nitrate, to come in contact with the tissue. Injuries of this nature are usually transient, but may contribute to the destruction of the periodontium.

6. *Excessive occlusal force.* See Chapter 6 for a discussion of this type of trauma.

Neoplasms

There are numerous benign and malignant lesions that involve the tissues of the periodontium. It is not within the scope of this book to discuss the various neoplasms of the periodontium, and the reader is referred to a standard text in oral pathology for this information.

SUGGESTED READINGS

Annals of Periodontology. 1996 World Workshop in Periodontics Periodontal Diseases: Epidemiology, Vol. 1, Section 1A;1–36.

Daly CG, Seymour G J, Kieser J B. Bacterial endotoxin: a role in chronic inflammatory periodontal disease. J Oral Path 1980;9: 1–15.

Gher M, Vernino A. Root Morphology-Clinical Significance in Pathogenesis and Treatment of Periodontal Disease. J Am Dent Assoc 1980;101:627–633.

Lang NP, Kiehl RA, Anderhalden K. Clinical and Microbiological Effects of Subgingival Restorations with Overhanging or Clinically Perfect Margins. J Clin Periodontol 1983;10:563–578.

Loe H, Theilade E, Jensen SB. Experimental Gingivitis in Man. J Periodontol 1965; 36:177–187.

Saglie R, Newman M G, Carranza F A, Pattison G L. Bacterial Invasion of Gingiva in Advanced Periodontitis in Humans. J Periodontol 1982;52:217–222.

Saglie FR, Pertuiset JH, Rezende MT, Sabet MS, Raoufi D, Carranza F A, Jr. Bacterial Invasion in Experimental Gingivitis in Man. J Periodontol 1987;58:837–846.

Sandquist G, Carlsson J, Hanstrom L. Collagenolytic activity of black-pigmented bacteroides species. J Periodontol Res 1987;22:300–306.

Schwartz RS, Massler M. Tooth Accumulated Materials: A Review and Classification. J Periodontol 1969;40:407–413.

Slot J, Listgarten M A. Bacteroides gingivalis, bacteroides intermedius, and actinobacillus actinomycetemcomitans in human periodontal diseases. J Clin Periodontol 1988;15:85–93.

Socransky S, Haffajee A. The bacterial etiology of destructive periodontal disease. J Periodontol 1992;63:322–331.

Systemic Contributing Factors

Terry Rees

INTRODUCTION

It has long been recognized that periodontal diseases are caused by local oral etiologic factors, especially bacterial plaque. It is also well recognized, however, that a significant number of systemic diseases and disorders may reduce or alter host resistance or host response and predispose individuals to periodontal destruction or to atypical gingival reactions. For example, stress or other systemic disorders may play a role in necrotizing gingivitis, wheras physiologic alterations in steroid hormones during pregnancy can alter gingival response to the presence of plaque. Ingestion of certain medications may lead to gingival overgrowth. The periodontium is comprised of bone, tooth structure, connective tissue, and epithelium. Therefore, it is apparent that systemic conditions that affect any body tissues may also have an effect on periodontal tissues. This chapter will focus on systemic disorders that induce or influence gingivitis or plaque-related periodontitis and the possible role of advanced periodontal disease as a risk factor for systemic disease. The following factors will be discussed:

- Aging
- Emotional and Psychosocial Stress
- Genetic Disorders
- Endocrine Imbalances
- Hematologic Disorders
- Nutritional Deficiencies and Metabolic Disorders
- Drugs and the Periodontium
- AIDS-Related Periodontal Diseases
- Periodontal Infections and Systemic Disorders

AGING

Epidemiologic studies have established that the incidence of periodontal disease increases with age. However, although periodontal attachment and alveolar bone loss may increase in the elderly, severe loss is found in only a few sites in a minority of subjects. It is unclear whether these changes represent the cumulative effects of periodontal disease over many years or a reduction in host resistance as a function of the aging process. The increased incidence of systemic diseases and the medicaments used to treat these diseases may also adversely affect host resistance in the elderly. Some authorities consider increasing age as a risk factor for periodontal disease because aging is associated with alterations in the periodontium, which—at least in theory—may adversely alter host response. For example, bone density may decrease and healing capacity may be reduced owing to physiologic slowing of the metabolic processes. The role of some putative periodontal pathogenic organisms may change with increasing age although it is unclear whether this a result of the aging process itself. There is ample evidence, however, that periodontal health can be maintained throughout life in the absence of local etiologic factors.

EMOTIONAL AND PSYCHOSOCIAL STRESS

A relationship between emotional or psychosocial stress and oral disease has been proposed for many years. Several studies have indicated an association between severity of periodontal disease and work stresses, life event stresses, and psychological reactions to life events (especially depression). A recent long-term study of nearly 1500 adults indicated that life event stresses, such as financial strain and depression, were associated with more severe periodontal disease. The health habits of individuals under stress, however, may decline as reflected by increased smoking, use of alcohol and illicit drugs, sleeplessness, eating disorders, and inadequate oral hygiene. These factors could play an important role in the incidence and severity of periodontal disease. The data indicated, however, that positive coping skills to stressful events negated the harmful effects of stress on the periodontium. Further studies are necessary to determine if stress alone should be considered a risk factor for periodontitis.

GENETIC DISORDERS

Currently there is growing evidence that heredity plays an important role in patient susceptibility to plaque-related inflammatory periodontal conditions. For example, studies of identical twins raised in separate environments revealed similar patterns of periodontal disease. Epidemiological long-term studies of groups of individuals without access to oral hygiene measures or periodontal treatment suggests that innate host resistance may be the most important factor in determining which individuals experience severe periodontal destruction. More recently, an exaggerated monocyte or macrophage derived interleukin-1 (IL-1) reaction has been found among individuals susceptible to early onset or severely destructive periodontitis. These individuals appear to possess an IL-1 gene polymorphism that leads to more inflammation and severe periodontal destruction when exposed to dental plaque. Patients found to possess this genotype may require more rigorous preventive and therapeutic periodontal treatment than those who are do not possess this risk factor.

Several genetic disorders may exert adverse effects on oral and periodontal tissues. These effects are usually the result of deficiencies or dysfunctions of hematologic cells associated with host defense. *Papillon-Lefevre syndrome* is an autosomal recessive disorder characterized by hyperkeratosis of the palms of the hands and soles of the feet and rapidly progressive periodontitis. The condition is often associated with deficiencies in neutrophil phagocytosis and chemotaxis. Other inherited disorders result in diminished numbers of neutrophils or in faulty neutrophil function. *Down's syndrome, chronic idiopathic neutropenia, cyclic neutropenia, Chediak-Higashi syndrome* and *leukocyte adhesion deficiency (LAD) syndrome* are examples.

Acatalasia is a rare hereditary condition characterized by a deficiency of the enzyme *catalase,* which leads to accumulation of toxic substances such as hydrogen peroxide in tissues, and induces tissue damage and necrosis. It is associated with precocious destructive periodontitis in infants and children.

The *Ehlers-Danlos* phenomena are a group of eight related hereditary conditions that feature hypermobility of body joints and hyperextensibility and fragility of body tissues, including oral mucosa. Generalized extensive periodontal destruction and delayed wound healing have been reported in some subsyndromes of the condition.

Hypophosphatasia and *pseudohypophosphatasia* are familial disorders associated with rickets-like bone abnormalities despite normal vitamin D metabolism. The conditions result in a deficiency of alkaline phosphatase in plasma and bone matrix. Susceptibility to periodontal disease and premature loss of primary and secondary dentition may occur as the result of faulty cementum formation, faulty periodontal ligament fibers, abnormal formation of alveolar bone, and defective neutrophil function.

ENDOCRINE IMBALANCES

A number of endocrine abnormalities may affect the periodontium directly or result from neutrophil dysfunction or altered wound healing. For example, *hyperparathyroidism* is associated with excessive secretion of parathyroid hormone, which results in imbalanced mobilization of calcium from bone. This may lead to osteoporosis and exaggerated bone loss in the presence of plaque-related periodontitis. A similar response has been noted in individuals who cannot properly utilize vitamin D and among estrogen-deficient females. The resulting osteopenia or osteoporosis may serve as a risk factor for more severe periodontal destruction and tooth loss in the presence of dental plaque. Conversely, estrogen supplementation or the use of bisphonates (estrogen substitutes) may offer a protective effect on the severity of periodontal disease. These factors will be of greater importance as the American population ages with a resultant increase in numbers of postmenopausal females seeking dental treatment.

Diabetes Mellitus

Diabetes mellitus is an abnormality in glucose metabolism characterized by a decrease in insulin production or metabolism. According to the most recent classifications suggested by the American Diabetes Association, Type 1 diabetes represents insulin depletion resulting from destruction of the beta cells of the pancreas. Affected individuals require insulin supplementation to achieve metabolic control of their disease. It often develops early in life and is far less common than type 2 diabetes in which insulin resistance occurs with or without insulin depletion. Type 2 diabetics may be treated with oral hypoglycemic agents and/or insulin. The classic signs and symptoms of uncontrolled diabetes mellitus include excessive thirst, hunger, and urination, as well as fatigue, pruritus (itching), and glycosuria (glucose in urine). Long-term complications may include atherosclerotic cardiovascular, cerebrovascular, or peripherovascular disease; retinopathy that often leads to loss of vision; nephropathy; peripheral neuropathy; and periodontal disease. Elevated blood sugar levels (hyperglycemia) may suppress the host's immune response and lead to poor wound healing and recurrent infections. In the oral cavity, this may be reflected by multiple or recurrent periodontal abscesses and cellulitis. Patients suffering from undiagnosed or poorly controlled diabetes mellitus are susceptible to gingivitis, gingival hyperplasia, and periodontitis. In part, periodontal destruction is owing to the factors just described, but the diabetic state is also associated with decreased collagen synthesis and increased collagenase activity. Additionally, altered neutrophil function has been identified in some, but not all, diabetics. Diabetes-induced secondary hyperparathyroidism may predispose the individual to excessive alveolar bone loss in the presence of periodontal infection.

The effect of controlled diabetes mellitus on periodontal disease progression is somewhat controversial. The bulk of evidence suggests, however, that the incidence and severity of gingivitis increases in diabetic children, but teenagers and adults with diabetes experience an increased susceptibility to both gingivitis and periodontitis. Recent evidence indicates that meticulous control of the diabetic state is associated with periodontal health. Conversely, strong evidence suggests that control of infections, including advanced periodontal disease, may be essential to establishment of good metabolic control in diabetics. Consequently, the dental practitioner should make the patient's physician aware if severe periodontal disease is present.

Patients with diabetes should be treated with caution in dental practice. The dentist must seek medical consultation if there is evidence of poor metabolic control. Patients must be cautioned to take their medication and to follow their usual diet in conjunction with dental appointments, and they must maintain meticulous oral hygiene to assure periodontal health. Patients should be treated in a relaxed, nonstressful environment, and appointments should be short. Decisions regarding use of antibiotics for treatment procedures should be based on the patient's overall health status and the extent of the procedure to be performed. One must always remain alert for evidence of developing insulin shock or diabetic coma.

Several multicenter studies of patients with diabetes indicate that strict metabolic control of plasma glucose levels in both type 1 and type 2 patients results in fewer medical complications. These studies also suggest that maintenance of plasma glucose at near normal levels can lead to an increased incidence of hypoglycemia. Some diabetics experience severe hypoglycemia without displaying or sensing the common signs and symptoms. These symptoms may include mood changes, mental confusion, lethargy, bizarre activities, coma or even death. These symptoms may also be observed in individuals with hyperglycemia although onset of symptoms is more gradual. In most instances it is prudent to treat unexplained reactions in the dental office by diabetic patients as though they are experiencing hypoglycemia. This treatment should include the administration of oral carbohydrates such as soft drinks, candy, orange juice, or Glucola. The unconscious patient can be treated with intravenous administration of dextrose.

Imbalances in Sex Hormones

Imbalances in sex hormones may have an adverse effect on the gingiva. For example, *gingival inflammatory hyperplasia* has been reported during puberty, during pregnancy, and as a result of intake of oral contraceptives. Sex hormone-related physiologic changes lead to altered capillary permeability and increased tissue fluids, resulting in an edematous, hemorrhagic, hyperplastic gingivitis in response to dental plaque. Gingival changes have also been reported in males treated with androgenic sex hormones.

Increased susceptibility to gingival inflammation during pregnancy begins in the second month of gestation, peaks in the eighth month, and gradually diminishes in the ninth month and following parturition. These changes closely correlate with progesterone levels during those time periods. Some evidence suggests that increases in estrogen and progesterone during pregnancy promote the development of a more anaerobic crevicular microbial flora. *Pyogenic granuloma* (pregnancy tumor) formation sometimes occurs during pregnancy as a result of the exaggerated tissue response to local irritants induced by altered sex hormone levels.

Periodontal treatment during periods of elevated sex hormone levels is predicated on removal of local irritants and establishment of meticulous oral hygiene. Surgical correction of pregnancy-related gingival hyperplastic changes should be delayed, if possible, until after parturition. Dental treatment can most safely be performed during the second trimester but elective procedures should be deferred when possible.

Characteristics of hormonally deficient females have been discussed previously in this chapter.

HEMATOLOGIC DISORDERS

Gingival inflammation and chronic periodontitis are characterized by the histopathologic presence of an inflammatory cell infiltration of polymorphonuclear leukocytes, lymphocytes, macrophages, and plasma cells. Other blood cells (red blood cells, platelets) are intimately involved with periodontal nutrition, hemostasis, and wound healing. For these reasons, systemic hematologic disorders may have a profound effect on the periodontium. Blood dyscrasias, such as *polycythemia, thrombocytopenia,* or *clotting factor deficiencies,* may result in prolonged hemorrhage following periodontal treatment procedures. Red blood cell disorders such as *aplastic anemia* or *sickle cell anemia* may adversely affect the results of periodontal therapy and induce severe postoperative complications. *Multiple myeloma* is a plasma cell malignancy often associated with gingival bleeding and destruction of alveolar bone. The majority of hematologic disorders associated with periodontal disease, however, are related to white blood cell function or numbers.

Agranulocytosis represents depletion of all blood granulocytes whereas *neu-tropenia* connotes the absence of circulating polymorphonuclear neutrophils. *Cyclic neutropenia* is characterized by cyclic depletion of neutrophil numbers, typically in 3-week cycles. These conditions are associated with severe localized or generalized periodontal destruction.

Leukemia is a malignant disease characterized by proliferation of white blood cell-forming tissues and increased circulating abnormal leukocytes. Periodontal lesions, including gingival enlargement, are common in individuals with leukemia. Gingival changes may be the result of infiltration of leukemic cells into the tissues, of hemorrhage into the tissues, and of plaque-induced inflammation.

Periodontal changes may also occur in patients undergoing treatment for leukemia. A toxic reaction to chemotherapeutic drugs may directly induce severe gingival erosion and ulceration, whereas bone marrow suppression may lead to neutropenic ulcerations, anemic pallor of the gingiva, bleeding owing to platelet deficiency, and reduced resistance to infection. Meticulous oral hygiene is important in reducing periodontal complications but close medical-dental coordination is required prior to performing any periodontal therapy.

Functional leukocyte disorders—especially neutrophil dysfunction—are commonly associated with severe periodontal destruction. These disorders were discussed in "Hereditary Conditions."

NUTRITIONAL DEFICIENCIES AND METABOLIC DISORDERS

The relationship of nutritional deficiencies to progression of periodontal disease has been disputed for many years. Tissue-related nutritional deficiencies result not only from reduced intake of nutritional substances but also from disruption of proper digestion, absorption, transport, or utilization of the nutritional element. Nutritional disorders have profound effects on all body tissues, including the periodontium. Efforts to correlate periodontal disease progression with nutritional deficiencies have typically been equivocal; there is no evidence that nutritional supplementation alone will enhance periodontal health unless a deficiency is present.

Severe vitamin C deficiency (*scurvy*) is known to induce dramatic periodontal destruction in humans. Initial changes may manifest as mild to moderate gingivitis, followed later by acutely inflamed, edematous, hemorrhagic, gingival enlargement. The oral symptoms are accompanied by significant general physiologic changes, including lassitude, weakness, malaise, sore joints, ecchymosis and weight loss. If undetected, scurvy will ultimately lead to severe periodontal destruction and spontaneous exfoliation of teeth. Despite these profound effects, no evidence suggests that vitamin C deficiency alone will initiate inflammatory periodontal disease.

Vitamin D is a fat-soluble vitamin required for physiologic balance of calcium and phosphorus in the body. Deficiency in vitamin D may lead to the development of osteoporosis manifesting as rickets in children or osteomalacia in adults. Either condition may be associated with generalized periodontal ligament destruction and alveolar bone resorption as described in Hypophosphatasia.

Severe protein deficiency, such as *Kwashiorkor,* has been associated with necrotizing lesions of gingiva and other oral tissues and with increased gingival inflammation and periodontal bone loss. These effects may occur as the result of altered immune responses in the presence of plaque-associated periodontitis.

It must be emphasized that mild nutritional deficiencies do not induce periodontal inflammation and destruction. Periodontal changes may be exaggerated, however, when plaque-related infection is present. Nonetheless, it should be obvious that an adequate nutritional status will help ensure satisfactory patient response to periodontal therapy.

DRUGS AND THE PERIODONTIUM

Drugs have long been recognized as potential secondary etiologic factors in periodontal disease. For example, drug-induced *xerostomia* may result in increased plaque and calculus accumulation. The ensuing loss of salivary buffering capacity, as well as reduction in salivary immunoglobulins, may alter host resistance to local irritants. Xerostomic potential has been associated with at least 400 drugs, including diuretics, antipsychotics, antihypertensives, and antidepressants. A recent controlled study identified a direct relationship between xerostomia induced by Sjögren's syndrome and established periodontitis.

Various drugs and medicaments may have direct effects on periodontal tissues. Many substances can induce chemical reactions in oral soft tissues, including the gingiva. Reactions range from mild hyperkeratosis to severe burns. Topically applied aspirin, phenolic compounds, volatile oils, anesthetics, fluoride preparations, and astringents are among those agents capable of eliciting such reactions. It may be important to note that chemical burns have been reported with the use of hydrogen peroxide mouth rinses.

Smoking has been recognized for many years as a contributing secondary factor in necrotizing ulcerative gingivitis. More recently, it has been identified as a very potent risk factor for periodontal disease and for adversely altering the response to periodontal therapy. Smoking may effect the periodontium by inducing a transient vasoconstriction of the gingival blood vessels and increased levels of cytotoxic substances in gingival crevicular fluid and saliva. Additionally, it is associated with increased tooth surface debris and calculus formation, but the most profound effect appears to be suppression of the host immune system, especially the function of leukocytes and macrophages.

Tobacco products are strongly associated with development of oral leukoplakic lesions with or without epithelial dysplasia or malignant transformation and the use of smokeless tobacco may induce localized gingivitis, gingival recession, and periodontal attachment loss. Drugs of abuse such as *cannabis* (marijuana) and cocaine can induce gingival leukoplakia and erythema, and heavy intraoral use of cocaine may result in ulcerative gingivitis and alveolar bone destruction.

Drug-induced *agranulocytosis* may result in severe gingival necrosis resembling generalized *acute necrotizing ulcerative gingivitis* (ANUG). Drugs implicated in causing agranulocytosis include the phenothiazines, sulfur derivatives, indomethacin, and some antibiotics.

Hypersensitivity reactions to various drugs, dental materials, flavoring agents, and food products may induce inflammatory contact lesions of the gingiva and other oral tissues. Erythema multiforme, fixed drug eruptions, and lichenoid drug reactions may also significantly affect gingiva and alveolar mucosa in response to drug ingestion.

Drug-induced gingival enlargements have been reported since the 1930s. Phenytoin (Dilantin) was the first agent associated with this phenomenon. Gingival overgrowth occurs in approximately 50% of patients receiving phenytoin and the anterior facial gingiva is most often involved. The overgrowth usually becomes evident within 3 to 12 months after initiation of phenytoin therapy, and there is a strong correlation between inadequate plaque control and the tissue changes. Currently, other antiepileptic drugs are increasingly being used, and the overall incidence of phenytoin-induced reac-

tions may be decreasing. Some other antiepileptic agents (other hydantoins, barbiturates, and valproic acid), however, have occasionally been associated with gingival overgrowth.

Therapeutic intake of sex hormones such as *estrogen, progesterone,* and *androgens* has been occasionally reported to be associated with gingival enlargement, and most recently, gingival overgrowth has been identified in association with the drug cyclosporin and a family of drugs, the calcium channel blockers. Nifedipine is the calcium channel-blocking agent that most commonly induces this reaction. Gingival changes are very similar to those described with phenytoin and reported incidence is believed to be between 10 to 20% of those taking the drug. Incidence is less with the other calcium channel-blocking agents, and isradipine and amlodipine have been identified as rarely—if ever—causing gingival enlargement.

It is of interest that gingival enlargement has occasionally been reported in response to heavy use of *cannabis* (marijuana). Overall, approximately 20 drugs have been identified as capable of inducing this reaction in the presence of plaque accumulation.

AIDS-RELATED PERIODONTAL DISEASES

Acquired immunodeficiency syndrome (AIDS) is characterized by profound impairment of the immune system of affected individuals. A detailed discussion of this condition is beyond the scope of this text. It should be noted, however, that evidence of infection with the causative *human immunodeficiency virus* (HIV) may often manifest in the oral cavity as severe or recurrent *candidiasis, oral hairy leukoplakia, Kaposi's sarcoma,* or as atypical periodontal diseases. The dental health care provider must be alert for these and other manifestations of immune deficiency and be prepared to assist the patient in management of HIV-associated oral lesions. The terminology used for HIV-related periodontal diseases has been revised and evidence indicates that the incidence of such diseases may increase with increasing immune deficiency. However, the majority of individuals with AIDS manifest with periodontal health or conventional forms of gingivitis or periodontitis. Unusual periodontal lesions may occur more frequently in individuals whose immune system is compromised for any reason, and all types of periodontal diseases associated with HIV infection have been reported in HIV-negative patients.

Linear gingival erythema (LGE) is a localized, persistent, erythematous gingivitis that may or may not serve as a precursor to a rapidly progressive *necrotizing ulcerative gingivitis* (NUG) *or periodontitis* (NUP). The inflammation is often limited to marginal gingiva but may extend into attached gingiva as a punctate or diffuse erythema. Linear gingival erythema is often unresponsive to corrective therapy, yet the lesions may disappear spontaneously. Treatment is similar to that recommended for other marginal gingivitis.

An increased incidence of *necrotizing ulcerative gingivitis* (NUG) has been suggested among HIV-infected patients but the relationship has not been fully substantiated. When found in an HIV-positive patient, the condition should be treated as described elsewhere in this text.

A necrotizing, ulcerative, rapidly progressive form of periodontitis (necrotizing ulcerative periodontitis [NUP]) does occur more frequently among HIV-positive individuals than the general population. Lesions of this type were, however, described long before the onset of the AIDS epidemic in 1981. Necrotizing ulcerative periodontitis features soft tissue necrosis and rapid periodontal destruction. Lesions, which may occur anywhere in the dental arches, are usually localized. The condition is painful and bone may be spontaneously exposed. Some evidence suggests an increased incidence of NUP among individuals with severe immune depression. Treatment consists of gentle debridement and scaling and root planing. Meticulous oral hygiene must be established, including home and office use of antimicrobial mouth rinses such as chlorhexidine gluconate. Metronidazole is the drug of choice if systemic antibiotic therapy is indicated.

Necrotizing ulcerative stomatitis (NUS) represents an extension of NUP to involve mucosal tissue and bone. It occurs in only a relatively small number of HIV-positive individuals and it probably represents noma or cancrum oris, which was described many years ago. As mentioned earlier, most HIV-infected patients experience periodontal disease of the same nature and severity as the general population. With proper home care and appropriate periodontal therapy, these individuals can maintain good periodontal health throughout the course of their illness. In AIDS treatment centers, there is a clinical impression that the incidence of AIDS-related periodontal diseases has diminished since newer antiviral agents and drug combination therapies have been introduced.

PERIODONTAL INFECTIONS AND SYSTEMIC DISEASES

Although the potential for systemic conditions to contribute to plaque-induced periodontitis is well documented, a growing body of evidence suggests that the presence of generalized, severe periodontitis may also contribute to certain systemic disorders or adversely influence their control.

An association has been identified between infections, including advanced periodontitis, and premature births or delivery of low birth-weight infants. These events are believed to occur because accumulations of gram-negative microorganisms such as that found in periodontitis results in increased release of prostaglandins and cytokines, which may act on distant sites such as the placenta. A similar relationship has been suggested between acute systemic infections and the occurrence of cardiovascular disease to include myocardial infarction and stroke. This may indicate that excessive accumulations of gram-negative organisms contribute to atherosclerosis. The mechanism of action is not clearly defined although animal studies and some human studies indicate that gram-negative bacteremias may induce platelet aggregation, creating hypercoagulation and increased blood viscosity—all of which appear to be important features of atheroma formation.

Severe periodontitis has also been associated both upper and lower respiratory diseases such as hospital-acquired pneumonia. As discussed previously, periodontitis may create difficulty in establishing good metabolic control of diabetes mellitus.

The relationship between periodontitis and systemic disorders is an area of intense interest at present and several studies are underway to evaluate this relationship. To date, ample evidence exists to encourage the dentist to advise medical colleagues of the relationship and to encourage periodontal health as an important component in management of some systemic diseases.

Suggested Reading

American Diabetes Association. Expert Committee on the Diagnosis and Classification of Diabetes. Committee report. Diabetic Care 1997;20:1183–1198.

Ellen RP, ed. Periodontal disease among older adults. Periodont 2000 1998;16.

EC Clearinghouse on oral problems related to HIV Infection and WHO collaborating center on oral manifestations of the immunodeficiency virus: classification and diagnostic criteria for oral lesions in HIV infection. J Oral Pathol Med 1993;22:289–291.

Fridrich KL, Kempf KK, Moline DO. Dental implications in Ehlers-Danlos syndrome. Oral Surg Oral Med Oral Pathol 1990;69: 431–435.

Genco RJ, Ho AW, Kopman J, et al. Models to evaluate the role of stress in periodontal disease. Annals of Periodontology 1998;3: 288–302.

Holm-Pedersen P, Löe, H, eds. Geriatric dentistry: a textbook of oral gerontology. Copenhagen: Munksgaard, 1986.

The impact of estrogen deficiency and therapy on women's oral health. Compendium of Continuing Education in Dentistry 1998; 19(suppl. 22).

Laufer D, Benderly A, Hochberg Z. Dental pathology in calcitrol resistant rickets. J Oral Med 1987;42:272–275.

Leggott PJ, Robertson PB, Rothman DL, et al. The effect of controlled ascorbic acid depletion and supplementation on periodontal health. J Periodontol 1986;57:472–479.

Newman HN, Rees TD, Kinane DF, eds. Diseases of the periodontium. Northwood, CA: Science Reviews Limited, 1993.

Periodontal aspects of systemic health. Compendium of Continuing Education in Dentistry 1998;19(special issue).

Rees TD. Drugs and oral disorders. Periodont 2000 1998;18:21–36.

Rees TD. Periodontal management of the patient with diabetes mellitus. Periodont 2000 1999 (in press).

Rees TD, Cataldo E. Periodontal management of HIV infected patients. Clinical periodontology. 8th ed. Carranza FA Jr., Newman MG, eds. Philadelphia: WB Saunders, 1996, 530–537.

Seymour RA. Calcium channel blockers and gingival overgrowth. Br Dent J 1991;170: 376–379.

Stamm JW. Epidemiology of gingivitis. J Clin Periodontol 1986;13: 360–366.

United States pharmacopia drug information: type 2 diabetes. USPDI, 18th ed, vol. I, vol. II: 822–1028, 1998.

Waldrop TC, Anderson DC, Hallmon WW, et al. Periodontal manifestations of heritable Mac1, LFA1 deficiency syndrome. Clinical, histopathologic and molecular characteristics. J Periodontol 1987;58:401–416.

Yukna RA. Cocaine periodontitis. Int J Periodont Restor Dent 1992;11:73–79.

Plaque-Related Periodontal Diseases: Pathogenesis

Jonathan L. Gray

The pathogenesis of a disease refers to the biologic and histologic events that occur in the tissues during the process of conversion from a healthy state to a diseased state. Understanding the pathogenesis of periodontal disease will allow the clinician to make rational decisions regarding the most predictable methods to prevent or treat this widespread disease.

TYPES OF PLAQUE-RELATED PERIODONTAL DISEASE

Gingivitis

Gingivitis is inflammation of the gingiva. No loss of attachment is associated with this condition. The clinical findings may consist of redness of the gingival margin, varying degrees of swelling, bleeding on gentle probing, and alterations in physiologic gingival architecture. There may be increased probing depth (pseudopockets). Pain is not a common finding in gingivitis.

Most forms of gingivitis are plaque-related although secondary factors may alter the clinical manifestations and can result in subclassifications, such as:

1. Acute necrotizing ulcerative gingivitis (ANUG)—see Chapter 22

2. Periodontitis associated with a systemic disease—see Chapter 3
3. Hormonal-influenced gingivitis—see Chapter 3
4. Medication-influenced gingivitis—see Chapter 3
5. Desquamative gingivitis—see Chapter 24

The clinical and histologic features are summarized in Table 4-1.

Periodontitis

Periodontitis is inflammation of the periodontium characterized by apical migration of the junctional epithelium with associated loss of attachment and crestal alveolar bone. The clinical findings include increased probing depth, bleeding on gentle probing (in the active disease states), and alteration of physiologic contour. Redness and swelling of the gingiva may also be present. Pain is not a common clinical finding.

Pocket Formation

A pocket is a gingival sulcus pathologically deepened by periodontal disease. It is bordered by the tooth on one side and by ulcerated epithelium on the other, and it has the junctional epithelium at its

Table 4-1   Clinical Findings and Histologic Features of Gingivitis

Clinical Change	Underlying Histologic Change
Gingival bleeding	Ulceration of sulcular epithelium, with engorged capillaries extending near surface
Redness	Hyperemia, with dilatation and engorgement of capillaries
Swelling, puffiness	Infiltration of connective tissues by fluid and cells of inflammatory exudate
Loss of ginigival tone	Inflammation, with destruction of gingival fiber apparatus
Loss of stippling	Edema in underlying connective tissue
Firm, leathery consistency	Fibrosis associated with long-standing chronic inflammation
Gingival pocket	Inflammation, with ulceration of sulcular epithelium and gingival enlargement

POCKET FORMATION

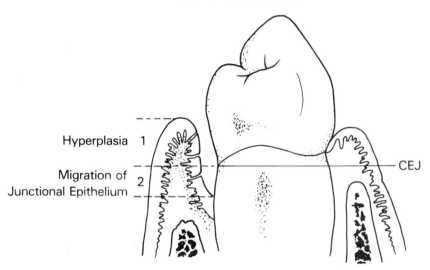

Fig. 4-1

base. Deepening of the sulcus can occur in the following three ways: 1) by movement of the free gingival margin coronally, as observed in gingivitis; 2) by movement of the junctional epithelium apically, with separation of the coronal portion from the tooth; and 3) by a combination of these two items (Fig. 4-1).

Classification of Pockets

Pockets may be classified as follows (Fig. 4-2):

1. *Gingival pocket (pseudo-pocket).* Deepening of the gingival sulcus as a result of an increase in the size of the gingiva. There is no apical migration of the junctional epithelium or loss of crestal alveolar bone (Fig. 4-2A).

2. *Suprabony pocket.* Deepening of the gingival sulcus with destruction of the adjacent gingival fibers, periodontal ligament, and crestal alveolar bone associated with apical migration of the junctional epithelium. The bottom of the pocket and the junctional epithelium are coronal to the crest of the alveolar bone (Fig. 4-2B).

3. *Infrabony pocket.* Deepening of the gingival sulcus to a level at which the bottom of the pocket and the junctional epithelium are apical to the crest of the alveolar bone (Fig. 4-2c). One, two, or three osseous walls, or various

combinations thereof, may exist, depending on the amount and pattern of bone loss (see Chapter 17 for classification of osseous defects).

Horizontal and Vertical Bone Loss

Horizontal bone loss refers to an overall reduction in height of the alveolar crest in which the crestal bone is generally at right angles to the root surface. Vertical bone loss refers to loss of bone at an acute angle to the root surface. Another term for vertical bone loss is angular bone loss. Suprabony pockets are associated with horizontal bone loss (Fig. 4-2B); infrabony pockets are associated with vertical bone loss (Fig. 4-2C).

Etiology of the Infrabony Pocket

Both suprabony and infrabony pockets are the result of plaque infection; however, some opinions differ as to the factors that influence the formation of the infrabony pocket. Most agree that vertical bone loss and subsequent infrabony pocket formation can occur whenever there is direct extension of inflammation into the periodontal ligament, in the presence of a sufficient thickness of bone. The controversy arises as to what factors

alter the pathway of inflammation from crestal bone to the periodontal ligament space. The etiologic mechanisms that have been proposed are as follows:

1. Large vessels that exit on one side of the alveolus may affect formation of an infrabony pocket.
2. The forceful wedging of food into the interproximal region may result in unilateral destruction of the attachment apparatus and downgrowth of the epithelial attachment.
3. Periodontal traumatism may produce crestal damage of the periodontal ligament (trauma from occlusion) that, in the presence of existing inflammation, can result in the migration of the junctional epithelium into the area of destruction (Fig. 4-3).
4. Plaque fronts on adjacent teeth advancing at different rates in an apical direction causing the alveolar bone destruction to occur at a more rapid rate on one of the two adjacent teeth resulting in vertical bone loss.

Classification of Periodontitis (Table 4-2)

A. Chronic Adult Periodontitis
B. Early Onset Periodontitis (EOP)
   1. Prepubertal Periodontitis

CLASSIFICATION OF POCKETS

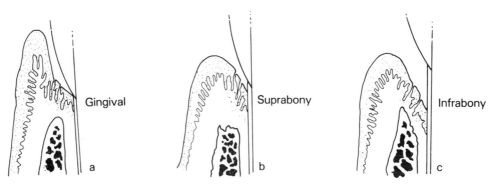

Gingival   a

Suprabony   b

Infrabony   c

Fig. 4-2

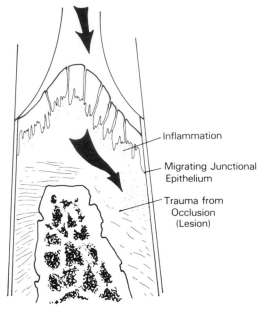

Inflammation

Migrating Junctional Epithelium

Trauma from Occlusion (Lesion)

Fig. 4-3

2. Juvenile Periodontitis (Periodontosis)
3. Rapidly Progressive Periodontitis
   a. Type A
   b. Type B
C. Refractory Periodontitis
D. Necrotizing Ulcerative Gingivo-Periodontitis (NUG-P)
E. Periodontitis Associated With a Systemic Disease

Chronic Adult Periodontitis

Adult periodontitis is a form of periodontitis that is usually slow-forming and appears to have an onset after the age of 35 years. Bone loss progresses slowly and is predominantly horizontal in nature. The etiological factors are local and primarily consist of gram-negative bacteria. Peripheral blood cell defects are not usually found in this form of periodontitis. Chronic adult periodontitis is the most common form of all the periodontal diseases involving bone loss.

Prepubertal Periodontitis

Prepubertal periodontitis is a term suggested for a type of periodontitis that starts soon after the eruption of the primary teeth. There appears to be a localized and generalized form of prepubertal periodontitis. These diseases do not occur on a wide spread basis.

Juvenile Periodontitis (Periodontosis)

Localized juvenile periodontitis (LJP) is a disease that primarily affects a small percentage of adolescents. It is a form of periodontitis that appears to have its onset at puberty. The classic appearance of LJP is characterized by severe vertical type bone loss about the permanent first molars. The permanent incisor teeth may also be involved. There is usually little (sparse) plaque accumulation, and there may be little or no clinical evidence of inflammation. The disease has a predilection for females with a 3:1 female-to-male ratio. There is a familial distribution of the disease, and evidence suggests that there are functional defects in either neutrophils or monocytes but not in both cell types.

Certain gram-negative anaerobic bacteria show a strong relationship to this condition. One of the microorganisms, *Actinobacillus actinomycetemcomitans,* strain Y4, produces substances that could play a prominent role in the extensive tissue destruction seen in LJP. These substances Include the following: a leukotoxin that is toxic to leukocytes, collagenase, endotoxin, and a fibroblast inhibitory factor. There is also a form of the disease called generalized juvenile periodontitis, which involves most of the dentition.

The treatment regimen should include initiation of an effective plaque control program, thorough root detoxification, and flap surgery to remove granulomatous tissue and to gain access to the root

Table 4-2 Classification of Forms of Periodontitis

	AP	LJP	RP-A	RP-B	PP	REF	NUG-P
Age (years)	35	12–26	14–35	26–35	Under 12	?	?
Sex ratio F:M	1:1	3:1	2–3:1	?	1:1	1:1	?
Lesions	Variable	1st molar/ incisor	General	General	General/ loc mixed dent	Variable	Variable
TAM	Yes	Minimal	Minimal	Yes	Minimal	Yes	Yes
Neutrophil chemotaxis	Normal	Depress	Depress	Depress/ normal	Depress/ normal	Normal	?

surface. In addition, there is strong evidence that 1 gram of tetracycline administered daily, in four equally divided doses, over a 10-to-21-day period will improve the clinical result.

Rapidly Progressive Periodontitis

Rapidly progressive periodontitis is a disease that usually begins between puberty and 35 years of age. The disease is characterized by severe generalized alveolar bone loss, which includes the majority of teeth present. The bone loss may be horizontal or vertical or a combination of both. The amount of bone destruction appears to be out of proportion to the amount of local irritants present. Rapidly progressive periodontitis may be associated with systemic disease (i.e., diabetes mellitus, Down syndrome, and other diseases), but the disease is found, also, in the otherwise healthy individual.

This entity can be divided into two subclasses:

- Type A: This form occurs between the ages of 14 and 26 years of age. It is characterized with rapid generalized loss of bone and attachment.
- Type B: This form is characterized by rapid general loss of bone and attachment during the ages of 26 and 35 years.

The treatment regimen should follow that prescribed for LJP. The disease may respond to this regimen, but it is known to be refractory to all forms of therapy.

Refractory Periodontitis

Refractory periodontitis is a condition in which multiple sites in patients exhibit continued attachment loss in spite of usual and customary periodontal therapy. The sites remain infected by periodontal pathogens.

Necrotizing Ulcerative Gingivo-Periodontitis

Necrotizing ulcerative gingivo-periodontitis is a form of periodontitis that usually follows long-term repeated episodes of untreated or incompletely treated acute necrotizing ulcerative gingivitis. The repeated insults to the periodontium causes destruction of the interproximal tissues, leaving interproximal crater formation in both soft tissue and alveolar bone. This form of periodontitis is cyclic, and maintenance is extremely difficult (see Chapter 22 for a more complete discussion of this disease).

Additionally, case classification may be related to the extent of periodontal involvement or destruction (see Chapter 11).

PATHOGENESIS OF PLAQUE-RELATED PERIODONTAL DISEASE

Plaque-related periodontal disease is characterized by inflammation. The inflammatory process is activated to limit the spread of the disease process; however, in addition to this beneficial effect, the inflammatory process also has a destructive component. The objective of treatment is to enhance the beneficial aspects of inflammation and to limit or control the destructive potential.

The inflammatory response in plaque-related periodontal disease can be initiated by a variety of factors. A number of the lytic enzymes produced by bacteria can cause direct tissue destruction in the periodontium. Other bacterial products (e.g., endotoxin) may activate the complement system, which results in the formation of biologically active proteins that stimulate an increase in vascular permeability with migration of inflammatory cells from the vascular channels, the chemotactic response, cell adherence, and phagocytosis. The end result of complement activation is cell lysis of both host and bacterial cells.

The immunologic response appears to affect the initiation, and probably the perpetuation, of the inflammatory response. The bacteria in plaque contain a multitude of antigens. The antigens can stimulate the B and T lymphocytes of the gingival connective tissues to proliferate and to contribute to both the humoral and cell-mediated immune response, respectively. To support this concept, evidence shows that patients with plaque-related periodontal disease have circulating antibodies to plaque antigens. In addition, cultures of peripheral lymphocytes from patients with plaque-related periodontal disease show a greater cell-mediated immune response to plaque-derived antigens than peripheral lymphocytes from periodontally healthy patients (see Chapter 5 for a more complete discussion of the role of the immune response).

Histopathology

The histologic picture of developing plaque-related periodontal disease has been divided into four stages at the light microscope level (the model proposed by Page and Schroeder).

Initial Lesion

The first microscopically observable tissue changes occur after *2 to 4 days* of plaque accumulation. There are small accumulations of polymorphonuclear neutrophils (PMNs) and mononuclear cells subjacent to the junctional epithelium. A decrease of perivascular collagen occurs in this area as well as a decrease of some of the collagen supporting the coronal portion of the junctional epithelium. Gingival fluid can be detected clinically in the gingival sulcus. No more than 5 to 10% of the gingival connective tissue is involved during this stage. Classic vasculitis of vessels subjacent to the junctional epithelium is present.

Early Lesion

The early lesion occurs after *4 to 7 days* of plaque accumulation. The changes observed in the initial lesion persist and are more severe at this stage. The major characteristic of the early lesion stage is the formation and maintenance of a dense lymphoid cell infiltrate within the gingival connective tissues. Numerous small-sized and medium-sized lymphocytes accumulate immediately below the junctional epithelium. These cells are the predominant inflammatory cells. The junctional and oral sulcular epithelium begin to form rete ridges (pegs). Numerous injured fibroblasts are observed in close association with lymphoid cells. The collagen content is reduced approximately 70% in the areas of inflammation.

The events in the sequence of developing plaque-related periodontal disease, thus far, have occurred at the microscopic and biochemical levels. In time, as the inflammatory cells and tissue fluids begin to accumulate, the gingiva will begin to show clinically detectable symptoms. Which brings us to the next stage.

Established Lesion

The established lesion is a progression of the early lesion and is observed after *2 to 3 weeks* of plaque accumulation. The destructive tissue changes noted in the first two stages persist. The plasma cell is now the predominant inflammatory cell type within the affected connective tissues.

The plasma cells produce immunoglobulins, primarily of the IgG class. The junctional and oral sulcular epithelium continue to proliferate and may now be considered pocket epithelium. This epithelium varies in thickness and shows areas of ulceration. The inflammatory cells accumulate along vascular channels and between collagen fibers deep in the lesion. The collagen loss persists at the site of active disease, but areas distant from the lesion show foci of collagen formation. The periodontal ligament and alveolar bone show no change at this stage. *Clinical manifestations of the disease can now be observed.*

Advanced Lesion

A varying amount of time elapses before the advanced lesion occurs. There are many cases in which the advanced lesion never appears. The area of the lesion enlarges. Strands of pocket epithelium penetrate deep into the connective tissue. There is extensive destruction of the collagen fiber bundles and of the gingiva; however, the transseptal fibers continually regenerate as the lesion moves apically. The plasma cell continues to be the predominant cell type. Many of these cells appear injured, and can be observed deep within the tissue. Crestal alveolar bone resorption occurs, especially in the area of the vascular channels.

Disease Progression

The initial, early, and established lesions represent varying severities of gingivitis. The advanced lesion can be considered periodontitis. All the events in one stage in the life cycle of plaque-related periodontal disease need not be completed before another stage begins. The stages are a continuum of the disease process, with considerable overlap between stages. Periodontitis must be preceded by gingivitis; however, all untreated gingivitis does not necessarily proceed to periodontitis.

Progression of periodontal disease is now considered by numerous investigators to be a cyclic process. There appear to be extended periods of quiescence with short episodes of disease activity. The attachment loss that occurs during these bursts of disease activity varies from minor loss to relatively extensive tissue loss.

Spread of Inflammation

Periodontitis usually develops as a sequel to persistent chronic gingivitis. Interdentally, inflammation and bacterial products spread from the gingiva to the alveolar process along the neurovascular bundle of the interdental canal at the crest of the septum (Fig. 4-4A.1). Inflammation spreads along the course of the vascular channels because the loose connective tissue surrounding the neurovascular bundles offers less resistance than the dense fibers of the periodontal ligament. The point at which inflammation enters the bone depends on the location of the vessels. In some instances, large vessels exit at one side of the alveolar crest, permitting direct spread of the inflammation into the marginal portion of the periodontal ligament (Fig. 4-4A.1A). After reaching the marrow spaces, the destructive process extends laterally into the periodontal ligament via the intra-alveolar

SPREAD OF INFLAMMATION

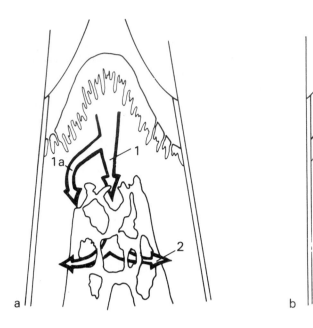

Fig. 4-4

opening (Fig. 4-4A.2). On the facial and lingual surfaces, the destructive process spreads along the supraperiosteal vessels and penetrates the marrow space via the channels in the outer cortex (Fig. 4-4B.1).

Extension of the chronic inflammatory process into the alveolar bone is marked by infiltration of the marrow by leukocytes, new blood vessels, and proliferation of fibroblasts. There is marked osteoclastic activity. Progressive extension is accompanied by destruction of the trabeculae and subsequent reduction in the height of the alveolar bone. This destruction is not a continuous process; it is accompanied by osteoblastic activity and new bone formation, even in the presence of inflammation. Likewise, constant reformation of the transseptal fibers occurs while the attachment apparatus is destroyed. Alveolar bone loss does not occur until the physiologic equilibrium of bone is disturbed to the point that resorption exceeds formation. The resis-

tance to disease of the individual plays an important role in governing the rate at which bone loss progresses in untreated periodontal disease.

Genetic Factors in Periodontitis

Familial patterns have been documented for LJP for decades. Studies of twins have had mixed results. Human leukocyte antigens (HLA) have been associated with various forms of periodontal disease. For example, HLA-A9 increases in the presence of severe adult periodontitis. All such data is premature and inconclusive. Nevertheless, commercial tests for genetic susceptibility for periodontitis are available. There is a great deal of promise in these new tools, but it remains to be seen how they will be applied in clinical practice. It is conceivable that the pathogenesis of periodontitis may differ in these patients and that different treatment modalities may be required.

Table 4-3   Clinical Findings and Histologic Features of Periodontitis

Clinical Finding	Histologic Feature
Bleeding and pain on probing	Ulceration of sulcular epithelium
Blue-red discoloration of gingiva	Circulatory stagnation of chronic inflammation
Smooth, shiny gingival surface with loss of stippling	Atrophy of the epithelium and edema
Flaccidity of gingiva	Destruction of the gingival fiber apparatus
Exposed root surfaces	Result of long-standing chronic inflammation, with progressive apical movement of junctional epithelium and gingival margin, and corresponding loss of alveolar process
Occassionally pink, firm, heavily stippled gingiva with deep pocket formation	Reparative phase of inflammation predominating over the exudate and degenerative phase; pocket wall, however, presents degenerative changes and ulceration
Suppuration	Ulceration of epithelium

Smoking and Periodontitis

Smoking is a major risk factor for periodontitis, and may alter its pathogenesis. One study showed an increased odds ratio of 2.0 to 5.0 using attachment loss as the measurement tool. Smokers appear to have different flora and do not respond as well to treatment as nonsmokers. When all other factors are eliminated, smoking is as destructive as bacterial plaque.

Linear Versus Burst Theories of Periodontal Disease Activity

Since the 1980s, it has been assumed that periodontal disease occurred in "bursts" of attachment loss at specific sites rather than in a linear fashion. This controversy is being revisited. At this time, there is no answer because our techniques for measuring disease activity—periodontal probing, bleeding on probing, and radiographic changes—are too crude. Much more specific and sensitive tests for disease activity are required to solve this problem.

Clinical Findings Correlated with Histologic Features (Table 4-3)

The significance of the clinical findings in periodontitis can be more easily understood if findings can be correlated with the histologic features of the disease.

Critical Pathway Theory of Periodontal Disease

It is no longer sufficient to consider periodontal pathogenesis primarily on a cellular level as we have in the past. The model developed by Page and Schroeder that was presented earlier in this chapter is still an excellent way to depict the transition from health to periodontitis, although one must keep in mind that it is occurring at different rates throughout the mouth. To fully understand this subject, one must be able to correlate the biochemical and cellular events. An excellent model, known as the Critical Pathway Model of Periodontitis© was published in the 1996 World Workshop in Periodontics. There were actually several variations on this model including therapeutic intervention and risk factors such as smoking. We will deal with the basic model.

As the result of poor oral hygiene or exogenous infection, normal flora is converted into pathogenic flora. Inflammation, chemotaxis, antibody production, phagocytosis, activation of the compliment system, production of PGE2 and leukotrienes, interleukins and other cytokines occurs. If the body has normal PMNs and antibodies, the invading bacteria will be cleared, and the patient will experience either no disease, or limited disease (gingivitis). If, on the other hand, the patient has defective PMNs, the disease process may progress. It may also progress if the bacteria possess virulence factors that enable them to inactivate compliment, PMNs, or simply bypass this step by tissue invasion. Porphyramonas gingivalis and Actinobacillis atinomyce-temcomitans are examples of bacteria with such capabilities.

Once this has occurred, the predominant cell is the plasma cell and attachment loss begins. Genetics may predetermine this step involving the monocyte and t cell response. This causes in the release of catabolic cytokines IL-1, TNF, and IL-6, and the mediator PGE2. Both host cells and bacteria are stimulated to produce substances that are destructive to the gingiva, such as collagenase and matrix metalloproteins.

Simultaneously, the body is attempting to heal itself. If the balance between catabolism and anabolism shifts in favor of the former, the disease process will continue in a circuitous manner.

SUGGESTED READINGS

Consensus report. Periodontal diseases: pathogenesis and microbial factors. Annals of Periodontology 1996;1:926–932.

Grossi SG, Genco RJ. Periodontal disease and diabetes mellitus: a two-way relationship. Annals of Periodontology 1998;3: 51–61.

Lamster IB, Grbic JT, Mitchell-Lewis DA, et al. New concepts regarding the pathogenesis of periodontal disease in HIV infection. Ann Periodontol 1998;3:62–75.

Landi L, Amar S, Polins AS, Van Dyke TE. Host mechanisms in the pathogenesis of periodontal disease. Curr Opin Periodontol 1997;4:3–10.

Lang N, Adler, R, Joss A, Nyman S. Absence of bleeding on probing—an indicator of periodontal stability. J Clin Periodontol 1990; 17:714–721.

Male D. Immunology: an illustrated outline. 3rd ed St. Louis: C.V. Mosby, , 1998. Offenbacher S. Periodontal diseases: pathogenesis. Ann Periodontol 1996;1:821–878.

Page R C, Schroeder H E. Pathogenesis of inflammatory periodontal disease. A summary of current work. Lab Invest 1976;33: 235–249.

Periodontal diseases: pathogenesis and microbial factors [Review] [45 refs]. J Am Dent Assoc 1998;129(Suppl):58S–62S.

Tonetti MS. Cigarette smoking and periodontal diseases: etiology and management of disease. Ann Periodontol 1998;3: 88–101.

Host Defenses and Periodontal Disease

Jonathan L. Gray

Bacterial plaque is the primary cause of inflammatory periodontal disease, but it does not sufficiently account for all periodontal destruction in multivariant studies. The host response plays a major role in the disease process. The human body has a complex array of interdependent defense mechanisms to eliminate infecting microorganisms, heal, and maintain health. We refer to these systems as the inflammatory response and the immune system. Paradoxically, these systems that are intended to protect and heal the body have been shown to be responsible for some of the destruction in periodontal disease.

Immunology is an extraordinarily complex subject. Furthermore, separating inflammation and immunity into distinct entities is difficult because there are many situations in which their activities overlap. This chapter presents an overview of the workings of the inflammatory response and the immune system, and discusses their role in periodontal healing and destruction. The following topics will be presented:

- Inflammation
- Cellular Components of Inflammation
- Molecular Components of Inflammation
- Acute Inflammatory Process in Periodontal Disease

- Phagocytic System
- Non–Oxygen Dependent Phagocytosis
- Oxygen Dependent Phagocytosis
- Destruction of Host Tissues
- Compliment System
- Immunology
- Cellular Elements of the Immune System
- Molecular Elements of the Immune System
- Cytokines
- Immunoglobulins (Antibodies)
- Immune Response in Periodontal Disease
- Summary

INFLAMMATION

Inflammation is an orderly sequence of events that occurs in response to any injury or infection; therefore, it is considered to be "nonspecific" in nature. Inflammation is the initial response, occurring prior to activation of the immune system. It occurs in three stages:

1. Increased vascular supply.
2. Increased vascular permeability.
3. Active migration of phagocytic cells into the affected area.

Before discussing the process itself, the major cellular and molecular components of inflammation will be described.

Cellular Components of Inflammation

The primary cells responsible for inflammation are the leukocytes (PMNs), which are formed in the bone marrow from the same stem cell that forms monocytes. Specific cell surface markers determine which promyelocytes will become PMNs and which will become macrophages. These markers are lost after cell differentiation.

The presence of a few PMNs in the junctional epithelium is considered to be normal. An increase in their number indicates the initiation of host defenses. PMNs are phagocytic cells that constitute about 70% of the white blood cells. The cytoplasm of PMNs also contains elements that are responsible for cellular movement during chemotaxis, and they also contain lysosomes that are responsible for killing invading bacteria. Killing of microorganisms by these cells usually, but not always, occurs after the microorganisms have been phagosotyzed (ingested) by the cells.

The next cell involved in inflammation, the macrophage is derived from the circulating monocyte and arrives at the site of inflammation after the PMN. It is a large cell with phagocytic capabilities similar to the PMN. It also plays a critical role in the immune response.

Lymphocytes arrive late at the site of inflammation, and are associated with chronic inflammation. Lymphocytes are also one of the principal cell types in the immune system.

Mast cells are similar to the circulating basophil. They release histamine, platelet activating factor (PAF), prostaglandin E2 (PGE2), and leukotrienes (LTB4) and (LTD4), all of which have profound inflammatory effects.

Platelets release serotonin, an important inflammatory mediator.

Molecular Components of Inflammation

Histamine is a potent agent that increases vascular permeability, thus permitting inflammatory cells easier access to the affected site. It is released from mast cells and basophils. Serotonin (5-hydroxy-tryptamine) also increases vascular permeability.

Basophils, neutrophils, and macrophages release platelet activating factor (PAF). PAF increases the release of serotonin from platelets. Neutrophil chemotactic factor (NCF) is released from mast cells and is chemotactic for PMNs.

Chemokines are released from leukocytes. They constitute a large collection of cytokines, which cause mast cell degranulation and chemotaxis of PMNs. (The terminology can be very confusing. All molecules that affect or control the immune or inflammatory responses are referred to as cytokines. Accordingly, all chemokines are cytokines, but there are many other cytokines that are not chemokines.)

Activated compliment C3a causes mast cell degranulation. Activated compliment C5a causes mast cell degranulation, phagocyte chemotaxis, activation of PMNs, and increased capillary permeability.

Bradykinin from the kinin system causes vasodilation and increased vascular permeability. Fibrinopeptides are by-products of the clotting mechanism, and are chemotactic for PMNs and macrophages.

Prostaglandin E2 (PGE2) is a product of the cyclooxygenase pathway and causes vasodilation while potentiating vascular permeability caused by histamine and bradykinin.

Leukotriene B4 (LTB4) has its origins in the lipoxygenase pathway. It stimulates PMN chemotaxis and is synergistic with PGE2 in increasing vascular permeability.

Leukotriene D4 (LTD4), which is also produced via the lipoxygenase pathway, aids in vascular permeability.

Neutrophil chemotactic factor (NCF) is released from basophils.

Selectins are a group of three molecules responsible for assisting with migration of PMNs and macrophages across vessel walls. E selectins and P selectins are specific for PMNs, and L selectins are selective for macrophages. They help slow the cells down prior to adhesion to the endothelial wall. There are at least 12 other molecules from three different families that perform similar functions, including a group known as ICAMS.

Acute Inflammatory Process in Periodontal Disease

As mentioned earlier, acute inflammation is a three-stage process. As bacterial plaque accumulates in the gingival sulcus, the following events occur.

The vascular supply is increased by vasodilation in the affected area. Mediators such as histamine and PGE2 are responsible for this process. Serotonin, C5a, bradykinin, fibrinopeptides, PGE2, LTB2, and LTD2 cause increased vascular permeability and retraction of the endothelial cells. Selectins and ICAMS slow the PMNs, permitting them to migrate into the connective tissue. Migration and phagocytosis of PMNs are mediated by chemotactic factors such as NCF, chemokines, C5a, fibrinopeptides, and LTB4 enhance phagocytosis and neutrophil chemotaxis. The principal phagocytic cells involved in the host response to infectious microorganisms are the polymorphonuclear neutrophils and the macrophages. Killing of microorganisms by these cells usually, but not always, occurs after the microorganisms have been taken up or ingested by the cells.

PHAGOCYTIC SYSTEM

Non–Oxygen Dependent Phagocytosis

This consists of a battery of degenerative substances contained in organelles located in the cytoplasm of the phagocytes. These organelles are referred to as granules or lysosomes. The degenerative

THE INFLAMMATORY RESPONSE

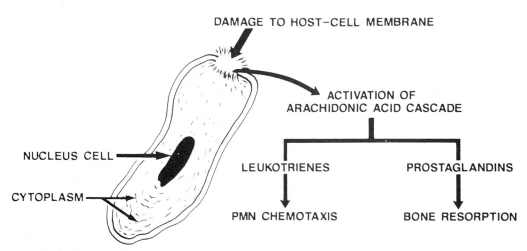

DAMAGE TO HOST–CELL MEMBRANE

ACTIVATION OF ARACHIDONIC ACID CASCADE

NUCLEUS CELL

CYTOPLASM

LEUKOTRIENES   PROSTAGLANDINS

PMN CHEMOTAXIS   BONE RESORPTION

DAMAGE TO CERTAIN CELL MEMBRANES CAN RESULT IN THE FORMATION AND LIBERATION OF FACTORS WHICH ARE RESPONSIBLE FOR THE CLINICAL SIGNS OF INFLAMMATION: ERYTHEMA, EDEMA, PAIN, AND TEMPERATURE ELEVATION. IN ADDITION, SOME OF THESE FACTORS ARE NOW KNOWN TO CAUSE BONE RESORPTION.

Fig. 5-1

COMPLEMENT

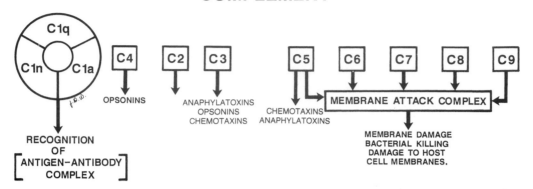

THE ELEVEN PROTEINS OF THE CLASSICAL COMPLEMENT SYSTEM ARE INDICATED AT THE TOP OF THE FIGURE.

THE ACTIVATION CASCADE PROCEEDS IN SEQUENCE FROM LEFT TO RIGHT. SOME OF THE BIOLOGICAL EFFECTS OF THE ACTIVATION OF VARIOUS COMPONENTS ARE DESIGNATED BY ARROWS.

Fig. 5-2

THE PHAGOCYTE (PMN)

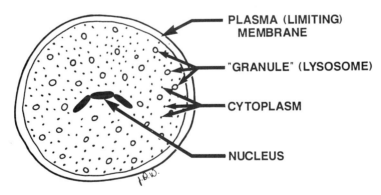

THE "GRANULE" IS ALSO CALLED THE LYSOSOME, ALSO REFERRED TO AS "SUICIDE PACKETS." THE ENZYMES THAT DAMAGE BACTERIAL CELL WALLS AND HOST CELL MEMBRANES ARE CONTAINED IN THE LYSOSOMES. THE CYTOPLASM CONTAINS THE "CYTOSKELETAL" ELEMENTS. WHEN STIMULATED THESE ELEMENTS BECOME ORGANIZED AND ARE RESPONSIBLE FOR THE CELLULAR MOVEMENT DURING CHEMOTAXIS.

Fig. 5-3

activities of enzymes carry out the granular contents and other factors broadly classified as cationic proteins, neutral proteases, acid hydrolases, and other constituents such as lactoferrin. The usual mode of killing by these enzymes occurs after the bacteria have been ingested. However, during the process of phagocytosis, these enzymes "leak out" of the phagocyte and enter the external environment of the cells. Possibly, this phenomenon is important in the sulcular, or pocket, fluid where bacterial killing, without prior ingestion, could be important to the defense of periodontal tissues. Furthermore, lysosomal enzymes may be important in neutralizing the actions of destructive enzymes and toxins synthesized and released by bacteria—whether or not the enzymes and toxins were first ingested into phagocytic cells.

Oxygen Dependent Phagocytosis

This system kills microorganisms inside the cell in an organelle called the phagolysosome. In this system, toxic oxidants and hydrogen peroxide are generated from oxygen radicals and a lysosomal enzyme, myeloperoxidase. The result of formation of these factors is extensive and lethal damage to bacterial cell walls.

The relationship of the polymorphonuclear neutrophil (PMN) to periodontal health and disease has been the subject of numerous studies. When humans or animals have defective neutrophils, such as in agranulycotosis or leukocyte adherence deficiency, periodontal disorders are common and severe. Animals depleted of or congenitally lacking PMNs undergo rapid periodontal destruction and tooth exfoliation. Extensive studies of humans with defects in

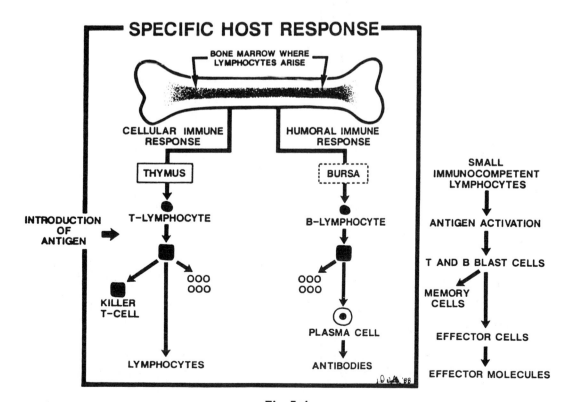

Fig. 5-4

PMN function have shown these individuals to demonstrate high susceptibility for periodontal tissue destruction. In the 1996 World Workshop in Periodontics, Offenbacker proposed that individuals with normal PMN function would have either gingivitis or periodontal health regardless of the bacterial challenge. Conversely, those with PMN deficiency or malfunction are much more likely to experience attachment loss. Conclusions from these studies indicate that the PMN is essential for the maintenance of periodontal health but can also be responsible for periodontal destruction.

Destruction of Host Tissues

It is well known that the body is responsible for much of the destruction that occurs during periodontal disease. This destruction can be viewed as an overreaction to a chronic infection. The following substances have the capability of destroying periodontal tissues during the process of defending against invading bacteria and their byproducts:

1. Colony-stimulating factors (CSFs).
2. Gamma interferon (IFN-γ).
3. Interleukin-1 (IL-1).
4. Interleukin-6 (IL-6).
5. Lymphotoxin.
6. Matrix metalloprotineases.
7. PGE-2.
8. Transforming growth factor-β (TGF-β).
9. Tumor necrosis factor (TNF).

These will be discussed in greater detail later in this chapter.

Serum Complement System

The *serum complement system* is composed of more than 20 serum proteins that, when activated, have potent biological activity. The system is important in both inflammation and immunity. There are two major pathways by which proteins of the complement system are activated. The first, the *classical pathway,* follows binding of antibody to bacterial cell wall surfaces. The second pathway, the *alternate pathway,* can be activated directly by constituents of cell walls of certain gram-negative bacteria. These constituents are called endotoxins. The following are some of the many effects of complement activation by both pathways:

1. Substances form that enhance the ingestion of microbial cells and microbial products by white cells (phagocytes). These substances are called opsonins. When activated, serum complement generates potent opsonic factors.
2. Activated serum complement induces mast cells to release substances such as histamine. These factors cause blood vessels to dilate and to become permeable, resulting in an influx of serum and serum factors into the local tissue spaces. Among the serum factors are antibodies and additional complement components.
3. A very powerful chemoattractant (for phagocytes) is generated when serum complement is activated. This chemoattractant, or chemotactic factor, causes neutrophils and macrophages to migrate toward a specific area in tissue.
4. Activated serum complement can result in factors that destroy microbial cell walls and cell membranes. This feature is important in killing certain bacteria. In the periodontal area, the large numbers of microbial cells and associated high levels of their metabolic products require that host responses consistently and efficiently control their concentrations and potential for invasion if serious infection is to be avoided.

The biologically active factors generated from serum complement probably play an important role in defense against microbial assault in periodontal tissues by directly destroying bacteria and by augmenting other host defense responses in controlling local concentrations of the microbial population.

As with all host responses, potential for periodontal tissue injury exists when complement activation occurs. Later, in this chapter, periodontal tissue injury from the influx of antibodies and phagocytes induced by complement will be discussed. In addition to these, however, host cell membranes can also be damaged by the direct action of complement activation, especially red cell membranes. As with all host responses, complement activation could be a factor in the periodontal tissue destruction that occurs in the clinical course of the disease.

IMMUNOLOGY

Traditionally, we have considered the immune system to have two parts, cellular immunity and humoral immunity. Although these designations are still useful, immunologists now tend to characterize the immune system into those components that recognize cell-associated antigens and those that recognize free antigens.

Cellular Elements of the Immune System

1. *B cells* (B lymphocytes) are produced in the bone marrow in humans and carry surface immunoglobulin (antibody) which reacts to antigens. Some B cells mature into plasma cells.
2. Plasma cells or *antibody-forming cells* (AFCs) are terminally differentiated B cells. They produce antibodies to specific antigens (invaders), and are divided into two groups, B-1 and B-2 cells.
   a. B-1 cells develop early in response to common bacteria.
   b. B-2 cells comprise the majority of all B cells and produce a greater variety of antibodies.
3. Produced in the thymus gland, *T cells* are responsible for the production of cytokines known as lymphokines. These cells play a dual role. First, they are tasked with killing virally infected cells and tumor cells. T cells also play a significant role in the modulation and amplification of the immune response. They are divided into two major subsets based on their cell surface markers, CD4 and CD8.
   a. T helper cells have CD4+ and CD8- cell surface markers. They are referred to generically as Th0 cells with two subsets, Th1 and Th2. The antigen is presented to them by the appropriate cell listed in the following, and cytokines necessary for continuation of the immune process are released: 1) Th1 cells interact with mononuclear phagocytes such as activated macrophages, and 2) Th2 cells release cytokines that are required for differentiation of B cells into plasma cells.
   b. T cytotoxic cells are CD8+ and are most effective against virally infected cells and tumors.
   c. T suppressor cells (Ts) have no unique cell surface marker. They are capable of increasing or decreasing the immune response in response to appropriate cytokines.
   d. Memory cells are populations of long-lived T cells and B cells that remain after exposure to an antigen. They provide a rapid response if that antigen is encountered in the future.
4. *Killer cells* are mononuclear cells that are capable of killing target cells, such as a tumor cell, sensitized with antibody.

5. *Natural killer cells* have the same ability as killer cells, except that the target cell need not be sensitized. These cells possess innate surface receptors to identify target cells.
6. *Monocytes* are circulating cells that can migrate into the tissues becoming macrophages. They have phagocytic capability, produce cytokines, and "present" antigens to B cells and Th1 cells for further processing. The B cells then produce antibody specific for that antigen, and the Th1 cells render the antigen for phagocytosis by macrophages.
7. *PMNs* are cells that phagosotyze antigens coated with antibody.

Cytokines and Other Molecular Components

Cytokines are non-antibody molecules that influence a wide range of activity in the immune and inflammatory systems as well as compliment, clotting, bradykinin, and arachidonic acid pathways. The most important cytokines are:

1. *Interleukins* are a diverse group of cytokines. Most are produced by and act on other cells in the immune/inflammatory response and have intertwining biologic activity.
    a. Lymphocytes, fibroblasts, and macrophages produce IL-1. It has the following functions: 1) stimulation of the production of endothelial adhesion molecules such as selectins to begin the inflammatory process; 2) production of prostaglandins by fibroblasts and osteoclasts; 3) activation of phagocytes that makes T cell surfaces more receptive to antigens; and 4) stimulation of the release of IL-2 by T cells, B cells, and NK cells.
    b. IL-1 stimulates prostaglandin synthesis.
    c. IL-2 enhances T cell and NK cell growth and activation.
    d. IL-4 causes B cells to activate and divide. It promotes immunoglobulin and is also a growth factor for mast cells.
    e. IL-6 is produced by macrophages and CD4+ T cells and stimulates the production of B cells and mast cells.
    f. IL-8 is an important cytokine. It is produced by fibroblasts, endothelial cells, and monocytes and stimulates activation and chemotaxis by macrophages, PMNs, and T cells.
    g. IL-10 is produced by CD4+ T cells and inhibits the production of cytokines by CD8+ T cells.
2. *Interferons* are cytokines usually associated with antiviral activity. Interferon-γ plays an important role in periodontal disease. It is released by the CD4+ T cells and enhances phagocytosis via a number of pathways.
3. *Migration inhibitory factor* (MIF) is produced by activated T cells and prevents the migration of macrophages from an area of inflammation or infection, thereby increasing the population of macrophages in that area.
4. *Tumor necrosis factor* (TNF) aids in the formation of selectins and ICBMs on endothelial walls, thus aiding in migration of leukocytes.
5. *Lymphotoxin* (LT) is produced by activated T-cells. It works together with IFN-γ to activate leukocytes.
6. *Transforming growth factor-β* (TGF-β) is a group of cytokines produced by macrophages and platelets. Its primary role appears to be the inhibition of the immune system.
7. *Prostaglandins* and *leukotrienes* were discussed earlier in this chapter.
8. *Matrix metalloproteins* (MMPs) are a group of enzymes that degrade collagen, the ground substance, and other structures. The nine that have

been identified have been classified into four groups based on the substrates upon which they act.

9. *Elastase, glucoronidase,* and *hyaluronidase* are lysosomal enzymes produced by the destruction of PMNs and fibroblasts.
10. *Colony-stimulating factors* (CSFs) exist for granulocytes, lymphocytes, and macrophages. They are cytokines derived from T cells that control hematopoiesis.

Immunoglobulins (Antibodies)

1. IgM is the first antibody on the scene. It initiates the complement cascade and is the main antibody in response to T independent antigens.
2. IgG is the next antibody to arrive; it remains longest. Having several subclasses, IgG is also the most predominant antibody. It coats antigens (opsinization) for destruction by phagocytes, prepares other antigens for destruction by killer cells, and also activates the compliment cascade.
3. IgA is found in the saliva (secretory IgA) and other areas where there is mucous membrane.
4. IgD is a trace antibody on differentiating B cells. It disappears after differentiation.
5. IgE binds to mast cells and basophils stimulating the release of vasoactive substances such as histamine, prostaglandins, and leukotrienes.

Immune Response in Periodontal Disease

If bacterial plaque is permitted to collect in the gingival sulcus, a lag period of several days occurs, during which there is no detectable antibody. After several days, the body responds to the presence of the bacteria and their byproducts. Fibroblasts, macrophages, and lymphocytes release IL-1, IL-2, IL-6, and IL-8. Selectins and ICAMs are activated, beginning the process of PMN diapedesis (movement through the vessel wall), migration, and chemotaxis. The process of diapedesis is enhanced, and the PMNs are followed by macrophages. Both are activated and enhanced by cytokines. This produces the initial redness of gingivitis.

Antigens are "presented" to B cells and monocytes with the aid of T helper cells. The latter release cytokines that cause the production of B cells which produce antibody specific for the antigen. The antigens are opsinized and phagosotyzed, and in the process, substances that are harmful to collagen and the ground substance are released. C3a and C5a cause mast cells to release histamine, which increases vasodilation and allows more protective cells to migrate into the area. Eventually, the sulcular epithelium becomes ulcerated, permitting more rapid ingress of the bacterial antigens. At this point, the gingiva is swollen, bleeding, and may be slightly painful.

Cytokines produced by fibroblasts, PMNs, and other host cells are both helpful and harmful in the protective process. The area becomes infiltrated with lymphocytes and finally by plasma cells. If treatment is not provided, or if the host defenses are insufficient, attachment loss will occur both as a result of the bacteria and the body's response to the bacteria.

Summary

Bacteria and host defense mechanisms are in balance in health. In disease, an imbalance exists, in which both the bacteria and the body's attempts to kill the bacteria and heal itself actually contribute to the destruction of periodontal tissue. This imbalance may be a result of bacterial virulence factors, altered host defenses, or external modifying factors such as tobacco smoke.

SUGGESTED READINGS

Gallin JI, Goldstein IM, Synderman R, eds. Inflammation: basic principles and clinical correlates. New York: Raven Press, 1988.

Korman K, Page R, Tonetti S. Host response to the microbial challenge in periodontitis Periodontology 2000 1997;14:33–53.

Landi L, Amar S, Polins AS, Van Dyke TE. Host mechanisms in the pathogenesis of periodontal disease [review] [47 refs]. Current Opinion in Periodontology 1997;4:3–10.

Male D. Immunology: an illustrated outline. 3rd ed. London: Mosby-Year Book Europe Limited, 1993.

Miyasaki KT. The neutrophil: mechanisms of controlling periodontal bacteria. Journal of Periodontology 1991;62:761.

Offenbacher S. Periodontal diseases: pathogenesis. Annals of Periodontology 1996;1: 821–878.

Roitt I, Brostoff J, Male D. Immunology. 3rd ed. London: Mosby-Year Book Europe Limited, 1993.

Diagnosis, Prognosis, and Treatment Planning

Jonathan L. Gray

The successful management of periodontal disease depends on the systematic conversion of examination data into a comprehensive, written treatment plan. Diagnosis, prognosis, and treatment planning are certainly three of the most important services performed in dentistry. To be a good diagnostician, one must gather all the facts, sort them, and then assimilate them into a step-by-step road map or treatment plan. The meticulous manner in which the clinician approaches the fact-gathering appointment(s) will determine the success or failure of case management. This chapter is designed to serve as a guide for the gathering of information and to discuss its use in the formation of a prognosis and treatment plan.

DIAGNOSIS

Limitations of Diagnostic Techniques

In the final analysis, periodontal diagnosis is more art than science. All periodontal diagnostic methods are surrogate methods. They measure or reveal the previous damage caused by periodontal disease without providing the clinician with data regarding the patient's current condition or future tendencies. At any given examination, it is virtually impossible to know with certainty whether a particular site is actively diseased. Only with the hindsight provided by radiographic bone loss or increased loss of clinical attachment can one be certain of disease activity. An observant and insightful practitioner may develop a "6th sense" regarding periodontal health, but research has proven that our diagnostic capabilities are a major shortcoming in periodontics. Advances in molecular biology, immunology, bacteriology, and radiography offer promising new alternatives for periodontal diagnosis and will be discussed later in this chapter.

Another limitation is our inability to use diagnostic information to develop a treatment plan and prognosis that can be relied on with any degree of certainty to achieve the desired result, even with compliant patients. As recent studies have shown, the standard clinical examination and treatment do not correlate well with the long-term survival of teeth. Unquestionably, other significant factors that we are as yet unable to measure need to be included in our examination and treatment planning. These will be discussed in greater detail later in this chapter.

The Periodontal Chart

The practitioner's approach to periodontal diseases will be more productive and less frustrating if information is recorded on a form that serves as a fact-gathering guide, allows brief shorthand notations, and provides space in which to formulate the treatment plan.

The basic means of gathering data that precede periodontal therapy may be considered as a series of surveys. As these surveys are completed, it may be helpful to estimate the comparative influence of each survey area on the patient's condition. The survey areas are as follows:

1. Health survey.
2. General dental survey.
3. Periodontal survey.
4. Occlusal survey.
5. Radiographic survey.
6. Deposits survey.

Stated simply, virtually all periodontal disease is an infection and is a struggle between the patient's resistance factors and bacterial plaque. Every single factor surveyed simply modifies the influence of either the disease agent or the host resistance.

Health Survey

The health survey includes a medical and a dental history.

Medical History

A medical history should be obtained first by a written questionnaire. After its completion, the written questionnaire should be reviewed with the patient so that a thorough explanation of any areas of concern may be provided. This is the appropriate time to refer patients for a medical consultation if any condition exists that might affect the progression of the periodontal disease and/or the management of the patient. A written consul-

tation report from the physician rather than a telephone report is essential.

The medical history is vital for three major reasons:

1. To detect oral manifestations of certain systemic conditions. These may include leukemia, diabetes mellitus, hormonal disturbance, etc. An alert diagnostician, in addition to ensuring good management for the patient, may detect conditions having important health implications.
2. To ascertain systemic conditions, such as pregnancy, diabetes mellitus, dyscrasias, nutritional deficiencies, and hypertensive cardiovascular diseases that may alter the response of the host to the bacterial insult.
3. To determine certain systemic conditions that require modification of both primary and supportive periodontal therapy. These include allergic conditions, rheumatic fever syndrome, diabetes mellitus, endocrine disorders, cardiovascular diseases and valvular prostheses, drug therapy (endocrine, corticosteroid, anticoagulant), physchologic problems, and use of tobacco products.

An example of the medical history's importance is in providing dental care for patients at risk of developing endocarditis. Endocarditis is a relatively uncommon life-threatening condition. Endocarditis usually develops in individuals with existing structural cardiac defects who develop bacteremia with organisms likely to cause endocarditis.

It is imperative that the therapist recognize patients at risk for endocarditis. Some surgical and dental procedures, and instrumentation use involving the mucosal surfaces or contaminated tissue can cause transient bacteremia. These rarely last more than 15 minutes. Any probing or manipulation of the gingival tissue (periodontal examination, scaling, root planing, curettage, root canal treatment, extraction, periodontal surgery, etc.) that causes bleeding can cause transient bacteremia, which could result in bacterial endocarditis in these patients. Note that most cases of endocarditis are not attributable to an invasive procedure. Patients who have cardiovascular problems should be managed in coordination with a physician, preferably a cardiologist. A written consultation should be obtained and retained as a permanent part of the patient's record. Occasionally, patients who claim a history of rheumatic fever are reported by their cardiologist to be free from valvular damage or associated sequelae, thereby negating the need for antibiotic coverage. However, it is extremely important that all patients with a history of rheumatic fever be carefully evaluated by a physician before any dental treatment is rendered. Consultation in writing—not by telephone—is preferred.

Antibiotic prophylaxis for at-risk patients is recommended for dental and oral procedures likely to cause bacteremia. The American Medical Association, the American Heart Association, and the American Dental Association have endorsed the following regimens (JAMA 1997;1794–1801). Cardiac conditions are divided into high-risk, moderate-risk, and negligible-risk categories based on potential of developing endocarditis.

Antibiotic prophylaxis is recommended with all dental procedures (including routine professional cleaning) likely to cause gingival bleeding in the high-risk and moderate-risk categories. Because alpha-hemolytic (viridans) streptococci are most commonly implicated in endocarditis following dental procedures, antibiotic prophylaxis should be specifically directed against these organisms.

A greater and more detailed explanation of the recommendations of the American Heart Association (AHA) for the prevention of endocarditis can be found in the June 1997 issue of the *Journal of the American Medical Association* or from their World Wide Web site at http://www.americanheart.org/. The American Dental Association has a more concise statement on the Internet at http://www.ada.org/.

The potential risk of dental treatment to the patient with artificial replacement devices is unclear. Consultation with the patient's surgeon is recommended to determine the need and appropriate type of prophylactic antibiotic regimen prior to dental treatment.

Dental History

Before the intraoral examination is conducted, the practitioner should obtain a complete dental history. By doing so, the practitioner is afforded the opportunity to assay the patient's attitude, establish rapport, and learn of past dental disease and response to treatment. It is also important to determine what methods of home care the patient is presently using, as well as the patient's general dental IQ.

General Dental Survey

The overall impression gained by this survey will begin to establish the magnitude of the problem. The following points should be observed and noted.

1. *Soft tissue survey.* This is the oral cancer search. Other lesions must also be noted, but few have consequences as severe, especially if not detected early or if completely overlooked.
2. *Positioning.* Arch alignment, morphologic malocclusion, and migration of teeth.
3. *Caries.* Location, type, and extent.
4. *Restorative dentistry.* Adequacy of restorations and prostheses. These must be viewed in relation to plaque retention, prevention of plaque removal, traumatogenic occlusion, and excessive leverage from torquing forces. It is also necessary to consider

possible infringement of the restoration margin on the "biologic width," the junctional epithelium, and connective tissue attachment. This can result in serious iatrogenic injury to the periodontium.

5. *Habits.* Examples include smoking, tongue-thrusting, bruxism, clenching, and factitious disease.

6. *Pulpal status of teeth, especially those with advanced bone loss (particularly when associated with teeth that have deep restorations and/or furcation involvement).* The relationships between pulpal status and periodontal disease have become increasingly important and may alter treatment planning. "Cracked tooth syndrome" may mimic or cause pulpal problems. Fractures are relatively common, especially among posterior teeth, and should always be considered when dealing with a deep, narrow pocket.

7. *Mobility of teeth.* This is a critical diagnostic and prognostic consideration. Some mobility is normal and may vary during the day, according to diet and stress. Pathologic mobility has several principal causes:
   a. Gingival and periodontal inflammation.
   b. Parafunctional occlusal habits.
   c. Occlusal prematurities.
   d. Loss of supporting bone.
   e. Traumatic torquing forces applied to clasped teeth by removable dentures.
   f. Periodontal therapy, endodontic therapy, and trauma may cause transient mobility. Tooth movement is measured by applying force buccolingually between two dental instrument handles.

Mobility is usually graded as 1, 2, or 3 (Fig. 6-1):

Grade 1 represents the first distinguishable sign of movement greater than normal.

GRADES OF MOBILITY

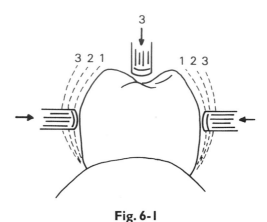

Fig. 6-1

Grade 2 is recorded if there is a total movement of approximately 1 mm.

Grade 3 is recorded if the tooth moves more than 1 mm in any direction and/or is depressible.

Reduction or control of pathologic tooth mobility may be achieved through removal or modification of the causative factors.

Periodontal Survey

This survey is a critical part of the diagnostic process. A calibrated periodontal probe, a furcation explorer, a front reflective surface examining mirror, adequate light, palpation, and air blast must all be employed to supplement visual examination of the periodontal tissues. Figure 6-2 demonstrates how information obtained from a periodontal survey may be recorded.

1. *Gingival color, form, and consistency.* These should be observed and recorded. Changes in any of these are suggestive of periodontal disease but cannot be correlated with the severity of the disease. For instance, one patient may have very red gingiva whereas another patient has only minimal color change.

It is possible that a biopsy of each would show that the patient with the least amount of color change actually has more severe destruction. However, gingiva that appears "normal" in color is usually healthy.

2. *Bleeding and purulent exudation.* These are clinical indicators of disease activity and should be noted. Exudation may be spontaneous or may be evident only on probing or palpation. Bleeding and suppuration are not indicators of the severity of the disease but may signify ulceration of the epithelial wall of the pocket. The presence of bleeding is not a reliable indicator of disease, but the absence of bleeding is a very reliable indicator of health.

3. *Pocket (probing) depth.* Measurement is taken from the gingival margin on all teeth with the aid of a calibrated probe. The instrument is held as close to the tooth surface as possible and is gently inserted into the sulcus or pocket until resistance is met. Any bleeding, suppuration, or subgingival calculus is noted and recorded. The probe is walked along the tooth surface, keeping it parallel to the long axis of the tooth. Three measurements are recorded on both the facial and lingual surfaces: distal, midfacial/midlingual, and mesial (Fig. 6-3). When a heavy calculus formation is present, it is often impossible to measure pocket depth accurately because calculus will impede the insertion of the probe. It may then be necessary to perform a gross debridement before pocket measurement is taken. The measurements are then recorded.

4. *Relationship of gingival margin to cementoenamel junction (recession).* This information is recorded as a continuous line on a chart. If this step is neglected, pocket measurements are meaningless. A 3-mm pocket, for example, on a tooth with a 5-mm gingival recession would signify greater destruction of the attachment apparatus than a 5-mm pocket on a tooth with hyperplastic gingiva (Fig. 6-4).

5. *Relationship of cementoenamel junction to the bottom of the pocket (attachment level).* This measurement should be recorded. The location of the base of the pocket in relation to the CEJ affects the prognosis of an individual tooth more than the pocket depth. For example, a tooth with 3-mm probing depth and a 5-mm recession has an attachment level loss of 8 mm, but a tooth with a 5-mm probing depth and no recession would have an attachment level loss of only 5 mm. This measurement is especially important when comparing with attachment levels at subsequent visits for reevaluation or maintenance. Attachment level loss may be an indication of disease activity.

6. *General width of keratinized gingiva, relationship of probing depth to the mucogingival junction, and influence of various frenal and muscle attachments on the gingival margin.* These should all be observed and recorded. The relationship between gingival width and health is very controversial. Many clinicians believe that 2 to 3 mm of attached gingiva is necessary if a subgingival restorative margin is planned. Numerous cases have been reported in which patients had little or no keratinized gingiva, yet remained healthy for long periods of observation.

7. *Pathologic invasion of furcation areas.* Careful probing with a curved furcation probe (e.g., a Nabors furcation probe) will make help this determination. The complicated anatomy of these regions presents diagnostic and therapeutic challenges. Furcations and classification are discussed in Chapter 18.

Occlusal Survey

Because occlusion may influence the progress and severity of periodontal disease, the occlusal status of every patient

Periodontics Chart

Patient Name: _Doe, Jane_

Patient Age and Sex: _40/f_

Doctor Name: _____

Date of Examination: _1988_

Date of Treatment Completed: _____

Case Type: _____

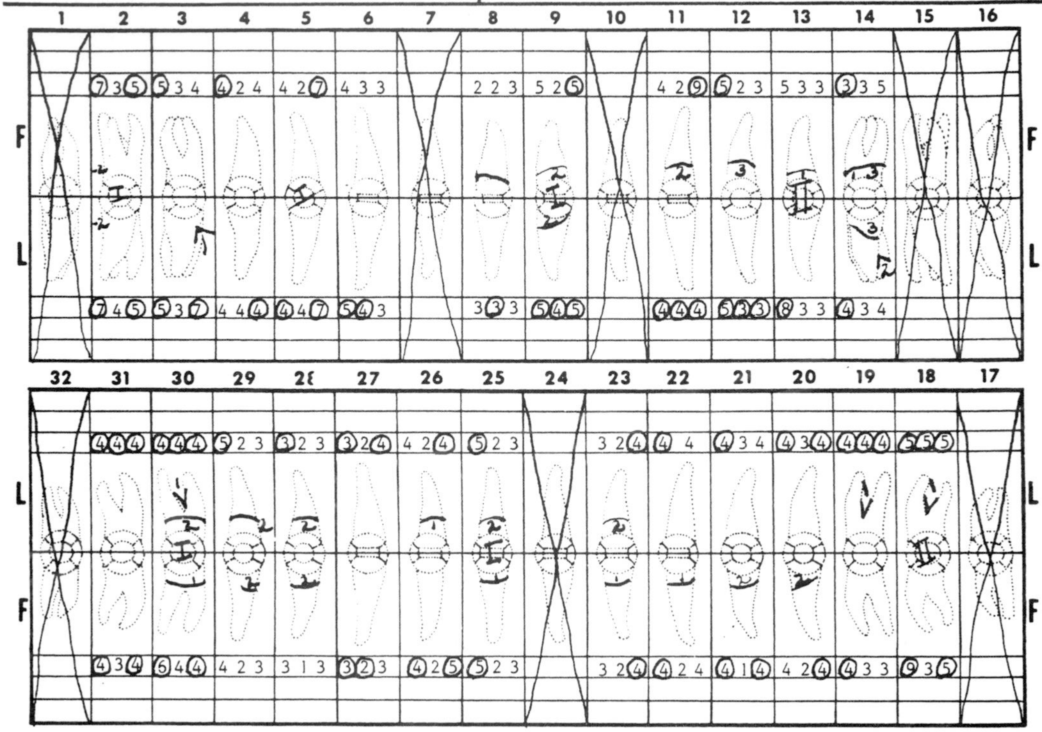

Mobility I, II, III	Furca Involvement 1, 2, 3	Food Impaction ↓	Missing Teeth X	Recession
To be Extracted = TE	Overhang ⌐ L	Inadequate Contact ‖	Mucogingival Involvement ≋	

INITIAL OCCLUSAL FINDINGS

CENTRIC RELATION OCCLUSION	1 ② 3 4 5 6 7 8	9 10 11 12 ⑬ 14 15 16	
	32 ㉛ 30 29 28 27 26 25	24 23 22 21 ⑳ 19 18 17	
RIGHT LATERAL	1 2 3 4 ⑤ 6 7 8	9 10 11 12 ⑬ ⑭ 15 16	CR = CO
	32 31 30 29 28 27 26 25←	24 23 22 21 ⑳ ⑲ 18 17	Hor. Vert.
LEFT LATERAL	1 ② ③ 4 5 6 7 8	9 10 ⑪ ⑫ ⑬ 14 15 16	
	32 ㉛ ㉚ 29 28 27 26 25→	24 23 22 21 20 19 18 17	
PROTRUSIVE	1 2 3 4 5 6 7 ⑧	⑨ 10 11 12 13 14 15 16	
	32 31 30 29 28 27 26 ㉕	24 ㉓ 22 21 20 19 18 17	

Occlusal Treatment Plan _____

Fig. 6-2

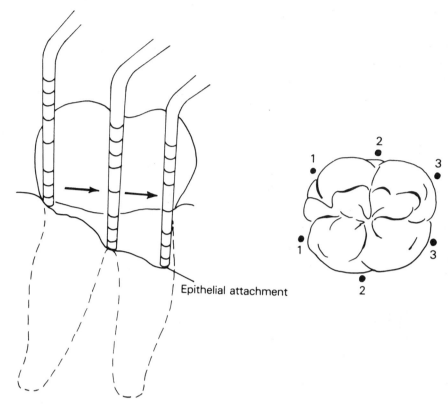

Epithelial attachment

Fig. 6-3

should be evaluated. An occlusal survey will enable the therapist to gauge the relative importance of occlusion in each individual case and to determine whether occlusal adjustment is indicated.

Analysis of the Occlusion

Certain information must be obtained before a final evaluation of the role of occlusion can be made.

Clinical Evaluation

The clinician must:

1. *Determine parafunctional habits (e.g., bruxing, clenching, doodling, and other factitious habits such as fingernail biting).* (The following information must be obtained with the patient in an upright position.)

2. *Identify the initial tooth contact in centric relation.* This is a reference point from which the occlusion can be adjusted. One way to find the initial contact in centric relation is to place gentle pressure against the center of the mandible and guide the mandible posteriorly (Fig. 6-5). Record the first contact in centric relation (first centric prematurity) by tapping the teeth into occlusal indicator wax or articulating ribbon.

3. *Determine the anterior slide of the mandible.* Have the patient slowly close the teeth completely from the initial contact in centric relation; observe anterior or lateral movement of the mandible. Also note any facial movement of the maxillary anterior teeth as the jaw closes from centric relation to functional (habitual) occlusion (fremitus).

4. *Determine prematurities in functional occlusion.* This is the position in which most tooth contacts occur (Fig. 6-6).
5. *Determine working contacts.* Working contacts occur when the mandible is moved laterally from functional occlusion with the teeth in contact. The patient is asked to glide the mandible right and left from the functional position. Working contacts are best recorded with ribbon.
6. *Determine balancing (nonworking) contacts.* When the mandible is moved to the right (right working), posterior teeth may contact on the left. These contacts are called balancing (nonworking) contacts. They are located by placing ribbon on the nonworking side and having the patient move the mandible into working position. Look for long, streaked markings on the teeth.
7. *Determine contacts in protrusive position.* Have the patient bite on the anterior teeth in tip-to-tip relation. Also note any posterior teeth that may contact in this position.
8. *Determine protrusive excursion.* Place the ribbon between the upper and lower anterior teeth and have the patient

close in functional position and then protrude the mandible until the teeth reach protrusive position.
9. *Check movement of teeth during chewing (fremitus).* Place the ball of the index finger on the teeth one at a time and determine if the tooth moves in habitual occlusion as the patient glides the mandible into working or protrusive position.
10. *Determine tooth/tooth relationships: open contacts, irregular contacts, food impaction sites, rough incisal/occlusal surfaces.* These may often be detected on the study casts.

Evaluation of Study Casts

The following occlusal information may be obtained from study casts:

1. Plunger cusps.
2. Wear facets.
3. Malposed teeth.
4. Abnormal marginal ridge relationship.
5. Condition of existing restorations (contour, buccolingual dimension).
6. First molar relationship (Angle's classification).
7. Overbite (vertical overlap of teeth).
8. Overjet (horizontal overlap of teeth).

Periodontal Trauma from Occlusion

Once the occlusal survey is complete, the clinician must relate the data to the existence or nonexistence of trauma from occlusion. The following outline of signs and symptoms will serve as a guide in diagnosis.

Clinical Signs

These include:

1. Passive mobility of teeth.
2. Fremitus.
3. Migration of teeth, especially "fanning" of anterior teeth.

RECESSION   HYPERPLASIA

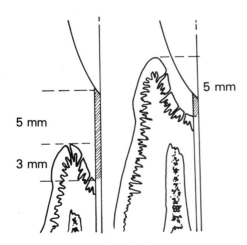

Fig. 6-4

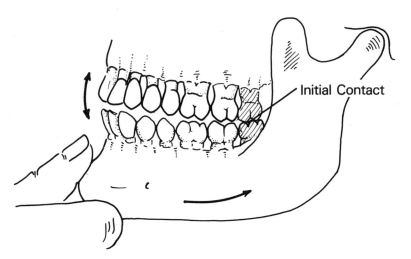

Initial Contact

Fig. 6-5

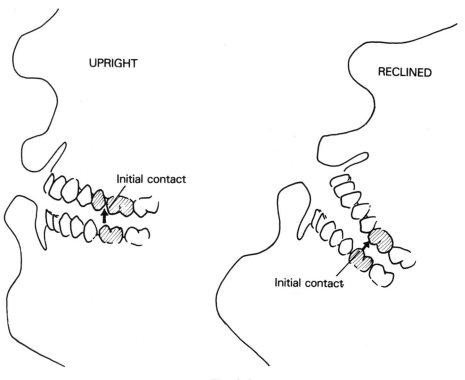

UPRIGHT

Initial contact

RECLINED

Initial contact

Fig. 6-6

4. Unusual wear patterns of teeth (facets).
5. Hypertonicity of masticatory muscles.
6. Periodontal abscess formation, especially in deep infrabony defects and furcas.

Symptoms

Trauma from occlusion is often asymptomatic, but the following symptoms maybe indicative of this condition:

1. Soreness on percussion and in function. This is often associated with new restorations and has a short-term history. In chronic periodontal traumatism, pain may be more vague and generalized.
2. Pain and spasm in muscles of mastication.
3. Food impaction caused by forceful wedging by opposing teeth.
4. Temporomandibular joint or myofacial pain/dysfunction syndrome.
5. "Looseness of teeth," vague "itching," and tendency to grind or initiate parafunction on certain teeth.
6. Thermal hypersensitivity of teeth.

Radiographic Signs

Radiography permits identification of characteristic evidence of trauma from occlusion.

1. Alterations in the lamina dura:
   a. Uneven thickening may be associated with tensional forces.
   b. Severe occlusal force may cause a complete loss of lamina dura.
2. Alteration in the periodontal ligament space. Widening may mean increased function or periodontal traumatism. The widening may be compensatory, especially if the lamina dura is thickened and intact.
3. Root resorption. This may be owing to excessive force in orthodontics, bruxism, or reconstruction therapy.

4. Hypercementosis. This may be a compensatory phenomenon to increase resistance to occlusal forces.
5. Osteosclerosis. Signs of this condition may occasionally be observed.
6. Angular bone loss and bone loss in furcation areas. These have been suggested in association with excessive occlusal force.
7. Root fracture.

Microscopic Changes

Various functional conditions, including trauma from occlusion, may produce changes within the periodontium that can be observed microscopically.

1. Changes that may result from non-function:
   a. Widened bone marrow spaces.
   b. Thin and disoriented trabeculae.
   c. Narrowed periodontal ligament, disoriented fibers.
   d. Cemental tears.
2. Changes that may be produced by over-function (within physiologic limits):
   a. Smaller than normal bone marrow spaces.
   b. Dense trabeculae.
   c. Wider periodontal ligament.
3. Changes that may be produced by overfunction on the pressure side (beyond physiologic limits):
   a. Compression of the contents of the periodontal ligament.
   b. Hemorrhage and concomitant hematoma.
   c. Thrombosis.
   d. Compression necrosis.
   e. Ischemic necrosis and rupture of vessel walls.
   f. Hyalinization.
   g. Undermining resorption of the alveolar process, starting from adjacent marrow spaces.
   h. Resorption of cementum.
   i. Root resorption.
4. Changes that may be produced by

overfunction on the tension side (beyond physiologic limits):

a. Widened periodontal ligament.
b. Hemorrhage and concomitant hematoma.
c. Thrombosis, hyalinization.
d. Apposition of alveolar process.
e. Hypercementosis.

Cemental and periodontal ligament tears (both may occur if occlusal force is of sufficient magnitude).

Prognosis

The accommodative capacity of the periodontium is the key to whether the resultant changes from occlusal trauma will be damaging. Certain factors may alter this accommodative capacity:

1. *Age of patient.* The accommodative capacity is at its highest in the young individual.
2. *Gingival inflammation.* The inflammatory process may hasten loss of the alveolar process and enhance the effects of excessive occlusal force on the periodontium.
3. *Systemic conditions.* These alter tissue responses to occlusal stress with the result that delayed healing may occur and the capacity to withstand forces is lessened.
4. *Amount of remaining alveolar process.* Loss of supporting bone may cause normal physiologic occlusal forces to become traumatic. The less remaining bone, the less the accommodative capacity of the periodontium.
5. *Force.*
   a. *Direction.* Those forces not directed along the long axes of the teeth are most detrimental (torquing forces).
   b. *Distribution.* Forces are more destructive when concentrated on a few teeth than when distributed over many.
   c. *Duration.* Forces that are continuous,

as in clenching and grinding habits, are potentially more destructive.
   d. *Frequency.* The more frequent the force, the greater is the opportunity for damage.
   e. *Intensity.* The clinician should always be mindful that, regardless of its direction, distribution, duration, frequency, or intensity, a force is traumatic depending on whether it produces destructive changes in the periodontium or within the stomatognathic system.

Radiographic Survey

Radiographs are indispensable aids in the diagnosis of periodontal disease, but they alone are not diagnostic. Radiographic interpretation should be considered along with clinical data to establish a final, accurate diagnosis. Each diagnostic regimen serves to monitor the accuracy of the other.

There are certain general requirements of a complete radiographic survey.

1. These film series should be included:
   a. Full-mouth periapical series.
   b. Four-film periodontal bite-wing series.
   c. Panoramic radiographs as an adjunct.
2. High-quality radiographs. Films should be technically adequate in density, contrast, and angulation, and should include all pertinent anatomic detail. Radiography will demonstrate the following information (Fig. 6–7 depicts many of the features).
   a. Root length and morphology.
   b. Clinical crown:root ratio.
   c. Approximate amount of bone destruction.
   d. Relationship of maxillary sinus to the periodontal deformity.
   e. Condition of interproximal bony crests, horizontal and vertical resorption. It should be noted that

the height of normal interseptal bone is usually parallel and 1 to 2 mm apical to a line connecting the cementoenamel junctions (CEJ) of adjacent teeth. When these landmarks are not on the same horizontal plane, the resulting angular appearance of a normal alveolar crest may resemble a pathologic infrabony defect. The astute diagnostician must be aware of these CEJ relationships, as well as of the dense appearance of healthy crestal lamina dura, to avoid unnecessary periodontal osseous surgery.

   f. Widening of periodontal ligament space on the mesial and distal aspects of the root.

   g. Advanced furcation involvement.

   h. Periapical pathosis.

   i. Calculus.

   j. Overhanging restoration.

   k. Root fractures.

   l. Caries.

  m. Root resorption.

Radiography will not demonstrate the following information (radiographs will not show disease activity, but the effects of the disease).

1. Presence or absence of pockets.
2. Exact morphology of bone deformities, especially tortuous defects, dehiscences, and fenestrations.
3. Tooth mobility.
4. Position and condition of the alveolar process on the facial and lingual surfaces.
5. Early furcation involvement.
6. Level of connective tissue attachment and the junctional epithelium.

Deposits Survey

A survey of the existing tooth-accumulated materials (TAM) is extremely important. To determine accurately the prevalence and distribution of plaque, it is necessary, even to the trained eye, to use disclosing solutions. For optimal usefulness in monitoring therapeutic progress, these accumulations should be measured and recorded repeatedly by using a plaque index. The deposits survey is conducted last because the dis-

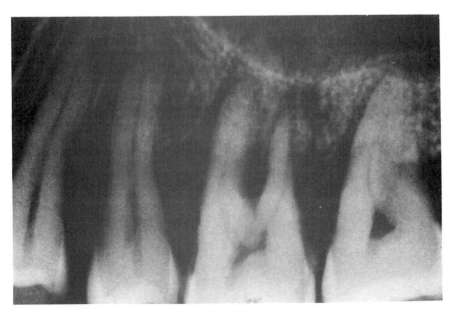

Fig. 6-7

closing media used in this examination mask other important clinical signs, such as changes in gingival coloring. Some clinicians prefer to question patients regarding their current tooth cleansing procedures at this time rather than during the dental history survey. The timing is unimportant as long as the information that permits the clinician to correlate technique with effectiveness is obtained.

Bacterial Analysis

Some practitioners may desire to identify the microorganisms in the periodontal pocket, especially in early-onset and refractory periodontal disease. A DNA probe or tests for monoclonal or polyclonal antibodies (such as a polymerase chain reaction test) are useful, especially to identify certain anaerobes. However, these tests do not reveal anything about antibiotic susceptibility. A bacterial culture and sensitivity test may provide information about which antibiotics are appropriate. Using a culture and sensitivity, coupled with a DNA probe, is probably the better combination to obtain the maximum amount of clinically relevant information.

Other Diagnostic Aids

Examination of the gingival crevicular fluid for catabolic enzymes, byproducts of bacterial lysis and periodontal destruction, gingival temperature changes, and other measures of tissue breakdown may prove to be valuable aids in the future. At this time, these tools require additional research and refinement.

PROGNOSIS

Prognosis is a forecast of the probable response to treatment and the long-term outlook for maintaining a functional dentition. Hopeless cases usually present few problems in establishing an accurate prognosis. Likewise, cases of simple gin- givitis, which can be expected to respond favorably when local and systemic factors can be controlled, present few problems in defining a prognosis. In borderline cases, however, the forecasting process becomes challenging. It remains to be seen whether tools and information derived from the basic sciences such as immunology and microbiology will improve our ability to predict which teeth will survive and for how long.

Problems are compounded when the prognosis concerns strategic, severely involved individual teeth on which a large and complex restorative treatment plan often depends. This situation places a heavy burden of responsibility on the diagnostician under any circumstance. No formula can be established for such situations. Rules of proportional bone loss (such as one-third or one-half of the supporting bone) have been expressed in the literature as condemning a tooth for extraction. In practice, such rules are of little value. If adhered to rigidly, such rules may lead to the sacrifice of teeth that might have been retained in health. The difficulty with any formula or rule is that there are many exceptions. The best way of meeting the problem is to establish certain basic principles, criteria of judgment, and probable behavior patterns of unrestorable teeth under the conditions in which they must function. There are two aspects of prognosis: the overall prognosis and the prognosis of individual teeth.

Overall Prognosis

Overall prognosis is concerned with the dentition as a whole and is the basic determinant of the extent of dental treatment to be provided. It includes consideration of the following factors.

1. *Attitude of the patient.* The success of periodontal treatment depends primarily on effective daily plaque control. With-

out patient cooperation and deep personal commitment and involvement in personal therapy, the prognosis is poor. This fact holds true no matter how skilled the managing practitioner.

2. *Age of the patient.* Usually, the younger the patient, the poorer the prognosis. Given two patients with periodontal involvement of the same degree, it is logical to assume that the younger has far less resistance because equal damage occurred in a shorter period. It follows that in a patient with weak resistance, healing, and repair may also be impaired.

   However, there is no causal relationship between age and periodontal disease, other than that older patients have been exposed to pathogenic bacteria for a longer time. Nor do all elderly patients in good health experience difficulty healing. One must evaluate the functional status, compliance, and general health geriatric patients rather than assessing them merely on age.

3. *Number of remaining teeth.* If the number and the distribution of remaining teeth are inadequate to support a satisfactory prosthesis, the overall prognosis is poor. Periodontal injury from extensive fixed or removable prostheses constructed on an insufficient number of natural teeth may hasten bone loss. Inability to establish a satisfactory functional environment for remaining natural teeth diminishes the likelihood of maintaining periodontal health.

4. *Systemic background.* The patient's systemic background affects the overall prognosis in several ways. When extensive periodontal destruction cannot be attributed to local factors, it is reasonable to assume a contributing systemic influence. The detection of systemic factors and the resolution of systemic factors may be extremely difficult. For these reasons, the prognosis in such patients is often poor. However, if patients have known systemic disorders that could affect the periodontium (e.g., use of tobacco, diabetes, nutritional deficiency, hyperthyroidism, and hyperparathyroidism), the prognosis improves on correction of the disorder.

   In the past few years two systemic conditions have been discovered to have unusually deleterious effects on the periodontium: smoking and leukocyte deficiencies.

   a. When all other factors are adjusted for, tobacco smoke is as harmful as plaque. A recently published study identified a subset of the smoking population who had attachment loss and recession in the absence of periodontal disease. Smokers also do not heal as well as nonsmokers after periodontal surgery. Clinicians and researchers are reassessing the treatment modalities. It may not be in a smoking patient's best interest to perform regenerative procedures or dental implants. However, too little data exist at this point to make a firm statement either way.

   b. It has shown that the polymorphonuclear leukocyte (PMN) is critical in the defense of the periodontium. Any patient with a qualitative (leukocyte adherence deficiency) or quantitative (agranulycotosis) defect in PMNs is likely to have severe, uncontrollable periodontal disease.

   If periodontal surgery is contraindicated because of the patient's health, the prognosis is uncertain. Incapacitating conditions that prevent adequate plaque control by the patient (such as Parkinson's disease) adversely affect the prognosis.

5. *Malocclusion.* Irregular alignment of the teeth, malformation of teeth and jaws, and disturbed occlusal relationships may be important factors in the cause

and the progression of periodontal disease. Correction by orthodontic or prosthodontic means is often essential if periodontal treatment is to succeed. The overall prognosis is poor when relevant occlusal deformities are not amenable to correction.

6. *Tooth morphology.* The prognosis is poor in patients whose teeth have short, tapered roots and relatively large crowns. The disproportionate crown:root ratio and the reduced root surface available for periodontal support render the periodontium more susceptible to injury by occlusal forces, and any loss of attachment apparatus has a more significant effect.

7. *Maintenance availability.* It is increasingly evident that overall long-term prognosis is dependent on the patient's availability and motivation to seek frequent maintenance recall visits, preferably at 3-month intervals. Patients who are unable to participate in a regular maintenance program, for whatever reason, are poor risks for periodontal therapy.

Prognosis of Individual Teeth

The following factors should be considered:

1. *Mobility.* Tooth mobility is caused by one or more of the following factors:
   a. Gingival and periodontal inflammation.
   b. Parafunctional habits.
   c. Occlusal prematurities.
   d. Torquing forces.
   e. Loss of supporting bone.
   Mobility is usually correctable unless it results solely from loss of attachment apparatus; this is not likely to be corrected. The likelihood of restoring tooth stability is inversely related, then, to the extent to which it is caused by loss of the attachment apparatus.

2. *Teeth adjacent to edentulous areas.* Abutment teeth are subjected to increased functional demands. More rigid standards are required in evaluating the prognosis of teeth in such locations.

3. *Location of remaining bone in relation to individual root surfaces.* When extensive bone loss has occurred on only one root surface, the center of rotation of that tooth is more coronal than if all root surfaces were extensively involved (Fig. 6-8). Thus, leverage on the periodontium is more favorably tolerated than would be expected given the extensive bone loss on the one root surface.

4. *Relation to adjacent teeth.* When a tooth has a questionable prognosis, the chances of successful treatment should be weighed against the effects on adjacent teeth if that tooth were extracted. Unsuccessful attempts at treatment frequently jeopardize adjacent teeth. Strategic extraction is often followed by partial restoration of bone, improving support of adjacent teeth (Fig. 6-9; with permission from Dr. Ronald L. Van Swoll). This result is enhanced if the adjacent teeth are scaled and root planed at the time of the extraction.

5. *Attachment level.* The location of the base of the pocket in relation to the CEJ affects the prognosis of an individual tooth more than the pocket depth. For example, a tooth with minimal pocket depth and extensive recession can present a poorer prognosis than a tooth with a deeper pocket and no recession and less bone loss. In addition, proximity of pockets to frenal attachments and to the mucogingival junction may jeopardize the prognosis unless corrective procedures are included in the treatment plan. When the periodontal pocket has extended to involve the apex, the prognosis is usually poor.

6. *Infrabony pockets.* The likelihood of eliminating infrabony pockets and their as-

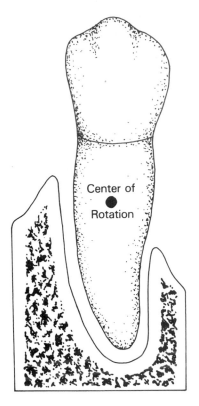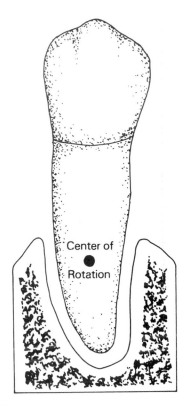

Fig. 6-8

sociated osseous defects is influenced by the number of remaining bony walls.

7. *Furcation involvement.* Bifurcation or trifurcation involvement does not always indicate a hopeless prognosis. Added support gives multirooted teeth an advantage over single-rooted teeth with comparable bone loss. Several factors influence the prognosis of teeth with attachment loss involving the furcation.

   a. Extent of furcation involvement (see Chapter 18).

   b. Access to the furca for surgical management. A narrow interradicular space offers a poor prognosis for new attachment procedures or root resection because of the close proximity of the adjacent roots. It also compromises the plaque control ef-

forts of the patient. Typically, the more divergent the roots, the better the prognosis; e.g., mandibular second molars have a poorer prognosis than mandibular first molars because the roots of the second molars are shorter and the interradicular space is more constricted.

   c. Access to the furca for plaque control. Usually, mandibular molars with furcation involvement have a better prognosis than maxillary molars with furcation involvement, because patients have better access to the furcas of the mandibular molars. Maxillary premolars with furcation involvement are poor candidates for therapy because of root morphology and poor access for plaque control before and after therapy.

8. *Caries, nonvital teeth, and root resorption.* In teeth mutilated by extensive caries, the feasibility of adequate restoration and endodontic therapy influences periodontal treatment. Extensive idiopathic root resorption jeopardizes tooth stability and adversely affects the response to periodontal treatment. The periodontal prognosis is not significantly affected in endodontically treated teeth.

9. *Developmental defects.* Developmental defects, such as the palatogingival groove observed on incisor teeth and molars, present a poor prognosis for successful management. Root concavities observed in some teeth, particularly the maxillary first premolar, complicate the prognosis for surgical success as well as for maintenance after surgery.

TREATMENT PLANNING

After the diagnosis and prognosis have been established, treatment is planned. The treatment plan is the road map for case management. It includes all procedures required for the establishment and maintenance of oral health.

Periodontal treatment requires long-range planning. The value of periodontal treatment to the patient is measured in years of healthful service of the entire dentition, not by the number of teeth retained at the time of treatment. The treatment plan, therefore, is concerned with the entire dentition as well as with the individual teeth. Its principal purpose is to provide a healthy foundation for the future rather than simply to salvage those teeth that were affected in the past. It is directed toward establishing and maintaining an atmosphere of health of the periodontium throughout the mouth, not solely toward spectacular efforts to "tighten" loose teeth.

The welfare of the overall dentition should not be jeopardized by heroic attempts to retain questionable teeth. The clinician should be concerned with practicing periodontics not "herodontics." The clinician is primarily interested in teeth that can be retained with maximal

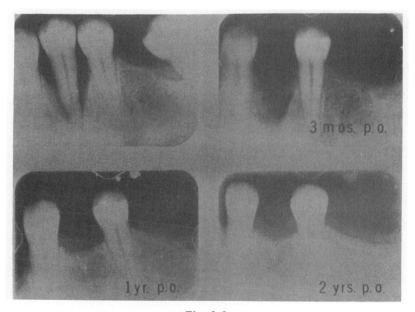

Fig. 6-9

longevity. Such teeth provide the basis for a constructive total treatment plan.

A treatment plan should be developed to achieve the following objectives:

1. Reduction or removal of all etiologic factors.
2. Reduction or elimination of all pockets and establishment of minimal sulcus depth.
3. Restoration of physiologic gingival and osseous architecture.
4. Establishment of a functional occlusion by restorative procedures and occlusal adjustment.
5. Maintenance of periodontal health through adequate plaque control by the patient and regular visits to the dentist.

If the clinician can successfully attain these objectives, most cases of periodontal disease can be arrested on a long-term basis.

Order of Treatment

The detailed treatment plan must be based on the patient's dental and medical histories, emotional status, clinical and radiographic examinations, and to the other factors that have been mentioned. Treatment plans, therefore, have many variations, but typically may consist of four phases: 1) bacterial plaque control, 2) surgical therapy, 3) restorative treatment, and 4) maintenance.

Bacterial Control

This phase has also been called "initial preparation" or "phase I therapy" and usually includes the following steps.

1. *Premedication.* Attention must be given to the need for premedication for subacute bacterial endocarditis, heart disease, hypertension, and other systemic conditions; in addition, when indicated, preoperative sedation should be implemented.

2. *Emergency care.* Immediate treatment of periodontal abscesses, acute necrotizing ulcerative gingivitis (ANUG), large carious lesions, tooth pain, etc.
3. *Patient instruction and motivation.* The patient's learning of personal bacterial plaque control procedures. *Success depends primarily on the patient's willingness to participate seriously as a cotherapist.*
4. *Extraction of teeth.* Teeth having a hopeless prognosis and those that removal of will improve prognosis of adjacent teeth are extracted.
5. *Scaling and root planing.* Removes calculus and contaminated cementum, enabling the patient to begin a program of personal plaque control as early as possible.
6. *Removal of overhanging restorations and other plaque-retentive areas.*
7. *Minor tooth movement.*
8. *Temporary stabilization.* Possibly required to facilitate overall treatment or to aid in determining the prognosis of certain teeth.
9. *Preliminary occlusal adjustment and odontoplasty (if indicated).* Obvious gross occlusal abnormalities (plunger cusps, initial prematurities, defective marginal ridges) should be evaluated early in treatment and corrected, if necessary.
10. *Evaluation of results.* Elimination of etiologic factors may produce sufficient improvement to permit modification of the original treatment plan. In this sense, the infection control phase may actually be complete and satisfactory therapy. The patient's attitude toward plaque control responsibility is also evaluated. Additional instruction may be required—even though the patient is making a sincere effort to practice recommended techniques. On the other hand, a patient's failure to cooperate in this critical area should prompt the clinician to modify, limit, or terminate the course of treatment.

Surgical Therapy (Phase II Therapy)

This phase of treatment includes procedures designed to reduce or eliminate the pocket by resection, the relocation of the gingival margin, or the use of new attachment procedures. This phase may also include surgical procedures for the correction of mucogingival defects or placement of dental implants.

Restorative Treatment (Phase III Therapy)

The restorative phase usually involves definitive occlusal adjustment, operative dentistry, replacement of missing teeth by fixed and/or removable prostheses, and permanent splinting, when indicated.

Maintenance (Phase IV Therapy)

Patients continue in the maintenance phase for a lifetime. Most patients who have been treated for moderate-to-advanced periodontitis require maintenance at least every 3 months. The length of time between recall appointments is dictated by the level of disease control accomplished by patients during the interval between recall visits. This phase of therapy is often downgraded by both the patient and the practitioner, yet it spells the difference between long-term success and failure (see Chapter 23).

SUGGESTED READINGS

Armitage GC. Periodontal diseases: diagnosis. Ann Periodontol 1996:1;37–215.

Giargia M, Lindhe J. Tooth mobility and periodontal disease [Review] [65 refs]. J Clin Periodontol 1997;24(11):785–795.

Hurt WC. Periodontal diagnosis—1977: a status report. J Periodontol 1977:48;533.

Lamster IB. In-office diagnostic tests and their role in supportive periodontal treatment. Periodontol 2000 1996;12:49–55.

Lang NP, Tonetti MS. Periodontal diagnosis in treated periodontitis. Why, when, and how to use clinical parameters. J Clin Periodontol 1996;23(3 Pt 2):240–250.

Listgarten M. Periodontal probing: what does it mean? J Clin Periodontol 1980;7:165.

Mandel ID. Overview of clinical trials of periodontal diagnosis methods and devices. Ann Periodontol 1997;2(1):98–107.

McGuire MK, Nunn ME. Prognosis versus actual outcome. II. The effectiveness of clinical parameters in developing an accurate prognosis. J Periodontol 1996;67:658–665.

McGuire MK, Nunn ME. Prognosis versus actual outcome. III. The effectiveness of clinical parameters in accurately predicting tooth survival. J Periodontol 1996;67:666–674.

Menassa G, Van Dyke TE. Periodontal diagnosis: current status and future directions. Int Dent J 1998;48(Suppl 1):275–281.

Proceedings of the World Workshop in Clinical Periodontics. Princeton, New Jersey. July 23–27, 1989.

Williams RC. Paquette DW. Periodontal disease diagnosis and treatment: an exciting future. J Dent Ed 1998;2(10):871–881.

CHAPTER

7

The Role of Occlusion in Periodontal Health and Disease

Marlin Gher

The one area that all dental clinical disciplines have in common is in the area of occlusion. Earlier investigators have stated that the most important function of the oral system was mastication. Articulators were developed that would allow these early clinicians to duplicate jaw movements. There was great concern over the role that TMJ and occlusion played in the stomatognathic system, and concepts were developed to stabilize condylar movements and wear on the teeth. The primary concern, for the early clinicians, was with complete denture stability. Because of this concern, the occlusionists developed occlusion that had bilateral balance (where the working side and the balancing side were in contact when the jaw moved in lateral excursions). This developed into the concept of group function occlusion. When a researcher who was studying the skulls of California Native Americans wrote a paper stating that those skulls showing the least amount of alveolar bone loss had an occlusion that was protected by a canine rise (cuspid protected occlusion) during lateral excursions, the dental community quickly changed direction and developed occlusions with cuspid protec-

tion. Adding to the confusion of the time, an Australian orthodontist studied the skulls and the dentition of living Australian aborigines and determined that the occlusion that created the least amount of periodontal tissue loss was a group function occlusion.

A more recent epidemiological study on a North American population indicates that 46% of the population exhibited bilateral group function, 21% exhibited bilateral canine guidance, and 27% of the population exhibited canine guidance on one side and group function on the other side. The investigators also found that there was no significant relations between centric relation or nonfunctional contacts and pocket depths. It appears that the older the patient, the more apt the patient is to have group function.

Occlusal concepts are developed and accepted, based on research that is conflicting in both design and conclusions. Current research on occlusion has been mostly performed on the animal model, primarily on the dog and monkey. The problem is that it is difficult to extrapolate the results to the human because these animals do not have lateral movement during mastication. Because of this, elaborate schemes and devices were developed to simulate the human condition. It is no wonder that the dental community is wary of the findings on occlusion.

Fortunately, some short-term and long-term studies on humans have shed some light on the role that occlusion plays in periodontal health and disease. More needs to be accomplished before occlusal concepts are set in stone. This chapter will attempt to clarify the role of occlusion on the periodontium, based on current research, especially the research that has used the human model.

The stomatognathic (gnathostomatic) system consists of the temporomandibular joints, neuromusculature of the masticatory apparatus, and the teeth within the periodontium. Any causative agent that affects one of the components may also affect the other components. Treatment of one of the components may also affect the other components; therefore, care must be taken to identify the cause of the disease that is to be treated.

The primary causes of periodontitis are microorganic (bacterial plaque and their byproducts); the role that occlusion plays in the initiation and progression of the disease process is secondary. Trauma from occlusion may alter or modify the progress of periodontal disease but does not initiate the inflammatory lesion (Chapter 6 details the diagnosis of occlusal trauma). To help clarify the confusion in occlusion, a few terms are defined:

1. *Trauma from occlusion (occlusal trauma).* The injury produced in the periodontium by occlusal forces exceeding the adaptive capacity of the periodontium. The injury may manifest clinically by mobility, migration of the teeth away from the force, and pain during biting or percussion. With use of a radiograph, the injury may be identified by a discontinuity of the lamina dura at the lateral aspects and around the apices of the involved teeth. A widening of the periodontal ligament space may or may not be evident.

2. *Primary occlusal trauma (Fig. 7-1).* An injury from an excessive occlusal force acting on a periodontium that has not been altered by disease (a healthy periodontium). Primary occlusal trauma is usually a result of excessive occlusal forces associated with such factors as parafunctional habits, high restorations, and removable partial dentures. There is no attachment loss. The lesion is reversible and can usually be corrected by eliminating the local factors (i.e., bacteria and their byproducts) and/or adjusting the occlusion.

3. *Secondary occlusal trauma (Fig. 7-2).* An injury from a normal occlusal force placed on a weakened periodontium. This is often observed after treatment of advanced cases of chronic destructive periodontitis. The greater the loss of periodontal support, the more important the occlusal factors become in the prognosis and treatment of the disease.

4. *Combined periodontal trauma.* An injury from an excessive occlusal force on a diseased periodontium. In effect, inflammation is present, pocket formation is present, and excessive occlusal forces exaggerate and/or exacerbate the disease process. Trauma from occlusion may be a codestructive factor in combination with the existing active periodontal lesion. The resultant lesion is not reversible by occlusal adjustment.

Current research data provide overwhelming evidence that occlusal trauma will not cause periodontal pockets and is not capable of initiating marginal gingival inflammation. Trauma from occlusion will not affect the progression of gingivitis to periodontitis. When periodontitis exists and occlusal trauma is superimposed on the active lesion, clinical and re-

Primary Occlusal Traumatism

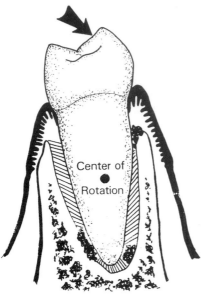

Fig. 7-1

Secondary Occlusal Traumatism

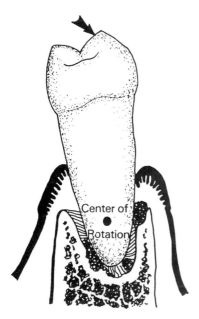

Fig. 7-2

search evidence leads us to believe that these excessive occlusal forces do not allow the periodontium to adapt.

Consequently, the rate of spread of the inflammatory process into the underlying tissues may increase. Trauma from occlusion, superimposed on the active inflammatory periodontal lesion, may act as a cofactor in the destruction of the periodontium and may result in deeper pockets and can contribute to angular bony defects. But, it is important to remember that this effect of trauma from occlusion on the periodontium must first have a plaque-associated inflammatory lesion.

The role that trauma plays in the destruction of the periodontium and the formation of angular bony defects is better understood if the periodontium is considered to consist of two zones, as described by Dr. Irving Glickman (Fig. 7-3):

1. *The zone of irritation.* Consists of the soft tissue coronal to the alveolar crest fibers and the transeptal fibers.
2. *The zone of codestruction.* Consists of the periodontium apical to the alveolar crest fibers and transeptal fibers.

The inflammatory lesion (gingivitis and periodontitis) starts in the zone of irritation and is caused primarily by irritation and infection from bacteria and their toxic products. Trauma from occlusion does not cause gingivitis or periodontal pockets. The marginal gingiva is not affected by trauma from occlusion and as long as the disease process is limited to the gingiva (zone of irritation), occlusal forces will not play a role in the pathogenesis of inflammatory periodontal disease.

When the inflammatory process extends to the alveolar process (to the zone of co-destruction), trauma from occlusion may play a role in the pathogenesis of the disease process. If the occlusal forces are unfavorable (excessive), occlusal trauma may alter the environment and the pathway of inflammation. These unfavorable forces may produce peri-

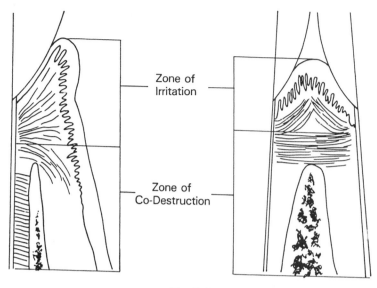

Fig. 7-3

odontal injury and thus become a code-structive factor that may affect the pattern and severity of tissue destruction. Substantial evidence indicates that increased loss of alveolar bone and altered osseous morphology occur when trauma from occlusion is superimposed on periodontitis. Evidence also indicates that trauma from occlusion will alter the healing rate during treatment and that teeth with periodontal mobility do not respond to treatment as do nonmobile teeth.

To briefly review the current concepts:

• Trauma from occlusion in the absence of gingival inflammation does not cause a periodontal pocket.
• Trauma from occlusion does not affect the loss of the connective tissue attachment.
• Teeth move in the direction of the occlusal force.
• Unilateral trauma may cause bone resorption on the pressure side and bone apposition on the tension side.
• Bone loss may occur on all sides of a tooth or may be extensive enough to cause tooth mobility.

• Trauma from occlusion, in the presence of inflammation, may contribute to angular alveolar bone loss.
• Trauma from occlusion may alter the healing response of the periodontium, following treatment.
• The less the tooth mobility, the more favorable the postoperative level of periodontal attachment.

Unless a traumatic injury (trauma from occlusion) is diagnosed, the occlusion should not be altered. If occlusal therapy is indicated, then it should be performed as part of the infection control (initial preparation) phase of periodontal therapy (prior to periodontal surgery). Occlusal therapy is indicated when:

1. The patient is in pain and trauma from occlusion has been identified as the causative factor.
2. There is increasing tooth mobility. It is incumbent upon the clinician to collect data on tooth mobility at each recall and maintenance visit to know if the mobility is increasing.
3. There is angular bone loss and pocket formation (infrabony pockets) and

trauma from occlusion has been identified as the causative factor.

4. Occlusal adjustments will aid in enhancing the masticatory function.
5. There is TMJ dysfunction and trauma from occlusion has been identified as the cause.

Various approaches to treating trauma from occlusion exist, and the most common methods are as follows:

1. Occlusal adjustment (equilibration).
2. Bite plates (night guards, bite guards).
3. Orthodontic tooth movement.
4. Splints (temporary, provisional, or permanent).
5. Reconstructive dentistry.

The primary goal of occlusal treatment is to establish harmony within the stomatognathic system. The overall primary goal of periodontal therapy, however, is to control the inflammatory response. Occlusal adjustment is the technique most often used when minor occlusal therapy is indicated. The goals of occlusal adjustment are:

1. To remove occlusal prematurities in maximal intercuspation and centric relation.
2. To eliminate balancing side interferences that act as torquing forces and prevent freedom of lateral movements of the mandible.
3. To adjust working side contacts to protect teeth with a weakened periodontium.
4. To eliminate protrusive interferences.
5. To direct occlusal forces in an axial direction.

Bite plates are most often used when patients present with signs of stomatog-nathic system breakdown caused by parafunctional habits (bruxism, clenching, etc.). Splinting may be necessary for patients who exhibit discomfort as a result of tooth mobility or hypermobility that interferes with masticatory function or increased mobility after periodontal therapy. Orthodontic treatment of the periodontal patient may be indicated to achieve a more acceptable occlusal relationship.

In most instances, it is desirable to perform occlusal therapy during the infection control phase (phase I), but following the control of periodontal inflammation. If extensive fixed prosthodontic dentistry is to be used as an occlusal corrective measure, these procedures should be postponed to at least 30 to 60 days after periodontal surgery has been completed.

SUGGESTED READINGS

Carlson-Mann LD. Recognition and management of occlusal disease from a hygienist's perspective. Probe 1996;30:196–197.

Gher ME. Changing concepts. The effects of occlusion on periodontitis. Dent Clin North Am 1998;42(2):285–299.

Gher ME. Non-surgical pocket therapy: dental occlusion. Ann Periodontol 1996;1:567–580.

Green MS, Levine DF. Occlusion and the periodontium: a review and rationale for treatment. J Cal Dent Assoc 1996;24:19–27.

Jin L, Coa C. Clinical diagnosis of trauma from occlusion and its relation with severity of periodontitis. J Clin Periodontol 1992;19:92–97.

Serio FG, Hawley CE. Periodontal trauma and mobility. Diagnosis and treatment planning. Dent Clin North Am 1999;43:37–44.

Serio FG. Clinical rationale for tooth stabilization and splinting. Dent Clin North Am 1999;43:1–6.

Plaque Control

Lorraine Forgas

Bacterial plaque is the primary cause of inflammatory diseases. Without plaque control, periodontal health can neither be achieved nor maintained. The success of virtually every aspect of clinical dentistry depends on plaque control, from the maintenance of a disease-free mouth to the maintenance of the most complex treatment involving dental implants.

Plaque control may be categorized into professional plaque control and patient plaque control. The clinician is tasked with the responsibility to render a patient as plaque-free and calculus-free as possible. Once this is achieved, the patient then assumes the major responsibility in maintenance. Professional visits remain important; however, the patient's daily plaque control routine remains the most important factor to success.

Too often, plaque control instruction is accomplished hastily, or not accomplished at all. Plaque control instruction is most likely the first component omitted from the appointment in an effort to save time. Informing and educating the patient are our first responsibilities. If the patient does not understand why plaque control is important, the patient's compliance is unlikely. It is surprising—indeed disappointing—the number of adult patients who have never been informed of proper home care and its direct relationship to the health of their teeth and gingiva.

Plaque control is an integral part of periodontal disease management. This message should be conveyed to patients. Otherwise, plaque control instruction has the potential to be interpreted by the patient as routine and mundane. Unfortunately, too many patients equate plaque control instruction with a nagging, "You need to floss more!" For plaque control to be effective, the patient must be informed, educated, and motivated. Once these criteria are fulfilled, the patient needs good manual dexterity. Absence of even one of these criteria will compromise success.

The most effective means to communicate the presence of disease and the need for improved plaque control is to show your patient the disease in his or her own mouth. Pamphlets, illustrations, and manikins are valuable adjuncts to instruction, but these alone have only a mild impact. You will gain your patient's attention when you point out the problem areas in his or her own mouth. For example, show your patient how deep the probe can be inserted subgingivally and how easily the gingiva bleeds. Point out color changes in the gingiva. The patient should be shown the plaque in his or her mouth. Disclosing agents are excellent tools for this purpose.

PLAQUE CONTROL PROCEDURES

Disclosing Agents

Patients cannot be expected to adequately remove plaque if they do not know where they are missing it in the first place. Disclosing agents are used to identify plaque for the patient, and they serve as excellent motivational educational tools. They may be incorporated into oral hygiene instruction for all patients, especially for children and for adults with inadequate oral hygiene.

Historically, iodine, food coloring, bismarck brown, mercurochrome, and basic fuscin have been used as disclosing agents. Today, erythrosin is the most widely used agent. The agents are available in either a liquid or chewable tablet form. The liquid is most convenient for dental office use and can be swabbed onto the teeth with a cotton-tipped applicator, or a few drops placed under the tongue can be swished by the patient and expectorated. The tablets work best for home use. The chewed-up tablet is swished and expectorated. Both liquid and tablets are available over-the-counter for patient use. Fluorescein disclosing agents are also available. These agents are barely visible under regular light, but fluoresce under blue light. They are ideal for adult patients who find the erythrosin staining objectionable.

Brushing

For a thorough discussion of the many different methods of brushing, the reader is referred to current periodontics and dental hygiene textbooks. The sulcular (Bass) method will be considered in this chapter as the preferred method because it is specifically designed to remove plaque adjacent to and within the sulcus.

The sulcular cleansing technique is usually recommended because of its effectiveness in controlling plaque at the gingival margin. It should be emphasized, however, that brushing instruction should be based on each patient's individual needs. More than one technique may be necessary for a patient to achieve acceptable plaque removal.

To cleanse the teeth using the sulcular technique, the toothbrush bristles should be placed at a 45° angle to the long axis of the tooth. When properly positioned, some of the brush's bristles will enter the sulcus. The brush is then gently moved in short, back-and-forth, almost vibratory strokes to disrupt the organized plaque. Each area is overlapped as the brush is moved.

The modified Bass technique is accomplished by including the rolling stroke following the vibratory stroke. The rolling stroke is designed cleanses the facial and lingual/palatal surfaces. The rolling stroke is accomplished by resting the toothbrush against the gingiva with the bristles directed apically. The brush is rotated coronally with a sweeping motion until the entire tooth surface is cleansed.

Manual Toothbrushes

A wide variety of toothbrushes are available to suit any patient's needs. Manufacturers are continually striving to improve brushes by altering size, overall shape, handle, bristle shape, and arrangement of bristles. Lack of conformity makes determining the most effective toothbrush difficult. Patient satisfaction should help dictate the type of brush used. The ideal toothbrush should be small enough to reach all areas of the mouth, have soft or extra-soft bristles, and effectively remove plaque without causing trauma to the hard and soft tissues.

Powered (Mechanical) Toothbrushes

Powered or mechanical tooth brushes can be especially useful for patients with limited dexterity, those who are physically or mentally disabled, those having poor motivation toward plaque control, those with orthodontic appliances, or those with implants. Several variations of brushes are available.

A variety of different powered brushes are available. Figures 8-1 and 8-2 are examples of the contrarotary and rotary type brushes, respectively.

Recently, different powered brushes have been introduced that produce sonic or ultrasonic vibrations. These vibrations produce a fluid cavitation that has the potential to disrupt plaque and its bacterial component. An example is shown in Figure 8-3. Studies show that all powered brushes achieve similar results removing plaque.

Manual Versus Power Brushes

Concerning the effectiveness of manual and powered toothbrushes, research has shown a distinct advantage of the powered brush over the manual brush.

The rotary brush has been shown to be significantly superior to the manual brush in reducing plaque and gingivitis. Research comparing the newer sonic and ultrasonic toothbrushes is not as conclusive.

When a patient demonstrates the ability to effectively use a manual brush in technique, switching to a powered brush is not necessary. When a patient has attempted a number of manual techniques and has been unsuccessful in controlling plaque, using a powered brush should be considered. It is often more rewarding, dentally and psychologically, to introduce an entirely new concept of tooth cleansing than to attempt to break bad habits that have developed over the years.

Proximal Cleansing

Interproximal plaque removal is crucial to periodontal health. The col, the saddle-like depression between the facial and lingual papilla, is non-keratinized. Because it is non-keratinized, the col is more susceptible to bacterial insult and breakdown. The anatomy of the col and the shape of the interdental gingiva cause plaque to harbor and proliferate. No toothbrushing technique, including mechanical toothbrushes, assures interproximal plaque removal.

Floss and Tape (Waxed and Unwaxed)

Many patients, when they hear the term dental floss, immediately think of food caught between the teeth. Being unin-

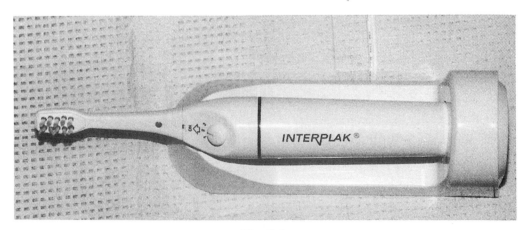

Fig. 8-1

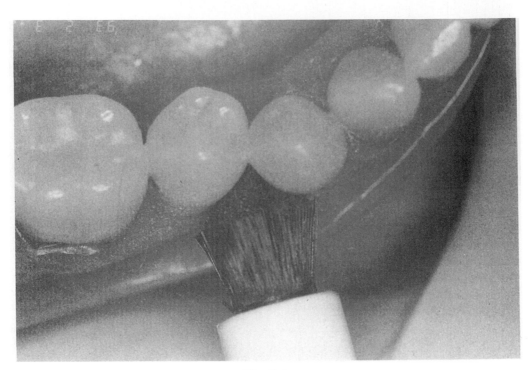

Fig. 8-2

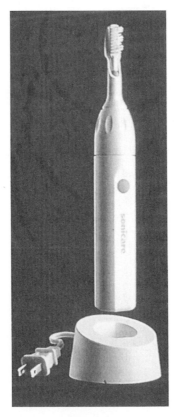

Fig. 8-3

formed, they have no concept of how to clean proximal surfaces and must be instructed in what they are to accomplish, why, how, and with what devices. Dental floss and tape—either waxed or unwaxed—are equally effective for cleansing proximal surfaces. Individual patient factors, such as contacts, restorations, tooth alignment, and manual dexterity should determine the type of floss used. Unwaxed floss may be recommended for a patient with adequately spaced contact areas, whereas waxed floss may be recommended to a patient with rough interproximal spaces. Flavored floss, floss with fluoride, and baking soda-coated floss are also available. More recently several brands of teflon-coated dental floss have been introduced to the market.

The use of floss presents certain dangers that should be explained to the patient. "Popping" floss between contact areas of adjacent teeth can lacerate papilla. Damage can be avoided by keeping one's hands close together, using only a very short zone of floss, exercising control, and sliding the floss back and forth between the contact areas while pressing apically. The floss-holding devices shown in Figure 8-4 have proven effective for some patients who have difficulty in guiding floss with their fingers. Others find it easier to tie the two ends of the floss together to form a circle, then taking up the slack by wrapping the floss

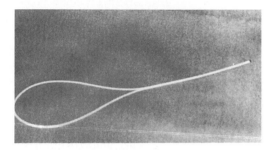

Fig. 8-5

around a finger. This technique improves the patient's ability to control the floss. Patients with fixed splinting of the teeth are faced with a difficult problem of access to the interproximal region. Floss can be threaded through embrasures by commercially available devices such as the one shown in Figure 8-5.

Removing floss in a straight occlusal direction can severely task the retention of restorations when contacts are tight. This problem can be alleviated if the patient either pulls one free end of the floss through the interproximal space or pull the floss through the contact laterally rather than occlusally.

In use, the floss is pressed closely against the tooth and wrapped slightly around the tooth as in Figure 8-6. The floss is then moved up and down against the tooth surface, cutting plaque from flat or convex surfaces. Problems arise when proximal surfaces are concave and inaccessible to the cleansing fibers (Fig. 8-7). Such surfaces require other devices.

Superfloss is a variation of dental floss. A strand of Superfloss is stiff on one end for ease of threading under bridge pontics or orthodontic wires. The remainder of the strand is unwaxed dental floss with a portion covered with a sponge-like material.

Gauze

Strips of gauze, in 1-inch or ½-inch widths, are particularly effective in removing plaque from proximal surfaces

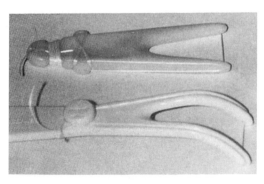

Fig. 8-4

adjacent to an edentulous space or the distal surface of the last molars.

Interdental Cleansers (Rubber, Plastic, and Wooden)

Rubber or plastic tipped interproximal devices can be used as aids to clean proximal surfaces. The plastic tipped devices may be too hard and can cause damage and discomfort. Some clinicians feel that these devices can be used to promote and maintain healthy interproximal gingival contours, if used as demonstrated in Figure 8-8. They may also be used for cleansing exposed furcations. Some clinicians prescribe these devices to clean within the gingival crevice by "tracing" each crevice along the gingival margin. Toothpicks and other wooden interdental cleansing devices can be used successfully by many patients who have been instructed in their proper use. Improperly used, they can damage the papilla. Some patients have difficulty using them in posterior areas, but these devices are convenient to carry, and their use readily becomes habitual.

Round toothpicks can be used very effectively when placed in a special holding device (Fig. 8-9). The Perio-Aid is one of these devices. The toothpick is moistened with saliva, then used to trace along the gingival margin to remove plaque and debris. Each facial, lingual/palatal, and proximal surface can be "polished" free of plaque with the wooden toothpick. These devices are especially effective in cleansing exposed furcations, crown margins, and areas of gingival recession. The toothpick may also be used to burnish fluoride or other desensitizing agents into the tooth.

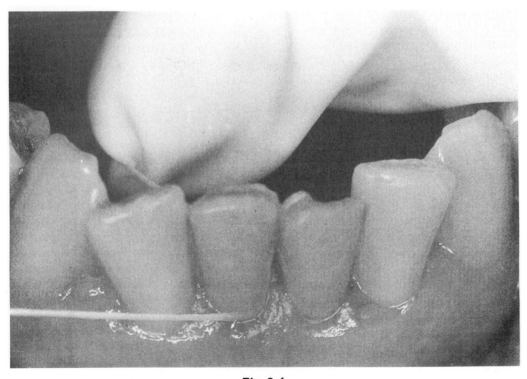

Fig. 8-6

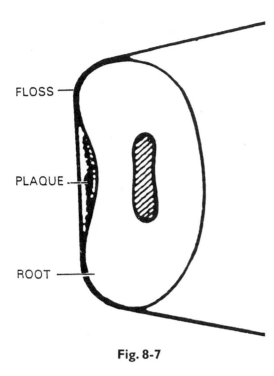

FLOSS

PLAQUE

ROOT

Fig. 8-7

Reasonable skill and effort are needed to use these rigid interproximal devices. The effectiveness of all rigid interproximal devices is in their plaque-removing potential rather than their gingival stimulation.

Aids for Cleansing Inaccessible Areas

Single-tufted (end-tufted) toothbrushes are highly effective, well-accepted by the patient, and safe in cleansing such areas as furcations (Fig. 8-10), concave surfaces, uneven gingival margins, malpositioned teeth, lingual and palatal surfaces, areas of erosion and abrasion, and around fixed prostheses. Patients are instructed to trace the gingival margins with the bristles directed toward the gingiva and to hold the brush in each interproximal area permitting the bristles to work interproximally and subgingivally. Inaccessible areas are dealt with individually. The

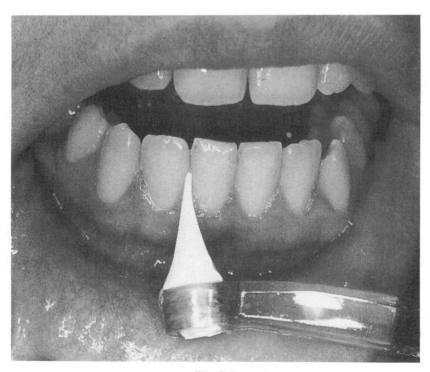

Fig. 8-8

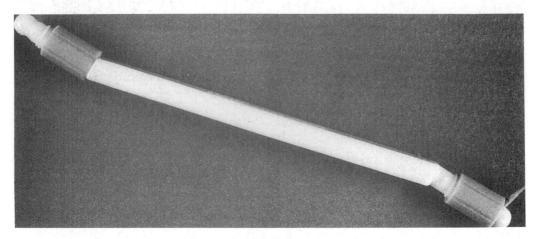

Fig. 8-9

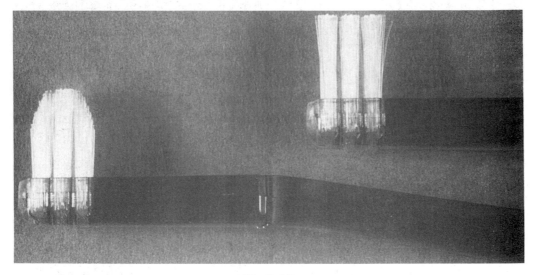

Fig. 8-10

powered rotary brush has tuft designs designed for inaccessible areas and furcations. The powered contrarotary brush will also reach these areas by altering the standard head design by removing the tufts in the second and fourth rows.

The interproximal brush is a small, spiral-type brush, resembling a miniature bottle brush, that is attached to a handle (Fig. 8-12). The brushes may be tapered or cylindrical. They are used in wide embrasures or open contacts and conform to concavities on the tooth surface to re-move plaque that flossing would not remove. The brush is inserted interproximally and moved in a facial/lingual direction. These brushes are especially useful in periodontal maintenance, implants, and orthodontic patients. Only those brushes with a teflon-coated wire core should be used with implants.

Oral Irrigating Devices

Oral irrigators, whether of the pulsating or steady-stream type, are considered

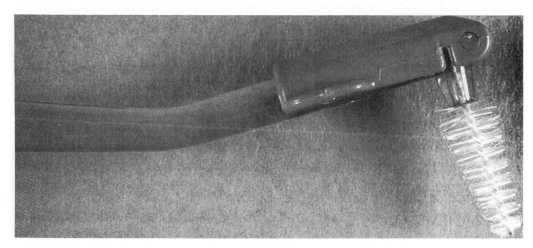

Fig. 8-11

useful adjuncts to the toothbrush for patients with poor oral hygiene, those with orthodontic bands, or those in fixation following orthognathic surgery. Irrigators do not remove attached plaque and, consequently, do not replace toothbrushes or interdental cleansing devices. Evidence suggests that irrigating devices may alter plaque by reducing its toxicity. The relationship of this alteration to oral health has not been fully demonstrated except in maintenance patients. Studies show that if used in the prescribed manner, the pulsating irrigator eliminates the motile forms of bacteria in 3-mm sulci and also significantly reduces the motile forms in sulci as deep as 6 mm. Irrigating devices are effective in removing loose debris from areas that cannot be cleansed by the toothbrush, such as around orthodontic bands, fixed bridges, and implants. It promises to be beneficial to gingival health that these devices are capable of reaching up to 6 mm subgingivally and displacing the unattached and motile microflora.

A multicenter multinational study demonstrated that it is possible to provide beneficial results to periodontal patients using irrigation as an adjunctive aid. The same study demonstrated that supragingival irrigation in periodontal maintenance patients provided additional benefits such as reduction of gingivitis and bleeding on probing.

Specifically designed subgingival tips that deliver solutions subgingivally have been developed. Subgingival penetration with these tips is greatly improved. Some studies have shown penetration of solutions in depths of 7 to 10 mm.

Some studies suggest that subgingival irrigation with antimicrobials, especially chlorhexidine, can result in a greater reduction of gingival inflammation.

Transient bacteremia may occur with the use of irrigators. The effect of such transient bacteremias in a healthy patient is unknown, but caution is urged in patients at risk for bacterial endocarditis. The potential for transient bacteremia is also associated with the use of all plaque control devices.

Mouth Rinses

In the past, mouth rinses were considered to be only flavored, breath-freshening solutions with little or no effect on oral health. Today, a number of antimicrobial mouth rinses are available, some of which help control the development of supragingival plaque and gingivitis. These mouth rinses can be valuable adjuncts for patients who are poorly motivated or patients whose physical disabilities make plaque control difficult or impossible.

Mouth rinses can be divided into two major categories. First-generation mouth rinses are capable of reducing plaque and gingivitis approximately 20 to 50% when used 4 to 6 times a day and have limited or no substantivity. Substantivity is the ability of an antimicrobial to bind to anionic groups on the tooth surface, on the oral mucosa, and on bacterial surfaces and—in effect—produce a sustained release of the active ingredients and therefore extend the antimicrobial effectiveness of the product. Second-generation mouth rinses are capable of reducing plaque and gingivitis by 70 to 90% when used 1 to 2 times a day and have an effective substantivity lasting 12 to 18 hours or longer.

Listerine, Cepacol, and Scope are considered to be first-generation mouth rinses because they lack substantivity. Of these products, Listerine (and its generic equivalents) is the only over-the-counter mouth rinse to receive the ADA seal of approval because of its ability to significantly reduce plaque and gingivitis. Listerine and its equivalents are phenolic compounds, containing three essential oils as their active ingredients: thymol, menthol, and eucalyptol. Alcohol content is 27%, and a cool mint version has an alcohol content of 21%.

These essential oil mouth rinses have demonstrated the ability to reduce plaque and gingivitis by approximately 18 to 25%. Some patients may experience a burning sensation. Slight staining is possible, but is not likely.

Chlorhexidine preparations containing 0.12% chlorhexidine gluconate are ADA approved and have substantivity lasting between 12 and 18 hours; these prep-

arations are available by prescription. Chlorhexidine has been intensely investigated and is currently the most effective agent available to reduce plaque and gingivitis, between 35 to 45%. Adverse side effects include stained teeth and composite restorations, a slight increase in supragingival calculus, and taste alteration. Chlorhexidine activity is decreased by blood and purulent material, as well as by toothpaste. Rinsing well with water prior to rinsing with chlorhexidine is suggested.

Prebrushing Mouthrinses

Some products are available as prebrushing mouth rinses. They claim to loosen plaque and therefore increase the effectiveness of tooth brushing. The products contain detergents. Numerous short-term and long-term studies have concluded that there is no advantage to using a prebrushing rinse.

TEACHING PLAQUE CONTROL

There are many approaches to teaching patients effective plaque control. No single technique has been devised that will satisfy the needs of every patient or that can be taught by every clinician.

There are certain fundamental principles that can be applied to virtually every patient. They are:

1. *Keep instructions simple.* Remember that practicing plaque control is an exercise in manual dexterity. The more complex the technique, the more skill the patient needs to learn.
2. *Do not teach too much at one time.* It is far better to introduce new techniques a few at a time over a longer period, than to expect the patient to remember and practice a long list of procedures that, after one exposure to them, appear very complicated.

3. *Encourage the patient.* Because varied personal abilities, not every patient will perform adequate plaque control at first. With further assistance and continued encouragement, almost all patients can be motivated to practice better oral hygiene. Do not, however, excuse lack of effort. One must differentiate between lack of willingness to improve and lack of knowledge and skill.

4. *Continue observation and supervision.* No matter how well the patient practices plaque control after the initial instructional program, repeated professional evaluation is required to help maintain a high level of performance. The interval between these supervisory evaluations will vary from patient to patient.

5. *Be flexible.* Although you may teach a specific technique to all patients, remember that not all patients have the same problems. Crowded or widely spaced teeth, lengths of crown, presence of fixed prosthetic appliances, and physical disabilities are only some of the variables encountered. Be prepared to alter techniques, and be knowledgeable about products available for use as adjuncts in controlling plaque. Finally, do not attempt to change patients to your technique if their present methods are effective.

SUGGESTED READINGS

American Academy of Periodontology Position Paper. American Academy of Periodontology Position Paper. 1995.

Christou V, Timmerman MF, Van der Velden U, Van der Weijden FA. Comparison of different approaches of interdental oral hygiene: interdental brushes versus dental floss. J Periodontol 1998;69:759–764.

Hancock EB. Periodontal diseases: prevention. Ann Periodontol 1996;1:223–249.

Lim LP, Davies WI, Yuen KW, Ma MH. Comparison of modes of oral hygiene instruction in improving gingival health. J Clin Periodontol 1996;23:693–697.

Prevention. JADA 1998;129(Suppl):15S–18S.

Silberman SL, Le Jeune RC, Serio FG, et al. A method for determining patient oral care skills: The University of Mississippi Oral Hygiene Index. J Periodontol 1998;69:1176–1180.

Westfelt E. Rationale of mechanical plaque control. J Clin Periodontol 1996;23:263–267.

Scaling and Root Preparation

Jane Amme

Scaling and root preparation are essential procedures in all phases of periodontal therapy. Mechanical tooth preparation usually includes scaling and root planing. It is often difficult to determine where scaling stops and root planing begins, and frequently, the two procedures cannot be dissociated.

Scaling

This is the initial procedure in which the crown and root surfaces of the teeth are instrumented to remove calculus, plaque, accumulated material, and stain.

Root Preparation

Root planing is a technique designed to remove cementum or surface dentin that has been altered by disease. It has been suggested that the term "root detoxification," which is more descriptive of the treatment attempted, supersede the often misunderstood and misinterpreted term of "root planing." Root detoxification is the procedure directed at rendering the diseased root surface free of plaque, cementum, surface dentin, and contaminated toxins or microorganisms. Root detoxification can be accomplished by mechanical means, chemical procedures, or a combination of these two. The use of chemical agents to treat the diseased root surface is under investigation. Some examples of these chemical compounds include chlorhexidine gluconate (Peridex7) irrigation, stannous fluoride, Betadine, and tetracycline hydrochloride. Future research may provide new and more effective products for root detoxification (see Chapter 11).

Rationale for Tooth Preparation

Supragingival Area

The goal is to obtain a tooth surface that does not encourage the accumulation of deposits and can be maintained by the patient. Scaling and polishing are the indicated procedures to achieve a clean, smooth supragingival tooth surface.

Subgingival Area

The objective of root preparation is to clean and detoxify the root surface to accomplish the following:

1. Minimize the toxic root contribution as an ongoing insult to the adjacent periodontal tissues.
2. Obtain a biologically acceptable root surface for tissue adaptation and potential new attachment.

INSTRUMENTATION AND ARMAMENTARIUM

Prerequisites for scaling and root planing are a thorough knowledge of root structure and effective basic instrumentation skills. The successful practice of periodontics centers on the skillful use of instruments during scaling and root planing (root detoxification). These instruments generally include scalers, curets, files, and sonic and ultrasonic scaling devices. Calculus deposits can be removed by any of these instruments. Curets, however, are the instruments of choice for root detoxification procedures because they are the most effective, causing the least amount of trauma to the hard and soft tissues. Ultrasonic and sonic instruments may be effective root detoxification instruments, especially with new improvements in their design, but need further testing to prove their efficacy.

PERIODONTAL EXAMINATION INSTRUMENTS

Periodontal Probe and Nabors Probe

Radiographs alone can not be relied upon to determine the attachment levels in a patient with gingivitis or periodontitis. The periodontal probe is the only reliable means of assessing periodontal pocket depths and attachment levels. It also is used to determine bleeding sites. The periodontal probe is manufactured with various designs: single-ended with multiple numerical markings and color-coded variations, working end sizes, and shapes. The Nabors probe is designed to assess the furcation areas.

Explorers

The successful clinician must have the ability to detect calculus and variations in root surfaces with an explorer during scaling and root planing procedures. This

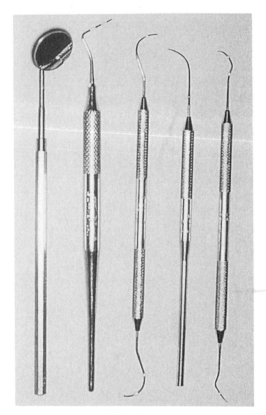

Fig. 9-1

important skill is as important as proficiency of root planing instrumentation technique. The development of tactile sensitivity is a key factor to becoming a competent clinician. The explorer is an extremely sensitive instrument because it is wire-like; this quality permits vibration for detection of tooth surface characteristics and the presence of calculus, caries, furcations, and root surface variations. Explorers are available in single-ended, double-ended mirror-image, and double-ended designs (Fig. 9-1).

SUPRAGINGIVAL DEPOSITS REMOVAL INSTRUMENTS

Scalers, Hoes, Files, and Chisels

Scalers are designed for supragingival deposit removal and are available in straight and curved sickle designs. The straight sickle scaler (the Jacquette Scaler is one example) has two cutting edges on a straight blade that ends in a sharp point and is triangular in cross section. The curved sickle has two cutting edges on a curved blade. Scalers feature a rigid shank and a thin face, which aids in chipping off calculus, especially in interproximal areas. The triangular shape or sharp back does not allow for deep submarginal instrumentation without trauma to the soft tissue. Scalers with straight shanks are designed for anterior teeth, while angled shanks are for use on posterior teeth (Fig. 9-2).

HOES
Used to dislodge heavy supramarginal calculus deposits.

FILES
Used to crush and remove heavy calculus deposits.

CHISELS
Used to dislodge bridges of calculus on Anterior Mandibular teeth.

Fig. 9-3

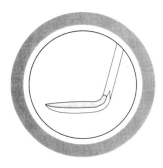

The Straight Sickle Scaler
Two cutting edges on a straight blade
that end in a sharp point.
Also known as a Jacquette Scaler

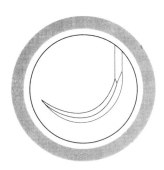

The Curved Sickle Scaler
Two cutting edges on a curved blade
that end in a sharp point

Fig. 9-2

Other instruments for supragingival deposit removal include hoes for dislodging heavy calculus, , and chisels for removal of calculus "bridges" from mandibular anterior teeth (Fig. 9-3).

SUBGINGIVAL DEPOSIT REMOVAL INSTRUMENTS

Universal and Area Specific Curets

Curets are the instrument of choice for hand root preparation. Curets have flexing shanks for tactile sensitivity and a face that ends in a rounded toe. They are moon shaped in cross section. The rounded back and toe allow for submarginal instrumentation without trauma to the surrounding soft tissues. Many types of universal and area-specific (Gracey) curets are available with variations to meet almost any clinician's needs. There are two basic curet designs. The universal curet has a blade with two cutting edges and is designed for general use. This curet can be used on the mesial and distal surfaces of the tooth and does not require changing the working ends of the instruments. The blade is not offset, and the face of the blade is beveled at 90 de-

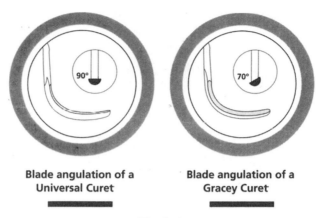

Blade angulation of a Universal Curet

Blade angulation of a Gracey Curet

Fig. 9-4

grees to the shank. Both cutting edges are used. The area-specific (Gracey) curet is designed for specific areas in the mouth. The Gracey curet is honed to offset the blade, and the face of the blade is beveled at 60 to 70 degrees to the shank. One cutting edge of this curet is used.

Several manufacturers make a rigid curet. The rigid curet features a larger, heavier, and less flexible shank than the standard curet. The rigid curet is designed to remove moderate to heavy calculus, but the heavier instrument design decreases the tactile sensitivity (Fig. 9-4).

AREA-SPECIFIC CURET MODIFICATIONS

After-Five Curets and Mini-Five Curets

The Hu-Friedy After-Five curets are modified area-specific curets. The terminal shank is elongated by 3 mm to allow access to deep periodontal pockets and root surfaces. The blade is thinned to ease gingival insertion and reduce tissue distention. These curets are available in the rigid and finishing designs.

The Mini-Five curets are a modification of the After-five design. The length of the blade is reduced by a half inch to allow ease of instrumentation and better adap-

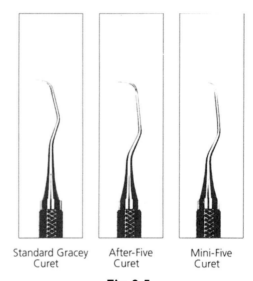

Standard Gracey Curet

After-Five Curet

Mini-Five Curet

Fig. 9-5

tation in areas that are difficult to instrument. They are available in finishing and rigid designs (Fig. 9-5).

Gracey Curvettes

The American Dental Instrument Gracey curvettes consist of a set of four instruments. The blade length has been reduced to half of the length of the Gracey curet, and the blade is modified to curve slightly upward. The shorter blade, upward curvature, and blunted tip allows for adapta-

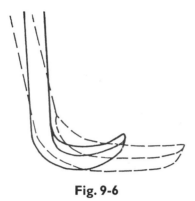

Fig. 9-6

tion in the deep anterior and premolar and line angle of posterior teeth (Fig. 9-6).

Langer Curets

The three Langer curets combine the advantages of the area-specific shank design with the versatility of the universal blade honed at 90 degrees. This allows for adaptation to both mesial and distal surfaces without changing instruments. The combination of shank design of the Gracey 5–6, 11–12, and 13–14 blade and the universal curet blade make up the basic Langer set of curets (Fig. 9-7). The Langer curets are also available with the After-Five and Mini-Five modifications, as well as with a rigid shank design and Pattison design. Plastic instruments designed for use on the dental implant surface are covered in Chapter 21.

TECHNIQUE FOR HAND INSTRUMENTATION

Basic Principles

Proficiency in instrumentation is obtained by adhering to general guidelines:

1. *Work comfortably.* Make the patient comfortable, but mainly you should make yourself comfortable.
2. *Follow an orderly sequence of instrumentation.* This avoids omitting a particular tooth surface.

3. *Operate with maximal visibility.* When possible, it is best to have direct vision of the operated areas. Also, have a good light source. Fiberoptics are helpful in obtaining direct visibility. They can also be used for transillumination and may show small deposits that might otherwise be overlooked.
4. *Obtain maximal accessibility.* Use mirror and fingers.
5. *Maintain complete control of instruments.* Stability is essential for effective controlled action of the instrument.

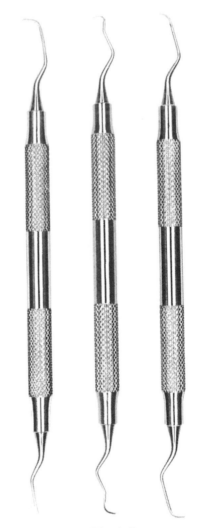

Fig. 9-7

6. *Maintain a clear field.* Gauze and cotton rolls, frequent flushing with water, and compressed air may be used. Flushing is helpful in ensuring that no calculus or tooth shavings remain in the gingival sulcus or pocket.

7. *Be certain that all instruments are sharp.* A dull instrument will merely slide over the thinner pieces of calculus, giving the impression that all calculus has been removed. Instruments must be sharp to be effective. Sharpen them after each use. Frequently, instruments require sharpening during the root preparation procedure.

8. *Be gentle and careful.* Do not confuse roughness with thoroughness.

9. *Know the function of each instrument.* Using the instrument correctly makes the job quicker and easier.

10. *Use as few instruments as possible.* You become more efficient and proficient when using fewer instruments.

11. *Know the relation of the instrument to the tooth and periodontal structures before activating it.* Put the instrument into place slowly and deliberately. This prevents undue injury to the tissues.

12. *Check for completeness.* Use explorers and probes for this purpose.

Basic Strokes

There are two basic strokes for scaling and root detoxification (Fig. 9-8):

1. *Exploratory stroke.* This is used to determine the topography of subgingival deposits. The blade of the instrument is passed along the root surface or calculus deposit, apically, to the depth of the pocket. If any apparent obstruction is encountered during exploration, the blade should be moved laterally from the root surface and, if possible, gently moved further apically. This movement aids in distinguishing between a ledge of calculus and the base of the pocket.

2. *Working stroke.* Once calculus or roughness is located, it is removed by engaging the root surface and calculus at an 80-degree angle and then deliberately moving the instrument along the root surface. This stroke is followed by a smoothing action done with absolute control. Use sharp curets with short strokes in a smooth, rhythmic, and continuous manner to accomplish root detoxification. The instrument should be placed at the edge of the deposit, and there should then be "stepping" or overlapping of areas around the tooth to cover the entire surface.

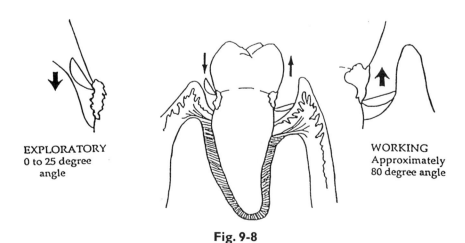

EXPLORATORY
0 to 25 degree
angle

WORKING
Approximately
80 degree angle

Fig. 9-8

ROOT PLANING STROKES

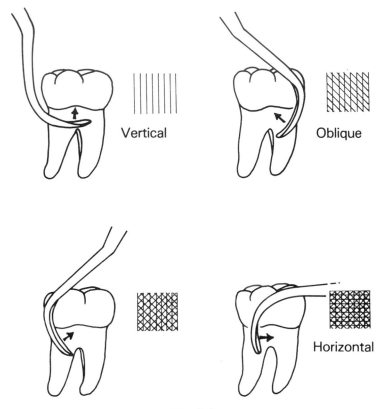

Fig. 9-9

Care must be taken to avoid scratching or gouging the root. The shaving action is continued until the root surface is completely smooth (Fig. 9-9).

Anesthesia

For most patients, supragingival scaling can be accomplished without anesthesia. Local anesthesia is indicated for proper scaling and root detoxification procedures performed on subgingival root surfaces. It is recommended that practitioners use block or infiltration anesthesia and limit the appointment to a segment, quadrant, or one-half mouth. The practi-tioner can adequately prepare the root with minimal discomfort to the patient.

ULTRASONIC AND SONIC SCALERS

The sonic and ultrasonic scalers provide a fast and easy means of debridement with a high degree of patient comfort. The combined effects of cavitation by the water and vibration by the instrument against the tooth surface provide the force necessary to dislodge debris and accretions. Soft and hard tissue will not be damaged if light pressure, constant motion of the tip, and adequate water spray are used. Several types of devices are available.

Magnetostrictive (Ultrasonic)

The Cavitron7 operates on the principle of magnetostriction: That is, if a bar of metal (or stack) is placed in a field of alternating current, the stack of metal vibrates at the speed generated by the field of alternating current. The Cavitron tips can vibrate at speeds between 25,000 to 35,000 cycles per second. The inserts commonly used for scaling are P-10 and the EWPP (Fig. 9-10). The P-10 can be used anywhere in the mouth and is effective on subgingival calculus. The EWPP is best suited for debridement of deep pockets. It can reach areas that other instruments cannot traverse because of its similarity in design to the periodontal probe. The newest addition of tip design is called "Slim Line" and consists of a set of slim tips that are designed for root preparation in deep pockets in all areas of the mouth (Fig. 9-11). The tip and corners of all Cavitron7 inserts are potentially dangerous. Even a dull insert will gouge teeth and restorations if used improperly.

A more recent development has been the introduction of the Cavimed7 instrument, which can deliver the operator's

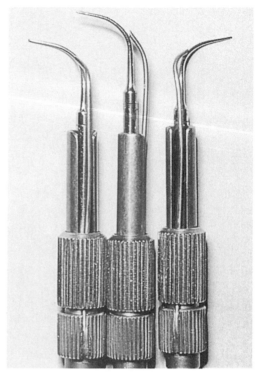

Fig. 9-11

choice of antimicrobial agent through a hollow tip while the instrument tip removes light deposits of calculus and plaque.

Piezoelectric (Ultrasonic)

The Odontoson is also a Piezoelectric ultrasonic scaler (Fig. 9-12) that is designed to deliver antimicrobial agents during subgingival scaling. The design of the scaling tips is similar to that of hand scaler tips.

SONIC SCALER

The Titan-S7 (Fig. 9-13) scaler tip vibrates at a range from 2000 to 6500 cycles per second. The sonic scaler is connected to the high-speed hand-piece hose and vibrates by air passing over the metal rod, which is contained in the Titan-S hand-

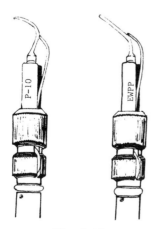

Fig. 9-10

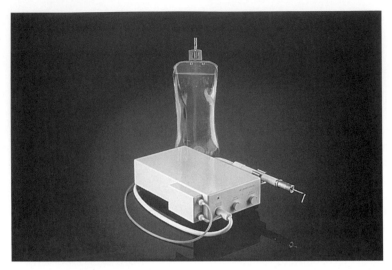

Fig. 9-12

piece. Three tips are available with the unit. The tip action is elliptical or orbital. The sonic scaler has less power for rapid calculus removal but is convenient because of its small size and ease of attachment. Other sonic scalers include Densonic, Orbison 30, and Lynx SM.

The ultrasonic and sonic instruments are highly recommended for use in gross debridement, particularly in cases of necrotizing ulcerative gingivitis or acute gingivitis. These instruments dislodge debris rapidly, while the water spray clears the operative site. Some clinicians advocate the use of the ultrasonic or sonic instruments for debridement during periodontal surgery. A washed field with improved visualization is helpful during the surgery; however, the water source from the unit often contains microorganisms that could be introduced into the surgical site. If these instruments are to be used during any surgical procedure, they should be used as a self-contained, sterilized unit with its own source of sterile, distilled water maintained in a sterile pressure tank. Even then, it is necessary to routinely check the tank and hoses leading to the instrument for possible contamination.

The ultrasonic and sonic scalers remove deep calculus with conventional tips, but gaining access to the calculus is difficult, and tactile sensitivity may be limited. The deeper the pocket, the greater is the chance of blockage of the water spray to the tip, and, consequently, the greater the possibility of patient discomfort and soft tissue damage.

Ultrasonic instrumentation removes the pocket lining if subgingival curettage is the objective, and healing of the wound is as rapid as after hand instrumentation. It must be emphasized that the ultrasonic and sonic scaler are not intended for root planing.

Heavy surface stain can be removed with these instruments. A great deal of time should not be expended in removing stain that could be removed quickly and more effectively with a rubber cup and polishing agent, or a Prophyjet7 polishing instrument.

The ultrasonic and sonic scalers are an excellent adjunct in periodontal therapy, but they are only an adjunct. One simply cannot perform effective root detoxification with these tips alone. It is extremely important that a face mask, gloves, and adequate eye protection be used by the

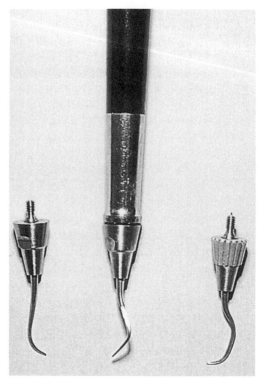

Fig. 9-13

dental team during the use of these instruments. It also is advisable for the patient to rinse with an appropriate mouth rinse before instrumentation. Routine use of the ultrasonic or sonic scaler in patients with contagious diseases is contraindicated. Extreme caution is indicated whenever an aerosol is produced.

POLISHING

Several low-abrasive, fluoride-containing agents are commercially available for polishing the supragingival tooth surface with a rubber cup after instrumentation. Care must be taken to select products that are minimally abrasive to avoid excessive loss of tooth surface. Other instruments that have been introduced for tooth polishing are the Prophyjet7 and the Young Dental Manufacturing polishing instruments. These instruments deliver a sodium bicarbonate and water mixture with a high volume of air and are effective in removing stain. They will not remove calculus. Precautions are necessary when using these instruments because of the aerosol contamination inherent with any instrument driven by high volumes of air. Gloves, masks, and protective eye gear are mandatory to protect both the operator and the assistant. Care should be exercised when treating patients who are on sodium-restricted diets, have respiratory problems, or wear contact lenses. Premedication is necessary before rubber cup polishing in patients requiring prophylactic antibiotic coverage.

Polishing with the rubber cup and Prophyjet may be contraindicated in the presence of severe inflammation, effects (caries and decalcification), and exposed root surfaces. Topical fluoride treatment is recommended after the polishing procedure.

SUGGESTED READING

Pattison GL, Pattison AM. Periodontal instrumentation, 2nd ed. Norwalk, CT: Appleton & Lange, 1992.

Wilkins EM. Clinical practice of the dental hygienist, 7th ed. Baltimore: Williams & Wilkins, 1994.

Wound Healing

John Rapley

Surgery disrupts the existing relationship of various cells and tissues of the body. Healing is the phase of the inflammatory response that leads to a new physiologic and anatomic relationship among the disrupted body elements. It generally includes all of the following:

1. Clot formation.
2. Granulation tissue development.
3. Epithelialization.
4. Collagen formation.
5. Regeneration.
6. Maturation

Understanding wound repair processes permits the operator to design and perform the proper surgical procedures to support overall therapeutic objectives and to ensure that the patient's healing period will be as brief and comfortable as possible.

Periodontal surgery can be broadly classified into two categories: procedures designed to correct soft tissue defects and those designed to manage defects of the alveolar bone.

HEALING OF SOFT TISSUE WOUNDS

Excision of Gingiva (Gingivectomy)

After excision of a portion of gingiva (Fig. 10-1a), a clot forms over the exposed connective tissue (Fig. 10-1b). Within hours, the connective tissue begins to produce granulation tissue (proliferating connective tissue characterized by increased mitotic activity in the fibroblasts, endothelial cells and capillaries, and undifferentiated mesenchymal cells) that buds out from the surface. This is soon covered and infiltrated by many neutrophils. The healing wound surface consists of a base of moderately inflamed connective tissue covered with granulation tissue, a layered zone of neutrophils, and a clot, in that order. Epithelium begins to proliferate from the margins of the wound and migrates cell by cell (at about 0.5 mm per day) under the clot, through the neutrophil zone, and over the granulation tissue (Fig. 10-1c). Epithelium continues to proliferate in a thin layer until it reaches the surface of the tooth. While this is occurring, fibroblasts in the granulation tissue begin to produce immature, incompletely polymerized collagen. By this time, the clot has been exfoliated, having served its function as a kind of bandage. Both the collagen and epithelium continue to proliferate and mature until a multilayered covering of epithelium overlies mature collagen. The gingival crevice is reformed after gingival excision by coronal growth of connective tissue and by apical migration of the junctional epithelium. If healing has progressed relatively free of destructive bacterial agents, the lining of the sulcus is composed of a flattened, intact, stratified

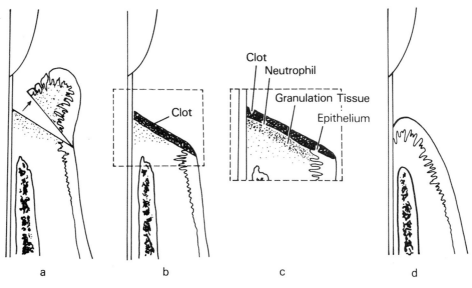

Clot
Neutrophil
Granulation Tissue
Clot
Epithelium

a   b   c   d

Fig. 10-1

squamous epithelium. If irritants have been present, rete pegs form along the basal layer of the epithelium.

The granulation tissue matures to the point at which the newly formed collagen is indistinguishable from the collagen fibers of the attached gingiva (Fig. 10-1d). The tissue clinically resembles normal gingiva within a few weeks, but it takes several months before the fiber bundles completely heal and organize.

Even though the gingival excision surgery has not directly involved bone, some osteoclastic activity on the cortical surface will occur, followed by rebound osteoblastic activity. This bone remodeling is on a microscopic level and is not usually of clinical significance as long as a sufficient thickness of connective tissue is retained over the bone.

Simple Incision

When a sharp instrument cuts into the gingiva, healing processes similar to those previously described occur. The slight differences are based on the architecture of the wound.

After an incision, if the cut edges are closely approximated, only a small space exists between the wound surfaces in which a clot can form (Fig. 10-2a). This clot serves only as a "plug" through which granulation tissue grows. It is advantageous to have minimal clot because the elements of the clot are ultimately resorbed, thus requiring cell effort. Healing by union of approximated granulating surfaces is termed *healing by primary intention.* This is the rationale of primary wound closure in gingival attachment procedures. The better the wound edge approximation and the smaller the clot, the more rapidly epithelial bridging between the cut soft tissue surfaces occurs, thereby sealing off the slower maturing connective tissues from the oral environment (Fig. 10-2b).

Clot absorption is concurrently occurring within the depth of the incision, as macrophages remove the fibrin and fibroblasts produce collagen. Collagen maturation occurs, and this is clinically indistinguishable from the collagen of the normal gingiva after a few months (Fig. 10-2c).

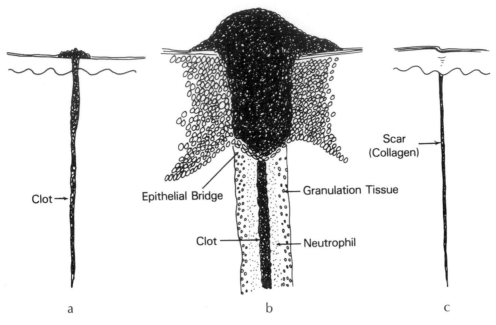

Clot

Epithelial Bridge

Clot

Granulation Tissue

Neutrophil

Scar
(Collagen)

a

b

c

Fig. 10-2

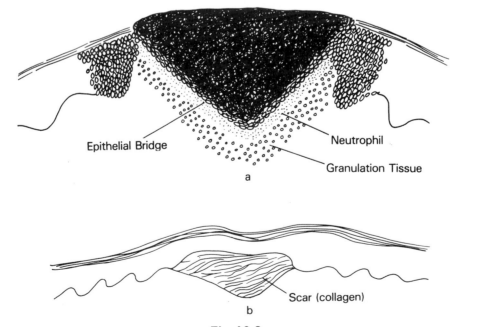

Epithelial Bridge

Neutrophil

Granulation Tissue

a

Scar (collagen)

b

Fig. 10-3

The epithelium will migrate farther into its depths along the cut surfaces in a poorly approximated wound, covering all exposed maturing granulation tissue and lining the wound (Fig. 10-3a). This is often termed *healing by second intention,* and eventually a relatively large mass of clot is sloughed (Fig. 10-3b).

Epithelial cells require energy for survival, proliferation, and migration. Their nutrients are derived by diffusion from the blood vessels. These cells can travel only a finite distance from the capillaries, beyond which they lose their source of nutrition. Therefore, the proximity of capillaries (granulation tissue) determines the route of epithelial proliferation.

Reattachment (Presurgical Level)

Reattachment is defined as the reestablishment of a soft tissue interface on the root surface after surgical detachment. When gingiva is surgically separated from a tooth surface, some collagen fibers remain embedded in and extend out of the cementum (Fig. 10-4a). If the tissue is intimately replaced onto the unaltered tooth surface, a small clot is interposed between the collagen fibers in the cementum and the collagen of the wound sur-

face of the gingiva (Fig. 10-4b). Forming granulation tissue penetrates the thin clot and permits the fibers extending from the cementum to unite with new collagen formed by gingival fibroblasts.

The epithelial attachment usually remains at its original position on the tooth, or it may migrate a few cells apically, depending on the clot size (Fig. 10-4c). If a large clot is formed (Fig. 10-4d), epithelium may migrate apically over the wound surface of the gingiva, resulting in a junctional epithelium that is considerably longer and more apically positioned (Fig. 10-4e). This occurrence is unlikely if appropriate end-of-surgery procedures, consisting of stabilization with sutures, application of gentle pressure applied for 2 to 3 minutes, and proper placement of a periodontal dressing, are performed if needed.

New Attachment

Soft tissue new attachment implies formation of new cementum, connective tissue fibers, and junctional epithelium at a more coronal level on previously diseased root surfaces. To achieve a more coronal attachment of connective tissue to the tooth, cells capable of producing new cementum and collagen must have

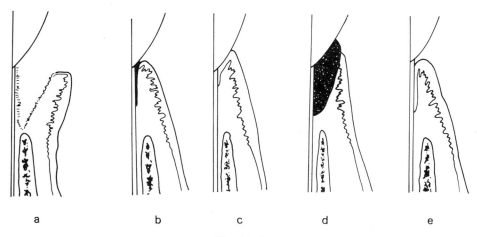

a   b   c   d   e

Fig. 10-4

access to the tooth surface coronal to the existing level of the junctional epithelium. The epithelium lining the pocket prevents such access and must be removed from the inner aspect of the soft tissue wall of the pocket (Figs. 10-5a and b).

The alveolar crest fibers and the transseptal fibers also prevent the fibroblasts and cementoblasts within the periodontal ligament from gaining access to the tooth surface coronal to the original position of the junctional epithelium. Removing the epithelial lining and the connective tissue covering the periodontal ligament space increases the access of cells capable of producing new cementum and collagen to the portion of the tooth that has been exposed to the periodontal pocket. If the root has been properly detoxified by careful mechanical root planing and possibly chemical treatment and if the wound surface is closely readapted to minimize clot size, cellular elements of the periodontal ligament may migrate coronally and may produce new cementum and new Sharpey's fibers, thereby establishing a new soft tissue attachment (Fig. 10-5c). However, considerable evidence suggests that repair after gingival new attachment procedures usually results in a long thin junctional epithelium adherent to the tooth (Fig. 10-5d). Clinical experience and longitudinal studies indicate that this epithelial adherence can be maintained with little or no change over time. Further evidence suggests that by demineralizing the toxic cementum or by physically excluding epithelial growth into the healing wound, a new connective tissue attachment is possible.

For years, confusion has existed over whether new cementum will form on pulpless teeth or teeth with root canal fillings. Animal studies indicate that new attachment can occur on pulpless teeth, teeth left open for drainage, and teeth with root canal fillings, with the same predictability as for teeth with healthy pulps.

Open Wounds

At the completion of certain surgical procedures (gingivectomy, gingivoplasty) some areas of the wound are denuded of epithelium and part of the mucosa. The type of tissue that will be produced during healing depends primarily on the type of tissue making up the wound and its borders. For example, a gingivectomy wound is usually bor-

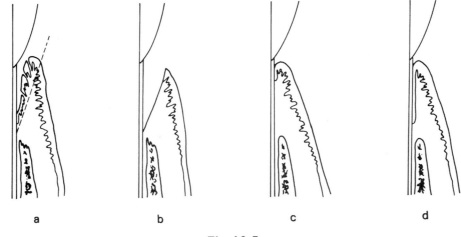

a   b   c   d

Fig. 10-5

dered by gingival tissue (dense collagenous connective tissue covered by keratinized epithelium); predictably, gingival tissue will re-form.

After certain flap procedures, areas of bone may be left with only a very thin covering of connective tissue. If gingiva originally covered the bone, then gingiva will re-form. If alveolar mucosa originally covered the bone, alveolar mucosa will usually re-form. Occasionally, and very unpredictably, an intermediate type of tissue that clinically resembles gingiva (transitional gingiva) may form. The formation of gingiva, however, can be predictably induced in an area of pre-existent alveolar mucosa if the apical and lateral borders of the wound are composed of mature gingiva.

Flaps

A flap is defined as the portion of the gingiva, alveolar mucosa, or periosteum that is elevated or dissected from the tooth and alveolar process and retains a blood supply. Many surgical procedures involve the use of flaps of various designs. There are two methods of raising a flap:

1. Blunt elevation (full-thickness or mucoperiosteal flap) exposing the bone surface (Fig. 10-6).
2. Sharp dissection (partial thickness or mucosal flap) leaving a varying thickness of connective tissue covering the alveolar process (Fig. 10-7).

When flaps are replaced to intimately cover the bone (whether in the original position or at a different location), healing

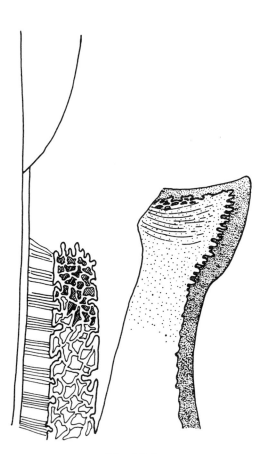

Fig. 10-6

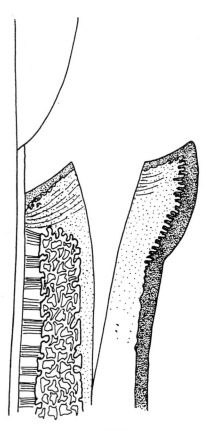

Fig. 10-7

is similar to that of a simple incision in that one connective tissue wound surface is placed against another with a small intervening blood clot. The rationale and technique for the full-thickness (mucoperiosteal) and partial-thickness (mucosal) flap are discussed in Chapter 14.

Free Gingival Grafts (Free Soft Tissue Autograft)

Free grafts in contrast to flaps are completely separated from their blood supply and are placed in a different recipient site. The vasculature at the recipient site provides all the nourishment for the graft.

The blood clot at the recipient site should be as thin as possible to permit ready diffusion of nutrients from the recipient site through the clot to the graft. Likewise, the inner surface of the graft should be as smooth as possible to reduce the "pooling" of blood and formation of thicker clots within the surface irregularities. Because the survival of the graft depends on revascularization, the graft must be immobilized at the recipient site.

Root Detoxification

Studies have shown that the removal of plaque, toxins, and calculus from exposed root surfaces results in beneficial changes in the periodontium. This sequence of events is depicted in Figure 10-8b. As an intact periodontium (Fig. 10-8a) progresses to pocket formation (Fig. 10-8b), chronic inflammation of the gingival results in depolymerization of some gingiva fibers, apical migration of the junctional epithelium, and some loss of crestal bone. The gingiva itself is somewhat enlarged as a result of edema. Young vascular connective tissue is present within the gingiva, as are many lymphocytes, plasma cells, fibroblasts, and neutrophils (all the elements of defense and repair).

This granulomatous tissue has little chance to repair because of continued tissue damage from products created by

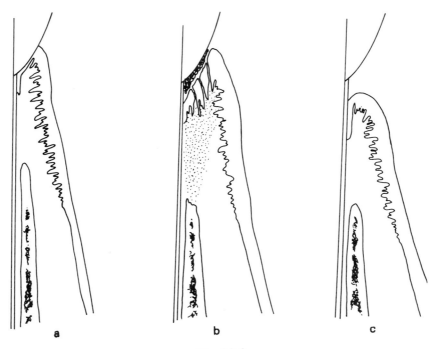

a   b   c

Fig. 10-8

and from the plaque microorganisms. If the local etiologic factors are removed by root detoxification procedures (mechanical root planing and, possibly, chemical treatment) and if effective plaque control procedures are established, the disease process will begin to resolve. The edema will subside and the granulomatous tissue will be converted to granulation tissue and can proceed to repair with regeneration of gingival collagen. As maturation progresses without the effects of plaque, further shrinkage will occur until a condition similar to that shown in (Fig. 10-8c) is reached.

HEALING INVOLVING BONE

General Principles

Bone undergoes remodeling throughout life. In health, osteoblastic activity and osteoclastic activity are in balance. This balance can be disturbed by changes in functional demands on the bone and by disease. Furthermore, any surgical procedure affects bone to some extent. The severity of the change depends on several factors, including the type of bone (cortical or cancellous), the thickness of bone, procedures done to the bone during the surgical procedure, and what type of covering it has after surgery. For example, if thin radicular bone overlying a maxillary canine were exposed during surgery and were left without soft tissue coverage after surgery, one could expect that during the healing process all exposed bone would be either resorbed or sequestrated, and that little of it would regenerate. However, if mostly cancellous interproximal bone were treated similarly, some resorption would occur during initial healing but the bone would then regenerate.

When performing periodontal surgery, one should remember the following:

1. Bone should be covered by soft tissue after surgery, if at all possible.

2. The thicker the soft tissue covering bone during and after the procedure, the less the bone is affected by surgery.
3. Thin bone will be permanently lost more easily than thick bone.

Thick, interproximal bone has sufficient intra-alveolar blood supply (cancellous bone) to withstand the loss of supply from the supraperiosteal vessels as a result of flap surgery. Conversely, thin radicular bone (minimal or no cancellous bone) is almost totally dependent on the blood supply from the supraperiosteal vessels and can be readily lost if this blood supply is compromised. Canines, first premolars, and the mesial roots of maxillary first molars usually have this thin bone. These teeth may even have bony dehiscences or fenestrations, as discussed in Chapter 1. The thickness of the radicular bone over all facial root surfaces should be considered carefully in the design and execution of surgical procedures.

Infrabony Defects

Many periodontal procedures are performed to stimulate new bone formation for repair of an osseous defect. Figure 10-9a represents a mesiodistal section through the proximal surfaces of two teeth and the interproximal bone and gingiva. A chronic infrabony defect is diagrammed to show three conditions common to most such chronic lesions:

1. Transseptal fibers are present as discrete bundles extending into the defect, and continuing to the cementum of the adjacent tooth.
2. A cortical surface may be present on the bony surface that forms the walls of the defect.
3. The junctional epithelium is apical to the crest of the bone and near the base of the defect.

If a new attachment is to form and provide increased support to the tooth, cells

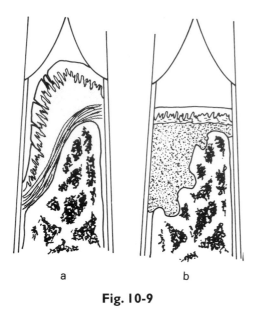

Fig. 10-9

must produce new cementum, new collagen fibers, and new bone. It may be necessary to remove the connective tissue portion of the pocket, the pocket epithelium, transseptal fibers, and the granulomatous tissue to give reparative cells access to the area involved.

After the soft tissue has been removed, any cortical bone lining the defect should be perforated (intramarrow penetration) to permit quick egress of pluripotential marrow cells for reformation of the attachment apparatus (Fig. 10-9b). Ideally, cementum, bone, and periodontal ligament are completely restored. Occasionally, however, only partial regeneration will result. The predictability of success for such new attachment procedures is discussed in Chapter 17.

Bone Replacement Grafts

Autogenous bone grafts have been used successfully for many years to manage osseous defects of the periodontium. The precise mechanisms by which these grafts contribute to healing and regeneration, however, remain unclear. It has been postulated that the primary effect of

autogenous grafts is osteogenic stimulation, but these grafts are believed to also act as actual bone producers as well as osteogenic stimulators.

Another possible benefit of autogenous grafts is that they act as a mechanical block or barrier to the downgrowth of epithelium into the wound. They are also thought to act as a trellis (scaffold) to guide and support the proliferation and migration of cells and vessels within the wound.

Fate of Bone Autografts

The fate of the calcified portions of autografts (and of other materials used) has been documented as follows:

1. The graft may retain vital osteoblasts and osteocytes and may be built upon by new bone. Such osteocyte viability is maintained only when the cells are close enough (within 1 mm) to a nutrient source; this suggests that osteocytes deep within a comparatively large fragment will die.
2. The graft may have no vital cells but may be built upon by new bone and later replaced by new bone.
3. The graft may remain as an inert, nonvital fragment, playing no apparent role in the healing process.
4. The graft may be completely resorbed during healing, acting as a scaffold for new bone formation.
5. The graft may be nonvital, playing no apparent role, and may be exfoliated during healing. Exfoliation may occur months after the surgical procedure.

Guided Tissue Regeneration Healing

Animal studies have suggested that the key aspect of wound healing depended on the cell type that initially repopulated the surgical area and their ability to progress. Different tissue types migrate into the surgical wound at different rates, and regeneration may occur if some tissue types (such as epithelium and connective tissue) could be delayed and other cell types (such as undifferentiated mesenchymal cells from the periodontal ligament and osteoblasts) could enter the progress in the surgical site. This concept was called *guided tissue regeneration,* and it used a barrier membrane to exclude the connective tissue and epithelium. Wounds healed in the protected area beneath the barrier membrane, as previously outlined

OTHER CONSIDERATIONS IN WOUND HEALING

Nutrition and Systemic Disorders

Healing occurs on a cellular-molecular level and requires the expenditure of energy and the utilization of nutrients, as needed for anabolic and catabolic activities. Any disorder that interferes with ingestion, digestion, absorption, or effective transport and use of foods will interfere with healing. Such disorders as diabetes; deficiencies in vitamins, minerals, and foods (especially protein); severe hormonal imbalances; and tobacco use can be expected to retard healing.

Age

Age by itself seems to have no effect on healing after periodontal surgery. General health seems to be of paramount importance.

Asepsis

Asepsis is a basic requirement for success in all surgery performed in the oral cavity. Periodontal surgery must be performed in a manner that will prevent introduction of foreign pathogens into the surgical field, which could cause infection and delay healing. In addition to

necessary infection control procedures, sterile gloves, instruments, and drapes should be routine in the performance of all oral surgical procedures.

Healing Rate

There seems to be a maximal speed at which various cells can clean up cellular debris, produce new materials, move through tissue, or perform reparative tasks. To date, there is no way to accelerate this process. Perhaps the best one can do is to avoid slowing the healing rate. To this end, factors such as nutrition, trauma, smoking, alcohol consumption, and other drug intake should be controlled during the healing period.

WOUND HEALING APPLIED TO PERIODONTAL SURGERY

A review of this chapter will be a reminder that many principles of wound healing apply directly to the success or to the failure of periodontal surgery. A summary of the more important principles that have been discussed follows:

1. A gingival wound may appear clinically normal within a few weeks, but many months will pass before healing is complete and fiber bundles have formed.
2. The better the approximation of two soft tissue wound edges and the smaller the clot, the more rapidly epithelialization occurs, thereby sealing off the slower maturing connective tissues from the oral environment.
3. In flap procedures, clot thickness should be kept at a minimum between tooth and wound surface to permit reattachment of connective tissue fibers at their original level or new attachment to occur at a more coronal level.
4. For predictable maturation of gingival tissue in apically positioned flaps,

gingival tissue should be maintained on the margin of the flap.

5. Relatively thin free soft tissue grafts on a recipient site with a thin intervening blood clot afford an excellent opportunity for graft survival.
6. Plaque, calculus, and contaminated cementum must be removed or detoxified for successful wound healing against the tooth surface.
7. Bone should be covered by soft tissue when the surgical procedure is completed.
8. The thicker the soft tissue covering over bone during and after the procedure, the less the bone will be affected.
9. Thin bone is permanently lost more easily than thick bone.
10. In the management of infrabony defects, all the soft tissue portion of the pocket (epithelium, transseptal fibers, granulomatous tissue) must be removed. In addition, any cortical bone lining the defect should be perforated to permit egress of pluripotential cells.

SUGGESTED READINGS

Egelberg J. Regeneration and repair of periodontal tissue. J Periodontal Res 1987;22:233.

Ramfjord SP, Engler WO, Hinkler JJ. A radioautographic study of healing following simple gingivectomy, II: the connective tissue. J Periodontol 1966;37:179.

Stahl SS, Wilkins G, Cantor M, Brown R. Gingival healing, II. Clinical and histologic repair sequences following gingivectomy. J Periodontol 1968;39:109–118.

Yumet JA, Polson AM. Gingival wound healing in the presence of plaque induced inflammation. J Periodontol 1985;56:107–119.

Principles of Periodontal Surgery

Arthur R. Vernino

The major goal of periodontal surgery is to create an oral environment that is conducive to maintaining the patient's dentition in health, comfort, and function for life.

REASONS FOR SURGERY

Provide Access

Surgery provides the clinician increased access to the root surface and alveolar bone. This access permits meticulous root preparation with the elimination of all hard deposits, contaminated cementum, and bacterial and tissue products from the root surfaces. Removal of toxic products from the root surface helps control the inflammatory process. In addition, the reduction in probing depths after surgical therapy allows the patient better access to all surfaces of the teeth for more effective plaque removal.

Repair the Periodontium

Other chapters in this book describe surgical methods designed to restore soft tissue and bone destroyed by disease. This surgery consists primarily of hard and soft tissue grafting techniques to restore the periodontium to a state that approaches the predisease level.

Modify Bony Architecture

Osseous defects and deformities create aberrations in the physiologic contour of the periodontium that contribute to plaque retention and are not consistent with a state of good health. Contouring the bone to eliminate osseous defects reduces plaque-retentive areas and allows the patient better access to the tooth surfaces for more effective plaque control.

Reduce Periodontal Pockets

Periodontal pockets may not always be totally eliminated, but they may be reduced by a variety of resective and regenerative techniques (Chapters 13 through 19). The primary goal is to reduce pocket depths to a manageable level for the dental team and for the patient.

PRESURGICAL CONSIDERATIONS

Patient Consent

When the periodontal treatment plan is presented to the patient, the patient should be informed that surgery may be a part of that plan. The patient should clearly understand the benefits and the possible risks or complications of any proposed procedures. The alternatives to surgery should be carefully explained to enable the patient to give an informed consent to the operative plan. A written entry of the discussion and patient agreement should be made in the dental record.

Contraindications for Periodontal Surgery

There are many reasons for not performing periodontal surgery. The existence of certain medical problems (such as uncontrolled diabetes or blood pressure) could make periodontal surgery inadvisable. A complete medical history must be taken before the performance of any periodontal treatment (see Chapter 3). Excellent plaque control is mandatory for success of periodontal surgery. The patient must be informed, at an early stage of the treatment, that no surgery will be performed unless the plaque is adequately controlled before surgery and until the patient understands and is committed to long-term maintenance care.

The magnitude of the existing periodontal destruction must be considered. Surgery performed in an attempt to treat severe periodontal destruction could result in further mutilation of the tissues, rather than restoration of the periodontium to health, comfort, and function. In many cases, extraction of teeth is the treatment of choice for a severely involved patient.

Some patients prefer to forego surgery, even after the advantages of surgery have been explained carefully. The best course of action with these patients is to cease further discussion of surgery and to determine an alternative treatment to maintain the existing dentition.

A practitioner who does not feel capable of the surgical management of the patient's condition or will not accept the responsibility of a satisfactory maintenance program for the patient should not attempt periodontal surgery. The dentist loses no status or prestige in the eyes of the patient in referring the advanced case to a trained specialist.

Infection Control/Phase I Therapy

Infection control (often called initial preparation or phase I) therapy should be completed before the final decision is made to perform surgery. Infection control therapy is one of the most valuable components of periodontal therapy. During this phase of treatment, it is possible to do the following:

1. Assess the patient's commitment to periodontal therapy.
2. Observe the patient's healing potential.
3. Reinforce plaque control instruction.
4. Reduce the need for surgery.
5. Improve tissue tone which facilitates soft tissue management at the time of surgery.

Three to six weeks after infection control therapy has been completed, the patient is re-examined thoroughly to determine what changes have occurred and what further periodontal therapy is required. On the basis of this examination, a decision about further treatment must be made. Table 11-1 is a decision matrix that considers the findings and the possible treatment alternatives one may make at this stage of treatment.

Anxiety Control

Most anxiety can be controlled by managing the patient in a kind and considerate manner. The periodontal surgeon should project a calm confidence in his or her ability to accomplish the surgical procedure. In a few patients, anxiety cannot be controlled without the use of some form of tranquilizing or sedative therapy. A variety of medications and methods are available for this purpose. Incumbent with use of sedation or drug therapy is

Table 11-1   Decision Matrix

Probing Depth Compared to Initial Exam	Bleeding	Localized	Generalized
Decreasing	No	Routine Maintenance Procedures	Routine Maintenance Procedures

	Yes	Consider:
		1. Reinforce oral hygiene
		2. Redetoxify roots
		3. Site specific treatment
		4. Shorten maintenance intervals
			Consider:
			1. Plaque control may be:
			  inadequate-retrain
			  If adequate, consider:
			1. Systemic antibiotics
			2. Refer to periodontist

Same	No	Routine Maintenance Procedures	Routine Maintenance Procedures

± 1	Yes	Consider:
		1. Reinforce oral hygiene
		2. Redetoxify roots
		3. Site specific treatment
		  (May include surgery)
		4. Refer to Periodontist
			Consider:
			1. Plague control may be:
			  inadequate-retrain
			  If adequate, consider:
			2. Systemic antibiotics
			3. Surgery
			4. Refer to periodontist

Increasing 2 mm and over	No	Consider: 1. Surgery 2. Refer to periodontist	Consider: 1. Systemic antibiotics 2. Surgery 3. Refer to periodontist
	Yes	Consider: 1. Surgery 2. Refer to periodontist	Consider: 1. Systemic antibiotics 2. Surgery 3. Refer to periodontist

the clinician's responsibility to be thoroughly familiar with all aspects of the regimen being considered and the knowledge and the equipment to manage the unexpected adverse reactions.

Antibiotics

Premedication with appropriate antibiotics must be provided for the first five systemic conditions listed:

1. Most congenital heart disease.
2. Rheumatic heart disease or other acquired valvular heart disease.
3. Idiopathic hypertrophic subaortic stenosis.
4. Mitral valve prolapse syndrome with mitral insufficiency.
5. Prosthetic heart valves.
6. Patients with joint prostheses (see below).
7. Patients with compromised immune systems (consult or refer to physician).

The recommendations of the American Medical Association, the American Heart Association, and the American Dental Association are discussed, in detail, in Chapter 6. Opinions regarding antibiotic coverage of patients with joint prostheses differ. The patient's orthopedist should be consulted to determine the choice of antibiotic.

A minimal amount of evidence supports the concept of antibiotic prophylaxis to prevent infection after periodontal surgery. The use of broad-spectrum antibiotics to suppress plaque and to improve healing after bone grafting procedures has considerable merit. Tetracycline is selectively excreted in gingival fluid in a concentration two to 10 times the concentration found in plasma. This high concentration in the target gingival sulcular area makes tetracycline particularly appropriate to prescribe after bone grafting procedures. The usual dosage is 250 mg four times per day, starting on the day of surgery and for 7 to 14 days thereafter. Tetracycline should not be taken with food because of the likelihood of impaired absorption. In addition, this antibiotic may cause discoloration of developing teeth; therefore, caution should be observed in prescribing it for pregnant women or for children with developing dentitions. Tetracycline is also contraindicated in patients with impaired liver and kidney function and those with known allergies to the medication.

Asepsis

It is imperative that periodontal surgery be performed under aseptic conditions. The oral cavity cannot be sterilized, but precautions should be taken to prevent cross-contamination and to preclude the introduction of extraneous bacteria into the patient's mouth. All instruments must be sterilized and placed on a sterile operating tray. The operator should wear a surgical cap and must wear a face mask and gloves. A sterile towel should be clipped to the front of the surgeon's clinic clothing. The patient should be draped with sterile towels, and the patient's hair and eyes may be wrapped with sterile towels. Great care should be taken to ensure that nonsterile items are not introduced into the operating field.

Emergencies

The clinician must know and take measures to minimize adverse patient reactions to any administered medication. All office personnel must have ready access to the emergency cart and be competent in the proper use of emergency equipment. Emergency equipment must be periodically inspected to ensure that the equipment is in good working condition. Each member of the office staff should be currently certified in basic cardiopulmonary resuscitation. It is good policy to have periodic drills in emergency procedures so that each staff member will have the confidence to perform effectively in an emergency situation.

Anesthesia

Periodontal surgery is usually performed under local anesthesia. The periodontal surgeon should use the minimum of local anesthetic required to keep the patient comfortable during the surgical procedure. The clinician should be aware that the dosage, the method of injection, and the vascularity at the injected site affect the patient.

The action and safe dose range of the anesthetic selected should be well known. The maximal dosage for lidocaine hydrochloride in a healthy person, when used with a vasoconstrictor, is 3.2 mg per pound of body weight. A 1.8-mL dental cartridge with 2% lidocaine hydrochloride contains 36 mg of lidocaine hydrochloride (20 mg per mL). By using this information, it is possible to calculate the maximal dose of lidocaine for a healthy patient. For example, 12 cartridges of 2% lidocaine hydrochloride (36 mg per cartridge) is the maximum that could be used for a 140-pound person (140 × 3.2 mg = 448 mg; therefore: 448 mg = 12.4 cartridges).

It is usually unnecessary for the epinephrine concentration to be greater than 1:100,000 (0.01 mg/mL) in local anesthetic agents used for periodontal surgery. The maximal dosage of epinephrine for a healthy adult patient is 0.2 mg of epinephrine per dental appointment (10 cartridges of lidocaine with an epinephrine concentration of 1:100,000). Patients with severe cardiovascular problems should receive no more than 0.04 mg of epinephrine per dental appointment (two 1.8-mL cartridges of anesthetic with 1:100,000 epinephrine concentration).

Caution: Any local anesthetic in dentistry should be injected with aspirating syringes and at a rate that approximates 1 mL/min.

SURGICAL CONSIDERATIONS

Surgical Plan

Before surgery, the clinician should carefully review the patient's radiographs and information regarding probing depths, amount of attached and keratinized tissue, and bony contours. These data are used to carefully plan the proper surgical procedure. Although a specific surgical plan is necessary, the clinician should be flexible enough to change the plan if an unsuspected problem is encountered during the surgery. In addition, the clinician must be aware of the anatomic structures that may influence the surgical plan.

Instrumentation and Flap Design

Cutting and root planing instruments must be sharp. Dull instruments traumatize tissue, complicate healing, and frustrate the operator. If dull instruments are found in a surgical set, a sterile sharp instrument should be obtained before proceeding. Extra scalpel blades should be readily available. Continuous awareness of the location of the cutting edge of a knife will prevent conversion of a flap into a free graft. Cells die when abused. This basic fact suggests a healthy respect for tissue during its manipulation. When a flap is being retracted after elevation, for example, there will be less trauma if the retractor is held gently but firmly against bone instead of against the undersurface of the flap.

Vertical relaxing incisions or access incisions extending toward the palatal vault or along the lingual alveolar plate in the mandible should be avoided. Incisions of this type, particularly in the palate, can interfere with the blood supply to tissue medial to the incision. In addition, the greater palatine artery may be severed if a vertical incision is placed in the posterior part of the palate. Hemorrhage from this vessel can be of major proportions. These incisions may be difficult to suture and often heal slowly with noticeable discomfort to the patient, especially those incisions in the mandible. These problems can usually be avoided by extending the initial flap incision to include a few teeth mesial or distal to the area of instrumentation. If vertical incisions are used on the facial side, they should be designed so as not to compromise the blood supply of the flap (Fig. 11-1). In addition, vertical in-

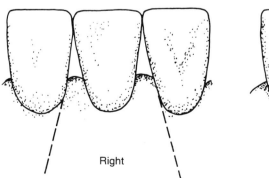
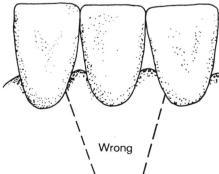

Right

Wrong

Fig. 11-1

INCORRECT VERTICAL INCISIONS

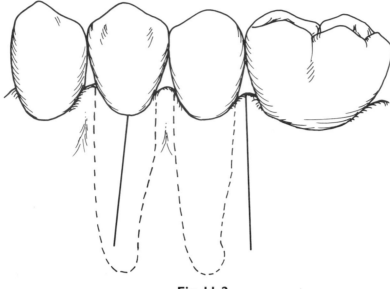

Fig. 11-2

cisions should be made at line angles to preserve the interdental papillae for suturing and to prevent necrosis of the wound edge; under no circumstances should vertical incisions be made over midfacial (radicular) surfaces of roots (Fig. 11-2). If a periodontally weakened tooth is used as a fulcrum for elevation of a flap (especially a palatal flap), a tooth can be accidentally removed.

It is essential that good visibility of the surgical site be maintained at all times. Blood and saliva may be eliminated from the operative area with good aspiration or by applying intermittent pressure with moist gauze sponges and using periodic irrigation. The gauze sponges should not have a cotton fiber liner.

Bone can be contoured with sharp chisels or rotating instruments. Caution should be exercised, especially if hand pressure is used, to prevent slipping of the instruments. If a handpiece and burs or stones are used, a sterile saline or water coolant should bathe the area. A fiberoptic handpiece is useful for im-proved visibility when bone is being contoured. Ultra-speed cutting should be done with the lightest pressure and intermittent contact.

Control of Bleeding

The amount of blood lost during periodontal surgery varies considerably. Studies have shown a range in blood loss of 16 to 592 mL per surgical procedure. The mean blood loss per tooth has been reported to be approximately 24 mL. Usually, a healthy adult can have a 1-L loss of blood before experiencing hypotension. However, an estimated loss of 500 mL of blood usually requires fluid replacement.

Bleeding may be controlled during resective procedures by putting pressure directly on the bleeding site with a saline-moistened gauze sponge. During flap surgery, bleeding may be controlled by replacing the flap and applying pressure to the flap with moistened gauze sponges. The pressure on the flap should be sufficient to overcome capillary or arteriolar pressure, but should not be so heavy as to damage tissue. Many times, heavy bleeding occurs from the interproximal tissues after flap elevation. This bleeding usually stops as soon as all of the granulomatous tissue has been removed. Bleeding from a nutrient canal in the bone can be controlled by crushing the adjacent bone into (swaging) the canal with pressure applied by a metal instrument.

Some substances are useful in areas where bleeding cannot be controlled by pressure. Thrombin-impregnated oxidized cellulose (Surgicel) strips may be placed over the bleeding site, with gentle pressure applied. These strips may be reapplied as necessary and will resorb over a short time. Microfibrillar collagen hemostat (MCH-Avitene) is another effective hemostatic agent. This material is a dry, sterile, shredded fluff, which is placed with a dry cotton forceps on the bleeding site as required. Microfibrillar collagen hemostat is resorbable and causes no adverse tissue or systemic reaction.

The use of topically applied epinephrine is not recommended as a hemostatic agent. Epinephrine is readily introduced into the systemic circulation and can cause significant elevation of blood pressure, cardiac arrhythmias, and possibly ventricular fibrillation. Patients with cardiovascular disease could be placed in an acute life-threatening situation from the use of topical epinephrine.

Bleeding should be stopped before the dressings are placed. The hemostatic effect of periodontal dressing is not great, nor are they adequate pressure dressings. Remember to strive for minimal blood clots in new attachment procedures. This goal is accomplished by applying gentle pressure to the flap or graft, with gauze soaked in sterile saline solution, for 2 to 3 minutes before the placement of the dressing. When the patient leaves the operative suite, there should be no bleeding from the surgical site.

Wound Closure

Wound closure is important to the success of new attachment procedures and bone grafting. The flap should be designed to permit maximal opportunity for primary closure in the interproximal region. As much interdental papilla as possible must be maintained; this is achieved by using a scalloped incision (Fig. 11-3). Proximal osteoplasty may be performed to improve approximation of the wound edges when new attachment procedures are being performed (Fig. 11-4a and b).

Suturing

Suturing is performed to:

1. Provide proper wound closure.
2. Position tissues.
3. Control bleeding.
4. Help reduce postoperative pain.

As stated above, primary wound closure is necessary for successful new attachment and bone grafting techniques. In mucogingival surgical procedures, precise suturing is imperative to maintain the tissues at the desired position.

Certain basic principles must be followed for successful suturing:

1. Use the fewest sutures necessary to accomplish the desired result.
2. Place tension on the suture sufficient to hold the tissue in place, but not so great that tissue necrosis may result. Too much tension may cause the suture to tear through the flap.

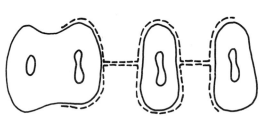

Fig. 11-3

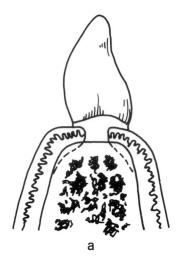
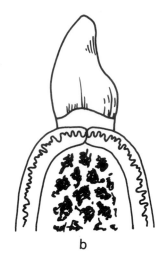

a   b

Fig. 11-4

3. Place the sutures in keratinized tissue whenever possible.
4. Take an adequate "bite" of tissue with the suture needle to prevent the suture from tearing through the flap.

A variety of suture materials may be used successfully. No suture material has all the desired characteristics. Monofilament and black silk sutures are used most often in periodontal surgery. The smallest suture material that is compatible with the surgical procedure performed should be used. Sterile (generally 0–4 or 0–5) prepackaged swaged 1/2 to 3/8 circle reverse cutting or tapered needles are recommended for most periodontal surgical procedures. Numerous suturing techniques apply to periodontal surgery. The four most common techniques are the interrupted suture, the sling suture, the continuous suture, and the mattress suture.

1. *Interrupted suture.* The interrupted suture can be used for almost all flap and graft surgeries. It has its greatest application when both tissue margins require the same amount of tension, as in interproximal tissue approximation (Fig. 11-5).
2. *Sling suture.* The sling suture encircles

the tooth and is used primarily when a flap has been raised on one side of the tooth and tying the flap to the opposite side is undesirable. These sutures are often used as suspensory sutures to hold a flap coronally, such as the laterally positioned flap (Fig. 11-6a and b).
3. *Continuous suture.* The continuous suture is similar to the sling suture. It is used when numerous teeth are involved in the surgery but a flap is elevated on only one side of the teeth. A variation, the double continuous suture, may be used to suture flaps that have been elevated on both the facial and lingual surfaces of the teeth (Fig. 11–7a and b).
4. *Mattress suture.* The mattress suture (vertical or horizontal) keeps the suture material out from under the margin of the flap. This suture is often used for interproximal tissue approximation over bone grafts, for excisional new attachment procedures, and for replaced flaps (Fig. 11-8a, horizontal mattress; Fig. 11-8b, vertical mattress).

Dressing the wound

Periodontal dressings are used after surgery for three reasons:

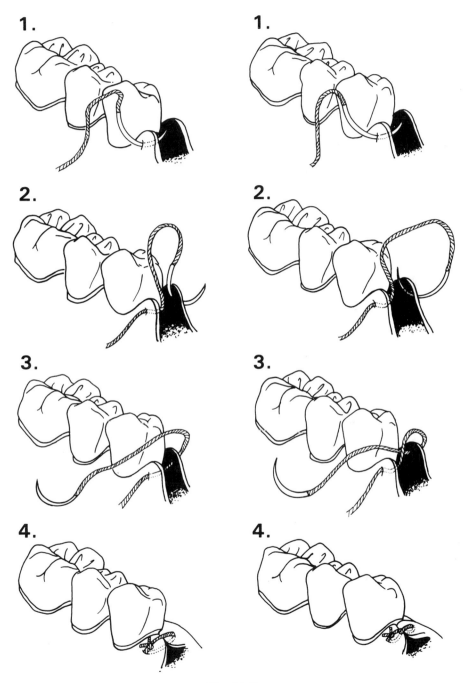

Fig. 11-5

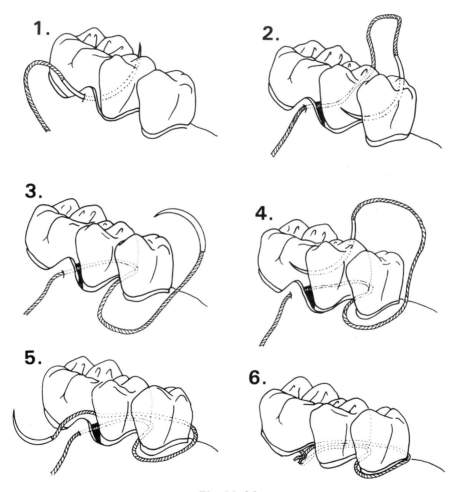

Fig. 11-6A

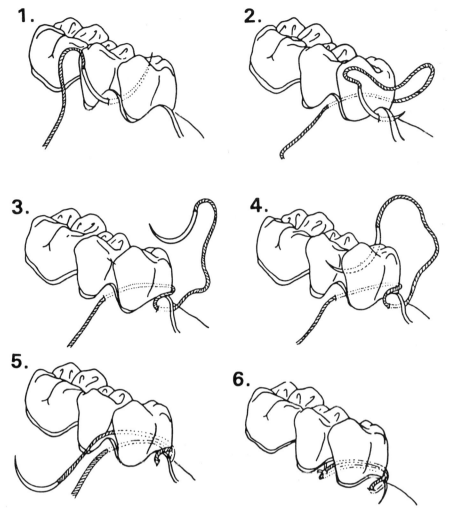

Fig. 11-6B

1. To protect the wound area.
2. To enhance patient comfort.
3. To help hold flaps in position.

The two dressings most commonly used are zinc oxide/eugenol dressings and zinc oxide/noneugenol dressings. The noneugenol dressings are the most popular; it is becoming more difficult to purchase eugenol dressings. Many clinicians believe that the use of periodontal dressing after flap surgery is unnecessary.

A variety of periodontal dressings are available commercially. These dressing materials should be prepared according to the manufacturer's directions. A lubricant should be placed on the gloved fingers before the dressing is handled. The dressing should be formed into small rolls approximately the same length as the surgical site. The dressing is adapted over the surgical area so that the apical one third of the clinical crown is covered, and it should be extended apically to ensure coverage of the surgical area without impinging on the mucobuccal fold or the floor of the mouth. A slightly dampened cotton-tip applicator is used to apply gen-

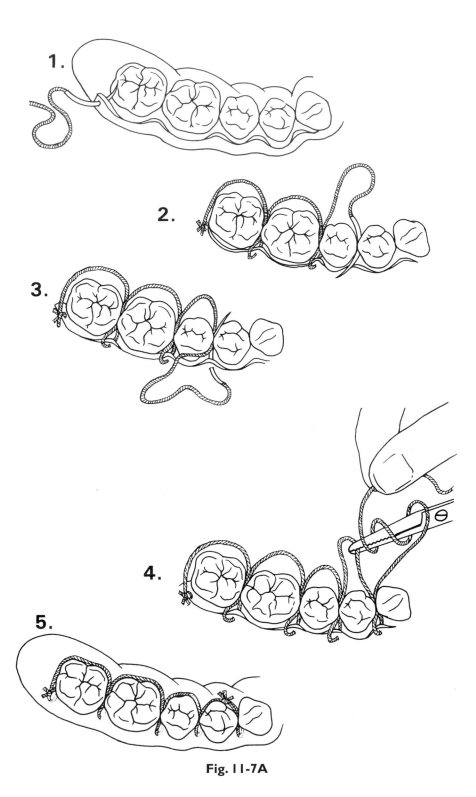

Fig. 11-7A

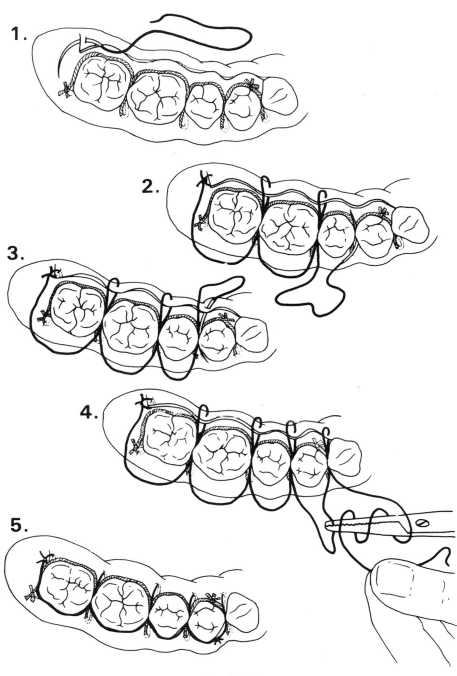

Fig. 11-7B

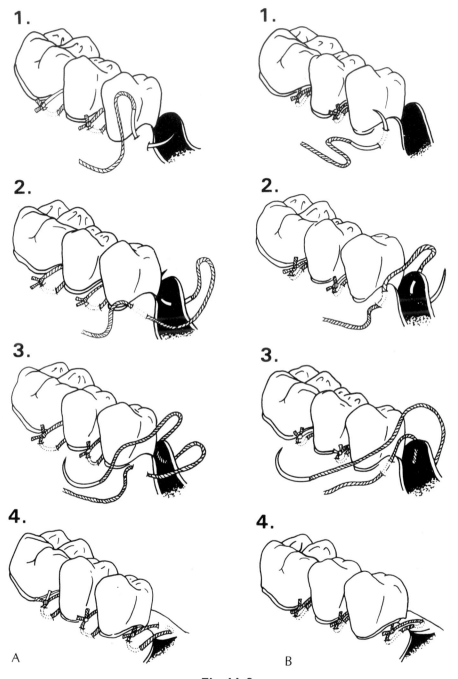

1.   **1.**

2.   **2.**

3.   **3.**

4.   **4.**

A   B

Fig. 11-8

tle pressure to the dressing interproximally. Care should be taken to ensure that the dressing is not forced under the flaps. A minimal amount of dressing material is used to cover the surgical site adequately.

The initial dressing is left in place for about 1 week. When it is removed, the entire area is cleansed with warm water or diluted hydrogen peroxide. Any dressing fragments found embedded in soft tissue or in interproximal areas are removed. The tooth surfaces are carefully examined, and any accumulated plaque, debris, or remaining calculus or dressing material is removed coronal to the gingival margins by using an appropriate low-abrasive prophy paste. The patient is instructed in plaque control. The principal criteria for replacement of the dressing are the patient's comfort and the ability of the patient to remove plaque without damaging the healing tissue. Ideally, the patient should receive weekly recalls for polishing and plaque control instruction during the first month after surgery.

The gelatin-base dressings, such as Stomahesive, are excellent for use after soft tissue augmentation procedures. This material has good stability properties and dissolves in 24 to 48 hours.

POST-SURGICAL CONSIDERATIONS

Postoperative Instructions

The patient should be given written postoperative instructions. These instructions must be carefully reviewed with the patient before dismissal from the dental office. Written instructions need not be elaborate and can be tailored to the individual patient. For example, a patient who has undergone surgery can be given the instructions listed in Figure 11-9.

Postoperative Problems

Bleeding and loose or lost dressings are infrequent problems after surgery, but they are the most common problems. When a patient returns to the dental office because of bleeding, the dressing should usually be removed entirely. The source of bleeding should be located by gently removing any clots that conceal it. Pressure applied to the site with saline-soaked gauze for about 5 minutes usually stops the bleeding. If it does not stop, another 5-minute application is indicated. Frequently, injection of the bleeding site with an anesthetic containing 1:50,000 epinephrine will stop the bleeding. If these procedures do not control hemorrhage, oxidized cellulose (Surgicel) or microfibrillar collagen hemostat (Avitene) may be applied to the bleeding site. Uncontrolled bleeding may indicate a deficiency in bleeding or clotting mechanism, and an evaluation of these systems may be required, including questioning the patient about aspirin intake. If the problem is a loose dressing, the dressing should be entirely removed and a new dressing should be placed after cessation of any resultant bleeding.

Tense swelling, severe pain, obvious purulence, or fever and malaise indicate infection, which should be treated promptly and vigorously. Infection rarely follows careful periodontal surgery; if it does, however, penicillin, erythromycin, or another appropriate antibiotic can be used effectively.

Postoperative root sensitivity may occur after dressings have been removed. It usually results from ineffective plaque control. Treatment of root sensitivity is discussed in Chapter 22. Because of greater emphasis on plaque control and on new attachment procedures rather than on resection, root sensitivity is not as common a problem as in the past.

LIMITATIONS OF SURGERY

Periodontal surgery is not curative. It provides access to the deeper tissues and to the root surface and allows restoration of

INSTRUCTIONS FOLLOWING PERIODONTAL SURGERY

Read and follow these guidelines for maximum comfort and fewer problems.

1. BLEEDING: We expect minor oozing for up to 24 hours after surgery, but if heavy bleeding occurs, contact us.

2. SWELLING: Some swelling is NORMAL after surgery. If swelling is expected, you will be given an ice pack to place adjacent to the surgery site(s) for the next 2 to 3 hours. Use the pack, 15 minutes on, 15 minutes off, and so on.

3. MEDICATIONS: Take your pills as instructed. Do not drink alcoholic drinks or take other medicine without checking with your doctor. Take pills with a full glass of water or juice to decrease the chance of becoming nauseous. If you do become sick and it continues, notify us.

4. FLUIDS: Drink plenty of fluids for the next few days. *DO NOT USE A STRAW!!*

5. DIET: Eat whatever feels comfortable, such as soups and soft foods, for a few days (e.g., instant breakfast foods).

6. ACTIVITY: Reduce your activities for the next few days. Avoid running or strenuous activity.

7. BRUSHING: A clean mouth heals faster! Exercise caution not to injure the surgery site(s).

8. MOUTHSOAKS: Gently rinse your mouth with warm water after each meal to keep the areas clean. You need not add salt to the water. **Use any prescribed mouth rinse as directed.**

9. AVOID: Smoking, alcoholic drinks, and peroxide rinses for at least 72 hours following surgery—ideally longer!

10. DRESSING: If a dressing was placed, it is intended to remain in place for 1 week. A few pieces may break off and is of NO concern. If the dressing seems loose or has come off, contact our office.

11. SUTURES: _ No sutures were placed.

12. PROBLEMS: If you have any problems about your healing:

Contact: Dr. _____ at _____

Additional Instructions: _____

Fig. 11-9

missing parts of the periodontium. When surgery is performed for motivated, cooperative patients by skilled, knowledgeable practitioners, it is an important part of periodontal treatment.

SUGGESTED READINGS

Baab DA, Ammons WF, Selipsky H. Blood loss during periodontal flap surgery. J Periodontol 1977;48:693–698.

Clarke MA, Buetelman KW. Anatomical considerations in periodontal surgery. J Periodontol 1971;42:610–625.

Davenport RE, Porcelli, RJ, Iacono VJ, et al. Effects of anesthetics containing epinephrine on catecholamine levels during periodontal surgery. J Periodontol 1990;61:553–558.

Malmed SF. Handbook of local anesthesia. St. Louis: C.V. Mosby Co, 1980.

Malmed SF. Sedation: a guide to patient management. St. Louis: C.V. Mosby Co, 1985.

Messadi D, Bertolami C. General principles of healing pertinent to the periodontal problems. Dent Clin North Am 1991;35:443–456.

Zinman EJ. Informed consent to periodontal surgery—advise before you incise [Abstract]. J Western Soc Periodontol 1976;24:101–115.

Nonsurgical Antimicrobial Therapy: The Role of Antimicrobial Agents in the Treatment of Chronic Adult Periodontitis

Peter F. Fedi, Jr. and William J. Killoy

Chronic adult periodontitis is a chronic disease that cannot be cured. The disease process can be arrested and controlled if treated properly, but this disease is similar to diabetes or hypertension: Once these diseases are diagnosed, treatment is rendered to arrest further progress and the patient then acts as a co-therapist to help control further breakdown.

This disease of the periodontium is the result of opportunistic microorganisms invading the sulcular area of the susceptible patient. Measures must be taken either to make the patient less susceptible or to reduce the number of pathologic microorganisms and their byproducts to a level that the patient's immune system can control.

Chronic adult periodontitis is primarily caused by bacteria that are usually incorporated in plaque. The plaque may be adherent plaque or loosely attached subgingival plaque. Bacterial plaque is a living, highly organized and complex microbial ecosystem. The mass of the bacteria within the plaque increase in number and activity until they reach a critical mass that the body can no longer control. This critical mass is different for each patient and for each location. The patient's immune system plays an important role in the defense mechanism, as do genetic factors, nutrition, local factors, and other systemic defense mechanisms (see Chapters 2, 3, and 4).

The primary goal in arresting the disease process is to reduce this critical mass of bacteria to a level that the body defenses can control. Many therapists use surgery, some use chemotherapy, and most use a combination of the two. The treatment of choice depends on several factors. Some of these factors are the severity of the disease present, the patient's defense potential, and the patient's ability and willingness to be a co-therapist in the control of the arrested disease process.

INDICATIONS

Some of the indications for a nonsurgical chemotherapeutic approach to treating early and moderate chronic adult periodontitis are the following:

1. The patient declines to have surgery.
2. The patient is unwilling or unable to practice good home care hygiene.
3. Probing depths are 5 mm or less.
4. Localized probing depths are 5 mm.
5. Surgery may fail because of anatomic considerations.

OBJECTIVES

The desired objectives are

1. To arrest the disease by reducing the bacterial mass to a level that is compatible with periodontal health.
2. To regenerate lost periodontium, if necessary, for the long-term survival of the dentition.
3. Once the disease is controlled, to maintain this level of health for an extended period (measured in years).

This chapter presents a six-step program for the general practitioner. This program can be used for managing most problems associated with chronic adult periodontitis. The program encompasses many of the procedures that have already been discussed in other chapters in this book.

The nonsurgical antimicrobial program is time-consuming, and attention to detail is mandatory if success is to be achieved.

The six phases of therapy are

1. Patient case analysis.
2. Patient education.
3. Professional bacterial control.
4. Personal bacterial control.
5. Reevaluation.
6. Maintenance therapy.

Clinical studies have shown that nonsurgical therapy for chronic adult periodontitis is highly effective. However, patients must be continually reevaluated and additional, more aggressive therapy is sometimes necessary to arrest and control some nonresponding or recurrent areas.

PHASE I: PATIENT CASE ANALYSIS

Patient case analysis includes all of the processes for

1. Diagnosis.
2. Determination of cause.
3. Determination of prognosis.
4. Development of treatment plan.

The parts of a case analysis have been discussed in greater detail in Chapter 6 (Diagnosis, Prognosis, and Treatment Planning). A reemphasis on what composes these portions of a case analysis may be in order.

The visual examination evaluates the color, contour, and consistency of the gingival tissues. Any change from normal should be noted and recorded.

Probing depth measurements must be recorded at six sites on every tooth. Probing depth by itself does not indicate disease; however, the deeper the probing depth, the more likely it is that an abnormality is present.

Bleeding or exudate after gentle probing must be recorded. This is often indicative of disease activity. It may take a short time for bleeding to occur after probing, and the patient may wipe these signs away when swallowing. Therefore, bleeding from pockets after 4 to 6 teeth have been probed should be identified. Bleeding upon gentle probing ranks among the most reliable clinical indicators of inflammation and should be considered a pathologic finding.

The adequacy of keratinized, attached gingival tissue should be determined.

Inadequate keratinized gingiva should be recorded.

Tooth mobility should be recorded and the findings recorded.

The teeth that appear to be in trauma from occlusion should be recorded.

Areas with plaque accumulation should be identified and the findings recorded. The simplest of the many plaque indices should be selected.

Several in-office tests are being developed. When they become commercially available, it will be necessary to incorporate them into the diagnostic armamentarium. Some of these diagnostic tests and devices are discussed in Chapter 6.

Once all the information has been gathered, a diagnosis can be made. The following classification can be helpful in determining a treatment plan:

Case type I: Gingivitis.
　　Color of gingiva: varies from pink to red.
　　Inflammation: superficial.
　　Bleeding: upon gentle probing.
　　Probing depths: usually 1 to 4 mm.
　　Bone loss: none.
Case type II: Early chronic adult periodontitis.
　　Color of gingiva: varies from pink to red.
　　Inflammation: Extends into the alveolar process and the periodontal ligament.
　　Bleeding: Upon gentle probing.
　　Probing depths: Usually 4 to 5 mm.
　　Bone loss: slight.
Case type III: Moderate chronic adult periodontitis.
　　Color of gingiva: varies from pink to red to purple.
　　Inflammation: extends deeper into the bone and periodontal ligament.
　　Bleeding: Upon gentle probing.
　　Probing depths: Usually 5 to 6 mm.
　　Bone loss: moderate.
Case type IV: Advanced chronic adult periodontitis.
　　Color of gingiva: usually red to purple.
　　Inflammation: severe to deep.
　　Bleeding: upon gentle probing.
　　Probing depths: 6 mm or greater.
　　Bone loss: severe; usually the furcations are involved.
Case type V: Unusual cases that do not respond to the usual treatment procedures, such as refractory periodontitis, localized juvenile periodontitis, rapidly progressive periodontitis, prepubertal periodontitis, AIDS.

Once an accurate diagnosis is made, a treatment plan can be developed on the basis of the identification of the case type.

Table 12-1 is a decision continuum that can be used to develop treatment plans for the various case types. Note that oral hygiene instruction is common to all case types and that maintenance is also common to all case type treatment plans.

PHASE 2: PATIENT EDUCATION

The dental profession has been very successful in relating to the public how and why the dentist repairs caries, replaces missing teeth, and makes a more aesthetic smile. The patient, however, has difficulty in accepting the fact that the treatment of periodontal disease does not cure or "fix" the disease. The result is that the patient does not appreciate the causes of periodontal diseases, the patient's role as a cotherapist, the limits of treatment, or the necessity for life-long preventive maintenance therapy to control the disease.

There is a time when the dental professional has the undivided attention of the patient. This, of course, is during the clinical examination. This time should be used not only for the examination but also for patient education. The patient has a right to know what is being done, the causes of the disease, the clinical findings, the overall and individual teeth prognosis, and the proposed solutions to the problems.

Table 12-1   Decision Continuum for Treatment Planning

Case Type I: Gingivitis	Case Type II: Early Chronic Adult Periodontitis	Case Type III: Moderate Chronic Adult Periodontitis	Case Type IV: Advanced Chronic Adult Periodontitis	Case Type V: Refractory Periodontitis, Localized Juvenile Periodontitis, Systemic Complications
1–2 appointments	2–4 appointments	4 appointments	4–6 appointments	4–6 appointments
1. Oral hygiene instruction 2. Scaling and polishing 3. Reevaluation 4. Prophylaxis and examination every 3 months	1. Oral hygiene instruction 2. Scaling, root planing, polishing by quadrant with anesthesia 3. Subgingival antimicrobial agents 4. Reevaluation 5. Maintenance therapy every 3 months therapy or	1. Oral hygiene instruction 2. Scaling, root planing, polishing by quadrant with anesthesia 3. Subgingival antimicrobial agents 4. Reevaluation 5. If necessary, site-specific adjunctive therapy or 6. Surgery or 7. Refer to periodontist 8. Maintenance therapy every 3 months	1. Oral hygiene instruction 2. Scaling, root planing, polishing by quadrant with anesthesia 3. Subgingival antimicrobial agents 4. Reevaluation 5. If necessary, site-specific adjunctive therapy or 6. Surgery or 7. Refer to periodontist 8. Maintenance therapy every 3 months	1. Oral hygiene instruction 2. Scaling, root planing, polishing by quadrant with anesthesia 3. Subgingival anti microbial agents 4. Reevaluation 5. If necessary, site-specific adjunctive 6. Microbial testing 7. Systemic antibiotic therapy or 8. Refer to periodontist 9. Maintenance therapy every 1–3 months

Phase 2 consists of educating the patient about periodontal infection and the role that the dentist and the patient must play in the control of the disease process. The patient must be motivated to want treatment and to become a co-therapist in the treatment of the chronic disease process. The patient must also be informed of alternative treatments and the consequences of no treatment.

PHASE 3: PROFESSIONAL BACTERIAL CONTROL

The professional bacterial control phase consists of treatment procedures that attempt to reduce or eliminate the primary and secondary etiologic factors associated with the disease process. As has been stated in Chapters 2 and 3, bacteria and their by-products are the dominating causative agents. There is, of course, an interaction of etiologic factors, including systemic and local factors such as smoking, trauma from occlusion, iatrogenic factors, and others. The primary objective of the bacterial control phase is to make the diseased tooth root and the environment of the pocket biologically acceptable to the surrounding tissues and the host.

Professional bacterial control consists of both mechanical and antimicrobial therapy. One-hour appointments are needed to treat a quadrant of teeth with moderate periodontitis; more time may be necessary in advanced cases. It is highly recommended that the quadrant be anesthetized before treatment.

Mechanical bacterial control consists of scaling, root detoxification (root planing), and polishing in an attempt to

1. Reduce the number of subgingival pathogenic microorganisms.
2. Remove accretions.
3. Detoxify the involved root surfaces.
4. Achieve a positive balance between the critical mass of pathogenic bacteria and the patient's defense mechanisms.

Meticulous attention to these procedures is mandatory (see Chapter 8 for a thorough discussion on scaling and root detoxification). Most studies show that scaling and root planing for a nonmolar required 10 minutes of instrumentation to achieve a state of biological acceptance. Clinicians generally spend between 2 and 6 hours diligently performing root planing procedures in treating early to moderate chronic adult periodontitis.

There are limitations to what can be accomplished in the mechanical phase of professional bacterial control. The curets used for these procedures are limited, by design, to effectively remove all plaque from all surfaces of involved teeth. Studies have shown that calculus and plaque were not completely removed, even though professionals were spending up to 30 minutes scaling and root planing a single tooth to achieve surfaces free of calculus and plaque.

After the scaling and root planing of the anesthetized quadrant, the teeth are polished with rubber cup and a polishing agent or with polishing devices such as the Prophyjet. The objective is to render the teeth plaque free. It is essential to polish all surfaces as far apically as possible without damaging the tissues.

Because it is almost impossible to completely remove all the plaque and calculus from the moderate to deep periodontal pockets with mechanical therapy, an additional procedure of antimicrobial agents should be used. This combination of mechanical and antimicrobial therapy will further reduce the critical mass of plaque to a level that the host defenses can effectively control.

ANTIMICROBIAL AGENTS

Antimicrobial therapy is synergistic with the mechanical removal of plaque and calculus. Effective antimicrobial agents meet the following criteria:

1. No harmful side effects to the host.
2. Effective against the subgingival and supragingival microflora.
3. Reach the bottom of the pocket.
4. Obtain an adequate concentration.
5. Remain in the pocket for an adequate duration to effectively reduce the microbial population.

Antimicrobial agents can be divided into two generations: first and second.

First-Generation Antimicrobial Agents

First-generation antimicrobial agents reduce plaque and gingivitis by 20 to 50%. They do not have substantivity (the ability to stick to the hard and soft tissues and release their beneficial effects over a long period). Therefore, the first-generation antimicrobial agents must be used frequently to achieve the desired results. The following are considered first-generation antimicrobial agents:

1. *Essential oils.* Thymol, eucalyptus, menthol, and methyl salicylate dissolved in a 26.9% alcohol base with a pH of 4.3. This antimicrobial agent alters the bacterial cell wall, and studies have shown that frequent daily use can reduce new plaque formation and gingivitis by 40 to 50%.
2. *Acetylpyridinium chloride.* Usually at a 0.05% strength in 18% alcohol base. Acetylpyridinium acts on the bacterial cell wall by altering its function. Short-term studies have shown an effectiveness in reducing new plaque formation by approximately 35%.

Second-Generation Antimicrobial Agents

The second-generation antimicrobial agents do have substantivity and can reduce new plaque formation and gingivitis by 70 to 90%.

Chlorhexidine digluconate is a second-generation antimicrobial agent that has been used safely and effectively for plaque and gingivitis control for more than 20 years. A 0.12% concentration of chlorhexidine in a 11.6% alcohol base is used supragingivally (as a mouth rinse) and subgingivally (in oral irrigators). It is a catatonic molecule that binds to the anionic compounds of the pellicle and salivary proteins. It therefore reduces pellicle formation. Chlorhexidine also alters absorption of bacteria to the tooth and is active against gram-positive and gram-negative microorganisms and yeast. It releases its beneficial effects from the salivary proteins over an 8- to 12-hour period. Chlorhexidine has been shown to reduce new plaque formation by 68 to 90% and to reduce gingivitis by 60 to 90%. Recently, a local delivery system containing chlorhexidine has been introduced to the dental profession. It will be discussed with local delivery systems.

Stannous fluoride (1.64%) is also considered to be a second-generation antimicrobial agent. A research team showed that a 2-day subgingival application of 1.64% stannous fluoride in nontreated periodontal pockets completely eliminates motile microorganisms in about 4 days. This study showed only a gradual increase in microorganisms over the next 10 weeks.

This long-term suppression of microbial growth enhances the professional and personal (patient) bacterial control and allows considerable resolution of the disease process. Second-generation antimicrobial agents are used at each patient visit. Chlorhexidine can be subgingivally irrigated by using a 25-gauge blunt canula

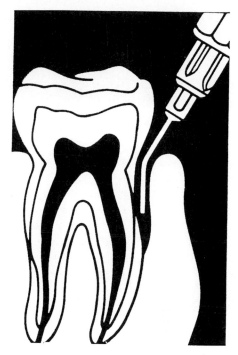

Fig. 12-1

(Figure 12-1) placed to the bottom of the pocket and "walked" around each tooth to be treated. Irrigating devices may include a variety of pumping devices or Luer-lock syringes (Figure 12-2). Modern ultrasonic units allow for an external source for a coolant and irrigation solution.

Betadine is an iodine solution that has been used successfully beneath the gingiva. It is most effective when used as the coolant and irrigation solution during ultrasonic root debridement.

Controlled Local Delivery of Antimicrobial Agents

Tetracyclines

Recent studies have used a controlled local delivery of tetracycline. The tetracycline is impregnated in a polyvinyl acetate fiber (Actisite; Alza Pharmaceuticals, Palo Alto, California; distributed by Procter and Gamble, Cincinnati, Ohio). After scaling and root planing, the tetracycline-

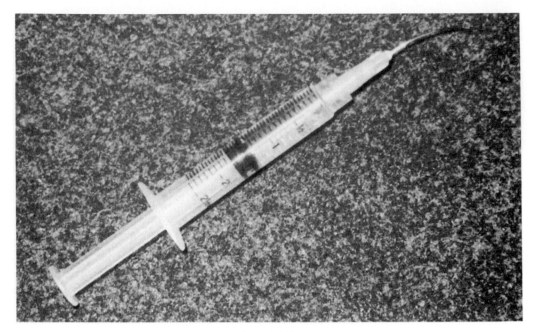

Fig. 12-2

impregnated fiber is placed subgingivally with a gingival cord packing instrument. The fiber slowly delivers high concentrations of tetracycline over a 10-day period. The fiber is removed 10 days later. The tetracycline fiber has been shown to significantly reduce pocket depth and bleeding on probing beyond that achieved with scaling and root planing.

A biodegradable polymer containing doxycycline hyclate (Atridox; Atrix Laboratories, Fort Collins, Colorado; to be distributed by Block Drug Corp., Jersey City, New Jersey) has been researched as a stand-alone (to be used without scaling and root planing) product. It is applied subgingivally by means of a syringe and cannula. The gel polymerizes on contact with moisture and provides high concentrations of doxycycline in the gingival crevicular fluid. It is retained by means of periodontal dressing or a tissue adhesive. Because it is biodegradable, it does not have to be removed. The retention system, however, should be monitored and removed at 7 to 14 days. Multicenter

clinical trials have shown that the subgingival application of the doxycycline polymer is as effective as scaling and root planing. Research is being conducted to test its effectiveness as an adjunct to scaling and root planing and without requiring a retention system.

A minocycline powder formulation consisting of minocycline hydrochloride in a biodegradable polymer has also been studied in Japan and Europe as an adjunct to scaling and root planing. This material is placed in the pocket by means of a cannula, is biodegradable, and requires no retention system. In these studies, the minocycline formulation has been placed many times. The results have been excellent.

Studies of a local delivery system using minocycline in microcapsules are being conducted in the United States.

Chlorhexidine

The most recent local delivery system to be approved for the treatment of periodontitis is the chlorhexidine chip, Perio-Chip (Atrix Laboratories, Fort Collins, Colorado; to be distributed by Block Drug Corp., Jersey City, New Jersey). This chlorhexidine chip is a 7.4-mg, $4 \times 5 \times 0.35$ mm rectangular chip rounded at one end. It consists of a biodegradable gelatin matrix containing 2.5 mg of chlorhexidine gluconate. The chip is inserted into 5-mm-deep pockets by grasping the flat end in a cotton forceps, inserting the rounded end into the pocket, and gently pushing it to the base of the pocket. The insertion procedure can be done in less than 1 minute. The chip is biodegradable and self-retentive and requires no postinsertion appointment for removal. Multicenter randomized clinical trials have shown that the chlorhexidine chip, when used as an adjunct to scaling and root planing in 5-mm-deep pockets, reduces pocket depth and maintains attachment level significantly better than do scaling and root planing alone. During these studies, the chip was placed every 3 months in pockets that remained 5 mm deep; this resulted in a continued improvement at each 3-month evaluation.

The development of many slow-release subgingival antibiotic formulations has been exciting. These products will add a new dimension to the treatment of early and moderate chronic adult periodontitis and give the dental therapist additional methods with which to control periodontitis.

PHASE 4: PERSONALIZED BACTERIAL CONTROL

Each patient's requirements for home therapy are different. The patient must be reminded that, like the hypertensive patient, he or she must follow a daily routine of home care. Just as hypertensive patients take medication daily to control their chronic condition, so must patients with periodontal disease "take medication" on a daily basis to help control the disease activity. This "medication" consists of various home care procedures.

Home care procedures vary. Certain basic home care procedures, such as brushing and flossing, are common to all patients. Many patients will require home irrigators, which may be used with or without antimicrobial agents. Some patients may require a powered tooth brush, and some may require interproximal cleaners. The prescription for personal home therapy is made on an individual basis and may be changed from appointment to appointment. For a thorough discussion of personal home therapy, see Chapter 8.

It must be emphasized that patient home bacterial control efforts are usually not effective in the nonsurgical antimicrobial therapy program until the professional bacterial control phase is accomplished.

PHASE 5: REEVALUATION

Reevaluation is the "major decision time." The patient's treatment has reached the crossroads of the therapy regimen. The goal of the periodontal treatment to this point has been to control the cause and thereby convert an active periodontal lesion to a controlled situation. Thus, the purpose of reevaluation is to see how well this goal has been accomplished. A further purpose is to determine what steps are necessary to control the infection if conversion from an active lesion has not been accomplished.

At reevaluation, the original treatment plan is modified. The patient's response to therapy (both professional and patient bacterial control therapies) is evaluated; depending on the findings, a new treatment plan may be developed.

The reevaluation appointment is conducted not less than 4 weeks after the last scaling and root planing appointment. The appointment consists of the same steps taken at the initial patient evaluation:

1. Visual examination.
2. Probing and attachment levels.
3. Bleeding and exudate upon probing.
4. Mucogingival involvement.
5. Mobility.
6. Occlusal evaluation.
7. Plaque control.
8. Microscopic evaluation.

Gingival color, contour, and consistency should return to normal. Probing depths may decrease, remain the same, or increase. Probing depth should be coordinated with bleeding upon probing. Table 12-2 is a decision matrix that coordinates probing depths, bleeding upon probing, and the procedure or procedures necessary to control any existing problem. Gingival margin location may change, and successful treatment usually results in an apical relocation of the gingival margin. Attachment levels may improve as a result of the attachment of the epithelium to a biologically acceptable root. Attachment levels provide a baseline with which to judge periodontal stability or instability. If attachments levels are stable, patients will retain their teeth.

Bleeding upon probing remains the most reliable indicator of inflammation. It generally disappears as the inflammation decreases and sulcular epithelium repairs. An abnormality must be considered present when bleeding upon gentle

Table 12-2   Decision Matrix for Reevaluation

| Probing Depth Compared To Initial Examination | Bleeding | Location of Problems Remaining | |
		Localized	Generalized
Decreasing	No	Routine Periodontal Maintenance	Routine Periodontal Maintenance

	Yes	Consider:
		1. Reinforcement of oral hygiene
		2. Re-root plan planing
		3. Local delivery of antimicrobial
		4. Short maintenance interval
			Consider:
			1. Plaque control may be:
			   Inadequate: Retrain
			   If adequate, consider:
			1. Diagnostic testing
			2. Systemic antibiotics therapy
			3. Referral to periodontist

Same ±1 mm	No	Routine Periodontal Maintenance	Routine Periodontal Maintenance

	Yes	Consider:
		1. Reinforcement of oral hygiene
		2. Re-root planing
		3. Local delivery of antimicrobial
		4. Possible surgery
		5. Referral to periodontist
			Consider:
			1. Plaque control may be:
			   Inadequate: Retrain
			   If adequate, consider:
			1. Diagnostic testing
			2. Systemic antibiotic therapy
			3. Surgery
			4. Referral to periodontist

Increasing 2 mm or more	No	Consider: 1. Surgery 2. Referral to periodontist	Consider: 1. Diagnostic testing 2. Systemic antibiotic therapy 3. Surgery 4. Referral to periodontist
	Yes	Consider: 1. Surgery 2. Referral to periodontist	Consider: 1. Diagnostic Testing 2. Systemic antibiotic therapy 3. Surgery 4. Referral to periodontist

probing remains. Appropriate aggressive treatment must be administered if the abnormality remains (Table 12-2).

Mucogingival improvement often appears as an apparent increase in keratinized gingiva. This appearance is usually due to a reduction in inflammation.

Mobility is caused by inflammation, trauma from occlusion, and loss of periodontal support. If inflammation has been reduced, mobility will be significantly decreased. Control of occlusal trauma will also decrease mobility. Increasing mobility should be considered pathologic and requires further treatment.

Occlusion is constantly changing. Control of the inflammation allows teeth to slightly reposition, thus altering the occlusion. Reevaluation and readjustment of the occlusion may be periodically necessary.

Plaque control is assessed at each visit. The disclosed plaque tells the clinician how well the patient is controlling plaque at that moment. It does not tell the clinician how well the patient controls plaque on a daily basis. If bleeding upon probing exists, especially in shallow sulci, with the absence of plaque, the clinician should suspect that the existing plaque control for that day was done for the benefit of the professional and is not a daily occurrence. Plaque control must be stressed at each visit.

At the reevaluation appointment, the clinician decides what must be done next. A maintenance interval may be established when the disease is under control. If the disease is not under control in one or more areas, more aggressive personal therapy should be instituted. The decision matrix (Table 12-2) is a guide for where and how to proceed.

Additional aggressive site-specific treatment is based on findings at the reevaluation appointment. Not all patients respond the same way, nor do all areas in a mouth respond equally well. A decision must be made as to whether the treatment to date has been or has not been successful. Where treatment has not been successful, additional (site-specific personalized) treatment must be instituted.

Many choices can be made for additional aggressive site-specific personalized treatment:

1. *Proceed to periodontal maintenance therapy.* When probing depths have decreased (or even if they remain the same and do not bleed upon probing), the clinician may consider that treatment has been successful. The patient will require thorough and frequent periodontal maintenance therapy (see Chapter 23). Reevaluation is a critical step in maintenance therapy because all areas do not always remain in a stable or controlled state.

2. *Re-Stress personal plaque control.* Retention of bacterial plaque, supragingivally or subgingivally, is the primary cause of persistent gingival bleeding upon probing. Personal plaque control should be re-stressed, retaught, and re-practiced with the patient.

3. *Repeat root planing.* Some teeth may not have responded as well as others in the same patient. Teeth that have not responded to the clinician's satisfaction may have residual plaque and calculus. Root planing must be done again. Despite only partial success in removing all the plaque and calculus from the roots of these teeth, with moderately deep pockets, some improvement often occurs. If the pocket is reduced, the clinician has another and improved chance of removing more of the offending etiologic factors.

4. *Controlled local delivery of antimicrobial agents at localized sites that have not responded may be used.* The placement of the subgingival tetracycline fibers, biodegradable chlorhexidine chips, doxycycline polymer, or minocycline polymer releases a sustained high dose of the antimi-

crobial agent to the diseased pocket. Recent studies have shown their effectiveness.

5. *Perform resective periodontal surgery.* In sextants or quadrants where pockets have deepened or remain the same depth but still bleed, resective surgery can gain access to the diseased root surface so that, with greater visibility, all or most of the plaque and calculus can be removed. If the clinician feels uncomfortable with performing resective surgery, referral to a periodontist is indicated.

6. *Perform regenerative periodontal surgery.* With proper case selection, a moderate amount of predictable success can be achieved by performing regenerative periodontal surgery. These procedures are indicated on teeth that have not responded and have deep infrabony defects. These regenerative procedures are technique sensitive. If the dentist is not proficient or comfortable with them, referral is in order.

7. *Prescribe systemic antibiotic therapy.* If, after the initial infection control procedures, severe generalized bleeding upon probing still exists, systemic antibiotic therapy should be considered. This therapy should also be considered for cases that worsen despite the clinician's best efforts or for cases whose severity far exceeds the amount of etiologic agents present. Bacterial tests are often necessary to help select the appropriate antibiotic. Once therapy is prescribed, the patient must be continuously monitored. Referral to a periodontist is often indicated.

8. *Refer the patient to a periodontist.* The general practitioner should treat only those patients he or she feels comfortable treating. The practitioner should obtain a good result and a good prognosis. Some clinicians are comfortable with treating advanced cases, whereas others are comfortable with treating only incipient or early cases. Under no

circumstance should a patient be allowed to become worse while under treatment. When the clinician becomes uncomfortable or uncertain, or if the patient is not responding to treatment, referral should be considered.

PHASE 6: MAINTENANCE THERAPY

Clinical investigations have clearly identified that success in treating patients with periodontal disease is not achieved unless a proper periodontal maintenance program is instituted. The proper interval between maintenance visits and the procedures involved are discussed in detail in Chapter 23. A proper maintenance program is of major importance for a successful nonsurgical antimicrobial therapeutic regimen.

Suggested Readings

Axelsson P, Lindhe J. The significance of maintenance care in the treatment of periodontal disease. J Clin Periodontol 1981;8: 281–294.

Badersten A, Nilveus R, Egelberg J. Effect of nonsurgical periodontal therapy. Moderately advanced periodontitis. J Clin Periodontol 1981;8:57–72.

Badersten A, Nilveus R, Egelberg J. Effect of nonsurgical periodontal therapy. Severely advanced periodontitis. J Clin Periodontol 1984;11:63–76.

Becker W, Becker BE, Ochsenbein C, et al. A longitudinal study comparing scaling, osseous surgery and modified Widman procedures. Results after one year. J Periodontol 1988;59:351–365.

Becker B, Becker W, Caffesse R, et al. Three modalities of periodontal therapy—five years final result [Abstract]. J Dent Res 1990;69(Spec Issue).

Buchanan SA, Robertson PB. Calculus removal by scaling/root planing with and without surgical access. J Periodontol 1987;58:159–163.

Caffesse R, Sweeney P, Smith B. Scaling and root planing with and without periodontal flap surgery. J Clin Periodontol 1986;13: 205–210.

Garrett S, Johnson L, Drisko CH, et al. Two multicenter studies evaluating locally delivered doxycycline hyclate, placebo control, oral hygiene, and scaling and root planing in the treatment of periodontitis. J Periodontol 1997;70:490–503.

Goodson JM, Cugini MA, Kent RL, et al. Multicenter evaluation of tetracycline fiber therapy: I. Experimental design, methods, and baseline data. J Periodont Res 1991;26: 361–370.

Goodson JM, Cugini MA, Kent RL, et al. Multicenter evaluation of tetracycline fiber therapy. II. Clinical response. J Periodont Res 1991;26:371–379.

Goodson JM, Haffajee A, Socransky SS. Periodontal therapy by local delivery of tetracycline. J Clin Periodontol 1979;6: 83–92.

Gordon J, Walker C, Murphy J, et al. Tetracycline: levels achievable in gingival crevice fluid and in vitro effect on subgingival organisms, I. Concentrations in crevicular fluid after repeated doses. J Periodontol 1981;52:609–612.

Greenwell H, Stovsky DA, Bissada NF. Periodontics in general practice: perspectives on nonsurgical therapy. J Am Dent Assoc 1987;115:591–595.

Hill RW, Ramfjord SP, Morrison EC, et al. Four types of periodontal treatment compared over two years. J Periodontol 1981;52: 655–662.

Jeffcoat MK, Bray KS, Ciancio SG, et al. Adjunctive use of a subgingival controlled-release chlorhexidine chip (PerioChip) reduces probing pocket depth and improves attachment level compared with scaling and root planing alone. J Periodontol 1998;69: 989–997.

Kaldahl WB, Kalkwarf KL, Patil KD, et al. Long-term evaluation of periodontal therapy: I.

Response to 4 therapeutic modalities. J Periodontol 1996;67:93–102.

Kaldahl WB, Kalkwarf KL, Patil KD, et al. Long-term evaluation of periodontal therapy: II. Incidence of sites breaking down. J Periodontol 1996;67:103–108.

Lindhe J, Westfel E, Nyman S, et al. Long-term effect of surgical/nonsurgical treatment of periodontal disease. J Clin Periodontol 1984;11:448–458.

Mazza JE, Newman MG, Sims TN. Clinical and antimicrobial effect of stannous fluoride on periodontitis. J Clin Periodontol 1981;8: 203–212.

Newman MG, Kornman KS, Doherty FM. A 6-month multicenter evaluation of adjunctive tetracycline fiber therapy used in conjunction with scaling and root planing in maintenance patient: clinical results. J Periodontol 1994;65:685–691.

Pihlstrom BL, McHugh RB, Oliphant TH, et al. Comparison of surgical and nonsurgical treatment of periodontal disease. A review of current studies and additional results after 6 1/2 years. J Clin Periodontol 1983;10: 524–541.

Ramfjord SP, Nissle R, Shick R, Cooper H, et al. Subgingival curettage versus surgical elimination of periodontal pockets. J Periodontol 1968;39:167–175.

Sherman P et al. The Effectiveness of Subgingival Scaling and Root Planing. I. Clinical Detection of Residual Calculus. J Periodontol 61: 3–8, 1990.

Soskolne W, Heasman P, Stabholz A, et al. Sustained local delivery of chlorhexidine in the treatment of periodontitis: a multicenter study. J Periodontol 1997;68:32–38.

Waerhaug J. Healing of the dento-epithelial junction following subgingival plaque control. II. As observed on extracted teeth. J Periodontol 1978;49:119–134.

Management of Soft Tissue: Gingivoplasty, Gingivectomy, and Gingival Flaps

Peter F. Fedi, Jr.

GINGIVOPLASTY AND GINGIVECTOMY

The chief purpose of gingivoplasty is restoration of physiologic gingival contours that will help prevent recurrence of periodontal disease. The restoration of an aesthetic appearance is also an important consideration. Gingivectomy is the excision of the gingival walls of a periodontal pocket; therefore, the purpose of gingivectomy is the elimination of a pocket. Both procedures should result in increased access for plaque control by the patient.

GINGIVOPLASTY

Indications

Gingivoplasty is usually indicated when physiologic contours are not present and the tissues are firm and fibrotic and are easily excised and contoured. This type of tissue most frequently results from chronic irritation.

Technique

Gingivoplasty entails the beveling of the gingival margin or interdental papillae with the creation of interdental spillways by blending the architecture of the interdental papillae with the interdental grooves (festooning). Gingivoplasty is usually performed with a periodontal knife or coarse diamond stones.

1. When a periodontal knife, such as the Kirkland no. 15/16, is used, the tissue is excised to establish the basic contours. The knife is then used like a hoe to scrape the tissues to achieve the final gingival architecture (Fig. 13-1).
2. Coarse diamond stones may also be used (Fig. 13-1). The stones may be of various shapes depending on the need and preference of the clinician. A steady stream of sterile saline solution or sterile water must be used to prevent burning of the tissue and clogging of the stone. When stones are used, the soft tissue often shows minute shreds or tags, which must be re-

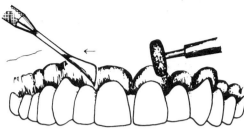

Fig. 13-1

moved. Fine scissors or nippers are usually used to remove tissue tags.

After the gingiva has been contoured by either of the techniques described, a periodontal dressing is placed over the surgical site. The dressing is changed weekly until sufficient healing has occurred to permit plaque control by the patient. At each dressing change, the operator should gently remove any accumulated plaque and debris with floss or tape and with a curet. The teeth in the operative site should then be polished with a low-abrasive polishing agent both facially and lingually, avoiding damage to the healing tissue. At the time of final dressing removal, all teeth are polished again, and the patient is reinstructed in plaque control procedures.

GINGIVECTOMY

Indications

Gingivectomy may be indicated for elimination of periodontal pockets when excision of the pocket wall will not cause an inadequate zone of attached gingiva. Some examples of disease entities that usually can be treated by gingivectomy are

1. Dilantin hyperplasia.
2. Chronic inflammatory hyperplasia.
3. Delayed passive eruption.
4. Hereditary fibromatosis.

Contraindications

Gingivectomy is not recommended in certain instances.

1. Where the pocket depths are at or are apical to the mucogingival junction.
2. Where the alveolar mucosa forms the soft tissue wall of the pocket.
3. When frenum or muscle attachments are in the area of surgery.
4. When treatment of infrabony defects is indicated.
5. When an aesthetic deformity may result.
6. When the amount of keratinized gingiva is inadequate (when gingivectomy is completed, a gingival margin composed of alveolar mucosa will remain).

Technique

1. Obtain satisfactory anesthesia by the block or the infiltration technique.
2. Measure the pocket depths in the surgical site with a calibrated probe. These levels are marked by puncturing the outer wall of the gingival tissue with the probe to establish bleeding points. When the entire area has been adequately measured and marked, the bleeding points will outline the required incision.
3. Make the initial incision apical to the bleeding points with a broad-bladed knife, such as the Kirkland no. 15/16 (Fig. 13-2). The incision should be beveled to about a 45-degree angle to the root of the tooth and should end on the tooth at a depth at or below the apical end of the epithelial attachment. Where the gingiva is thick, the bevel should be lengthened to eliminate a plateau or shoulder. Sometimes, access may be so limited or difficult that a proper bevel cannot be obtained with the initial incision. In this case, the bevel can be corrected later, either with a broad-bladed knife used as a

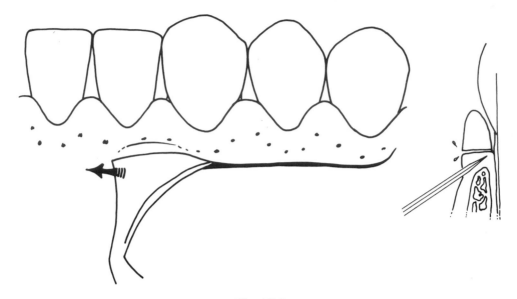

Fig. 13-2

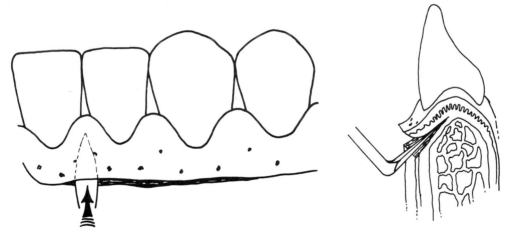

Fig. 13-3

scraper or with coarse abrasive rotary diamond stones.

4. Use narrow-bladed knives, such as the Orban no. 1/2, to excise the tissue interproximally (Fig. 13-3). Note that the angle of the blade is approximately the same angle made when the broad-bladed knife is used to make the initial incision.

5. Remove the incised gingival tissue with curets (Fig. 13-4).

6. Remove accretions from the root surfaces by scaling and root planing. Removal of the soft tissue walls of periodontal pockets renders the root surfaces more accessible and visible to the operator at this stage than at any other time during the procedure. Success or failure of the entire procedure depends on how well the operator performs root preparation.

7. Complete further contouring as needed

by using coarse diamond stones or a broad-bladed knife to scrape the tissue (Fig.13-5).

8. Remove tissue tags with scissors or nippers.

9. Flush the surgical site with sterile water or sterile saline solution to remove foreign particles.

10. Apply constant pressure against the wound for 2 to 3 minutes with cotton-free gauze sponges saturated with sterile water or sterile saline solution to stop the bleeding.

11. Apply periodontal dressing by ini-

tially placing small, pointed sections of the dressing interproximally with a plastic instrument. Next, place longer strips on the facial, lingual, and palatal aspects and join them to the interproximal sections. Cover the entire wound area with the dressing, taking care not to let the dressing interfere with occlusion or muscle attachments. A common error is to make the dressing too large.

12. Change the dressing and debride the wound weekly until the tissues have healed sufficiently for the patient to

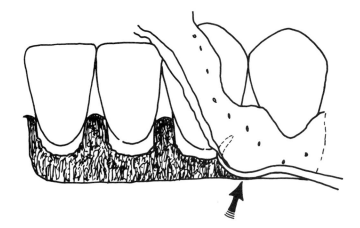

Fig. 13-4

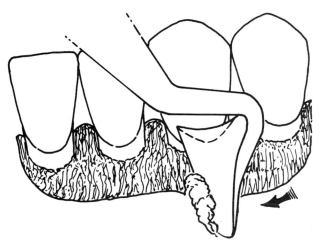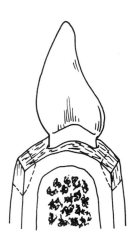

Fig. 13-5

accomplish plaque control. Epithelium will cover a wound at the rate of 0.5 mm per day after an initial absence of mitotic epithelial activity of 24 hours postoperatively.

13. After the dressing is removed, polish the teeth and instruct the patient regarding plaque control.

GINGIVAL FLAP

The gingival flap is subgingival curettage performed with a knife. The inner aspect (epithelium, epithelial attachment, and the granulomatous tissue) of the periodontal pocket is excised, and the remaining gingival tissue is closely approximated against and between the detoxified roots of the teeth, providing the potential for formation of a new attachment during healing. The gingival flap is never elevated beyond the mucogingival line. The gingiva is still attached to the alveolar bone.

Indications

The gingival flap is indicated for the following:

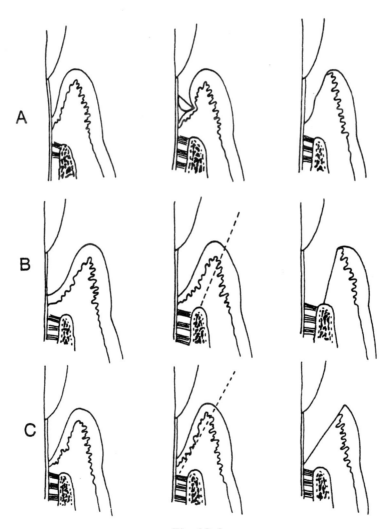

Fig. 13-6

1. Suprabony pockets of shallow to moderate depth (5 mm or less) that have an adequate width and thickness of keratinized tissue.
2. The anterior region, where esthetics is a consideration and access to the root for root planing is needed.

Contraindications

The gingival flap is contraindicated when the following conditions are present:

1. An inadequate zone of keratinized tissue.
2. Osseous defects that need correcting.
3. Pseudo-pockets that need correcting.

Objective

The objective of the gingival flap is pocket reduction by establishing a new attachment (epithelial or connective tissue) to the tooth at a more coronal level. There is little question that some shrinkage occurs in this surgical procedure, but clinical studies also indicate a more coronal attachment of soft tissue.

Surgical Procedure

Figure 13-6 illustrates the gingival flap technique. Once the patient has established adequate plaque control and the bacterial control phase is complete, the following should be done:

1. Anesthetize the area.
2. Make an internally beveled incision with a surgical blade from the margin of the gingival tissue apically to the crest of the alveolar bone (Fig. 13-7).
3. Carry the incision interproximally on both the facial and lingual sides, attempting to retain as much of the interdental papilla as possible (Fig. 13-8). The intent is to cut out the inner portion of the soft tissue wall of the pocket, all around the tooth. No attempt is made to elevate the flap completely

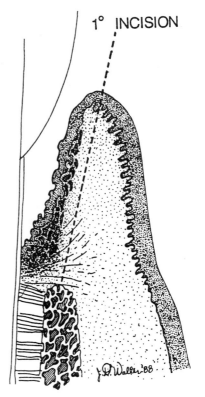

Fig. 13-7

away from its attachment to the alveolar bone (a gingival flap rather than a mucoperiosteal or mucosal flap).

4. A secondary incision is made from the bottom of the pocket through the alveolar crest fibers (and interproximally, through the transeptal fibers) to the crest of the alveolar bone (Fig. 13-9).
5. Remove the excised tissue with a curet.
6. Carefully detoxify all cementum that has been exposed to the environment of the pocket. Attempt to create a smooth hard root surface that is free of plaque and calculus (Fig. 13-10). Do not attempt to remove the connective tissue fibers that constitute the biological width and are still attached to the tooth about 1 to 2 mm coronal to the crest of the bone.
7. Rinse the area with sterile water or sterile normal saline solution and

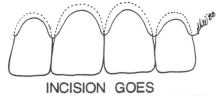

INCISION GOES
COMPLETELY AROUND TEETH

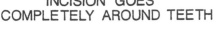

INCISIONS MEET
IN THE INTERPROXIMAL

Fig. 13-8

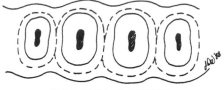

2° INCISION

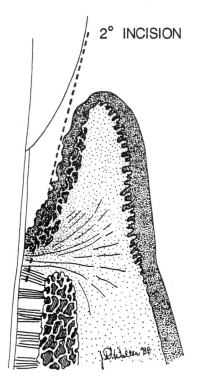

Fig. 13-9

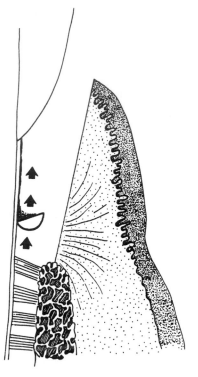

Fig. 13-10

examine the root surface to ensure that no calculus or plaque remains and that no large clots are present.

8. Approximate the wound edges. If the edges do not meet passively, contour the bone until good adaptation of the wound edges is achieved (Fig. 13-11).

9. Suture interproximally with interrupted or vertical mattress sutures.

10. For 2 to 3 minutes, apply pressure to the operative site from both the facial and lingual aspects. Use saline-soaked gauze to permit only a small blood clot to form between the tissue and the tooth.

11. Place a periodontal dressing over the site without forcing the dressing between the tooth and the tissue.

12. Remove the dressing and sutures in 7 to 10 days and polish the area.

13. Carefully review plaque control of the surgical site with the patient. Advise the patient to brush and to floss the area carefully and meticulously. A roll tooth brushing technique and use of interproximal flossing to the gingival margin during the initial period of

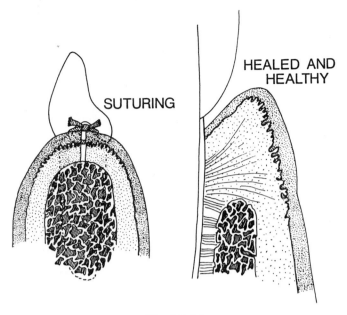

SUTURING

HEALED AND HEALTHY

Fig. 13-11

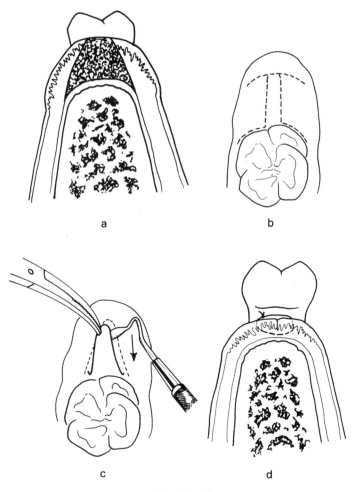

a

b

c

d

Fig. 13-12

healing will provide adequate plaque control without disrupting the healing process of the gingival tissue to the tooth surface. Success depends on controlling plaque formation during the critical first 4 weeks of healing.
14. Perform postoperative polishing once a week for 4 weeks.
15. Do not probe for 3 months to permit complete attachment of the epithelium and connective tissue fibers to the tooth.

DEEP POCKET RETROMOLAR AREA (DISTAL WEDGE PROCEDURE)

A deep pocket in the retromolar area may be corrected by a distal wedge or distal box procedure in conjunction with facial and lingual flap procedures.

Technique

There are various ways of performing the distal wedge procedure. One technique is as follows:

1. Use an undermining incision to prepare a partial-thickness flap on the facial and lingual surfaces of the retromolar area (Fig. 13-12a, with a no. 12-b (or d) scalpel blade. If desired, parallel undermining facial and lingual incisions may be used, followed by a connecting incision at the distal aspect of the two parallel incisions. This results in a rectangular box rather than a wedge (Fig. 13-12b).
2. Grasp the wedge of tissue at the distal edge with a curved hemostat and sever its connection from the bone crest (Fig. 13-12c).
3. Scale and root plane the distal surface of the molar.
4. Perform osseous surgery, if indicated. The distal surface of the second molar is a common area for a deep osseous defect, which may respond to bone grafting procedures.
5. Approximate the wound edges and suture with interrupted sutures (Fig. 13-12D).
6. Protect the area for 7 to 10 days, then remove the sutures and polish the teeth in the surgical site.

SUGGESTED READINGS

Grant D, Stern T, Listgarten M. Periodontics, 6th edition. St. Louis: C.V. Mosby Co, 1988.

Stahl S, Wilkins G, Cantor M, et al. Gingival healing II: clinical and histologic repair sequences following gingivectomy. J Periodontol 1968;39:109.

Wirthlin MR. The current status of new attachment therapy. J Periodontol 1981;5: 25–29.

Yukna R, Lawrence J. Gingival surgery for soft tissue new attachment. Dent Clin of North Am 1980;24.

Yukna R, Williams JE. Five year evaluation of the ENAP. J Periodontol 1980;51:7.

Management of Soft Tissue: Flaps for Pocket Management

Raymond A. Yukna

BASIC CONCEPTS AND CONSIDERATIONS

Objectives of Flaps

Periodontal flap procedures are designed to accomplish one or more of the following:

1. Provide access for root detoxification.
2. Reduce pockets that extend to or beyond the mucogingival junction.
3. Preserve or create an adequate zone of attached gingiva.
4. Permit access to underlying bone for treatment of osseous defects.
5. Facilitate regenerative procedures.

CLASSIFICATION OF FLAPS

A flap is defined as the portion of the gingiva, alveolar mucosa, or periosteum that retains its blood supply when it is elevated or dissected from the tooth and alveolar bone. Flaps may be classified on the basis of tissue components and the positioning of these components at the completion of surgery. The following section provides a classification and description of popular flap techniques for pocket management.

Classification Based on Tissue Contents

Full-Thickness (Mucoperiosteal) Flap

The full-thickness (mucoperiosteal) flap contains gingiva, mucosa, submucosa, and periosteum. It is prepared by bluntly dissecting the soft tissue from the bone. The technique is as follows:

1. Make a scalloped, internally bevelled incision from near the gingival margin to the crest of the alveolar bone, preserving as much keratinized gingiva as possible. Scalpel blades no. 11, 12b, 15, or 15c are commonly used to make this primary incision. The no. 11 or 15c blade in a modified handle works well on the lingual or palatal surfaces (Fig. 14-1A and B). The primary incision should extend around the necks of the teeth and interproximally, to preserve the height of the interproximal papillary tissue for primary wound closure.
2. Bluntly separate the tissue from the bone with a periosteal elevator or chisel to obtain sufficient flap reflection and mobility and adequate access to the underlying structures (crestal bone, osseous defects, contaminated

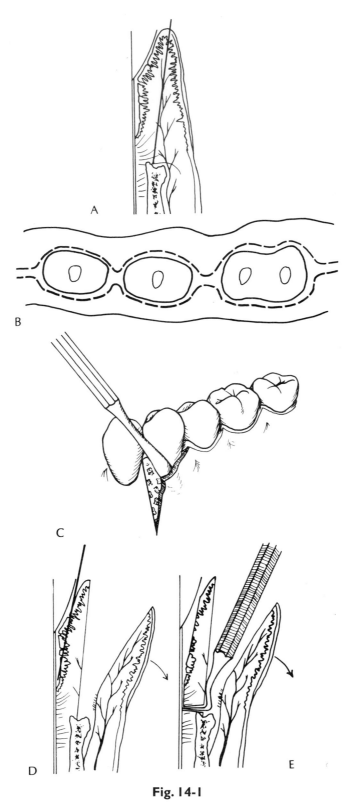

Fig. 14-1

root surfaces, and so forth) (Fig. 14-1C).

3. Make a second sulcular incision around each tooth to the bone crest or coronal aspect of the periodontal ligament with the scalpel blade, Fedi chisels, or Ochsenbein chisels. This secondary incision severs the supracrestal gingival fibers from the tooth (Fig. 14-1D).

4. The scalpel blade or gingivectomy knives are used to sever the remaining collar of tissue by cutting horizontally at the crest of the bone (Fig. 14-1E). This tertiary incision and the secondary incision facilitate easy removal of the excised pocket tissue.

5. Remove the excised collar of tissue with curettes, reverse-angle chisels, or hoes.

6. Debride the granulomatous tissue from any osseous defects.

7. Debride the root surfaces of calculus and plaque with ultrasonic, sonic, or hand instruments. Root plane the involved root surfaces until smooth and hard. Remember that the connective tissue fibers attached at the very apical portion of the exposed root surfaces should be left attached (about 1 mm coronal to the crest of the alveolar bone). Only the root surfaces that have been exposed to the environment of the pocket need be root planed.

8. Irrigate the surgical site and examine it for any residual root accretions or tissue tags.

9. Apply chemical agents (such as citric acid, tetracycline solution, and ethylenediaminetetraacetic acid) if desired to attempt to improve the biological condition of the root surfaces. Chemicals should be used only on portions of the root surface that will be covered with the flaps at the conclusion of surgery.

10. Treat any bony defects by debridement, grafting, guided tissue regeneration, or osseous resection as desired (see Chapter 16).

11. Depending on the surgical site and the surgical objective, replace the flap near its original position or position it apically at various levels with proper suturing.

12. Apply periodontal dressing (chemical cured or light cured) if desired. The clinician may desire to apply Orabase or another ointment to prevent wedging of the dressing beneath the flap and to prevent the dressing from binding to the sutures.

13. Remove dressing and sutures after 7 to 10 days. Carefully debride and gently polish the area. Instruct the patient in proper mechanical and chemical plaque control. See the patient again at about 20 and 30 days, then arrange for a proper supportive periodontal therapy schedule.

Partial-Thickness (Mucosal) Flap

The partial-thickness (mucosal) flap is composed of gingiva, mucosa, or submucosa, but not the periosteum. The partial-thickness flap is prepared by sharp dissection, close to the alveolar bone, with the intent of leaving the periosteum and some connective tissue attached to and covering the bone.

The technique for performing a partial-thickness flap is the same as that for performing a full-thickness flap except for the initial dissections and method of flap reflection.

1. Make a scalloped, internally beveled incision with a scalpel starting at the gingival margin parallel to and close to the outer surface of the bone, leaving about a 0.5- to 1-mm thickness of soft tissue attached to the bone. Scalpel blades no. 11, 12b, 15, or 15c are commonly used (Fig. 14–2a–d).

2. Sharp dissection with the scalpel rather than blunt dissection with an el-

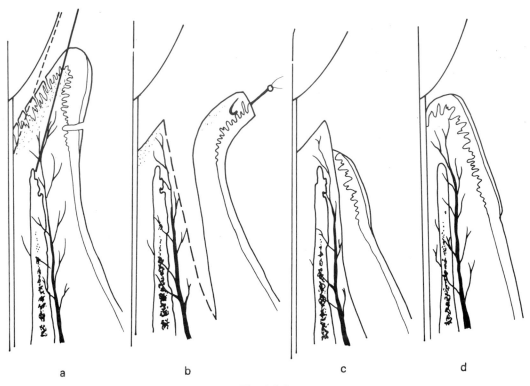

a   b   c   d

Fig. 14-2

evator is used. This often causes increased bleeding during surgery.

3 to 13. Essentially the same as for the full-thickness flap.

Comparison of Full-Thickness and Partial-Thickness Flaps

Opinions differ regarding the routine use of a full-thickness or a partial-thickness flap. Some clinicians believe that surgical bone loss is less likely to be permanent if partial-thickness flaps are used. Others have shown that full-thickness flaps actually cause less bone loss. Advocates of full-thickness flaps point out that necrosis of wound edges of the partial-thickness flap is more likely because of the possibility of blood supply compromise. In addition, surgical perforation is more likely in the partial-thickness flap. These complications could result in loss of tissue and delayed healing.

In practice, partial-thickness flaps are more difficult to perform, and true indications for their use are infrequent. Although this technique may seem to be indicated in areas of thin gingival or mucosal tissue (e.g., prominent roots), the thinness of the tissue presents technical problems at incision and there is increased possibility that the blood supply will be compromised. A preferable technique may be to perform a full-thickness flap, but not to instrument the connective tissue that remains attached to the root surface.

CLASSIFICATION BASED ON POSITIONING

The flap placements most frequently used in periodontal surgery for pocket management are the replaced flap and the apically positioned flap. Facial and lingual aspects of a surgical site may involve any combination of flap positioning, depending on therapeutic goals. Both full-thickness and partial-thickness flaps can be used, but in clinical practice partial-thickness flaps are usually not used when the tissues will be replaced.

Replaced Flap

Indications

A replaced flap (also called a repositioned flap and modified Widman flap) is one that is repositioned in or near its original position (Fig. 14-3a). A replaced flap is used to

1. Gain access to root surfaces for detoxification.
2. Allow access to and management of bone defects.
3. Achieve primary wound closure at the conclusion of the procedure.
4. Reduce pockets by establishing a new epithelial or connective tissue attachment at a more coronal level.
5. Provide closure over regenerative procedures.

The replaced flap is contraindicated if the zone of keratinized gingiva is inadequate. In this instance, a technique such as the apically positioned flap is indicated, not only to increase the width of the gingiva but also to dissipate the pull of the connective tissue and muscle fibers.

Technique

In the replaced flap procedure, a full thickness flap is usually employed for access to the diseased root surface and adjacent alveolar bone. At the completion of root preparation and osseous treatment, the flaps are replaced near their original position and are sutured (interrupted or vertical mattress sutures) interproximally. Every attempt must be made to approximate wound edges, create a seal around the tooth, and to obtain primary wound closure, particularly interdentally.

Apically Positioned Flap

Indications.

An apically positioned flap is placed apical to its original position at the completion of the surgical procedure. In addition to the access indications of the replaced flap, the apically positioned flap is also used to

1. Reduce pockets by positioning the gingival tissue margin apically.
2. Increase the zone of keratinized and attached gingiva.
3. Expose additional root structure for restorative dentistry.

The latter two objectives are accomplished by moving existing mature gingiva apically on the tooth or the alveolar process. Fibroblastic activity in the periodontal ligament and the retained connective tissue on the bone will form new connective tissue fibers coronal to the margin of the apically positioned gingiva. When mature, this new tissue will function as additional attached gingiva. The final posi-

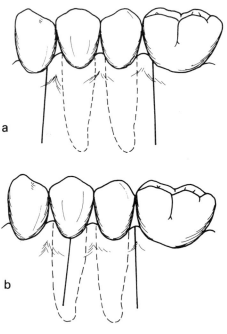

a

b

Fig. 14-3

tion of the flap margin may vary according to clinical conditions and the desired results of surgery. Flaps may be moved apically so that the margin is positioned:

1. On the tooth root 1 to 2 mm coronal to the alveolar crest (APF-T) (Fig. 14-3b).
2. At the alveolar bone crest (APF-C) (Fig. 14-3c).
3. Apical to the alveolar bone crest (subcrestal) (APF-SC) (Fig. 14-3d).

Technique

The apically positioned flap procedure may involve the use of a full-thickness or partial-thickness flap (Fig. 14-1 and 14-2). The following technique modifications and suggestions should be considered:

1. Because the interproximal apposition of wound edges is not a surgical goal, retaining all the interproximal tissue is not critical. A slightly scalloped incision is generally preferable to a straight-line incision, however, to retain a maximum amount of keratinized gingiva on the wound edge.
2. Reflect a combination full- and partial-thickness flap. It is common to begin the flap procedure by performing a partial-thickness flap in the gingiva and then to change to a full-thickness flap in the mucosa to achieve flap mobility and to preserve the maximum blood supply.
3. Acid or other chemical root treatment is not indicated for root detoxification in apically positioned flap procedures. Care should be taken to not overinstrument the root surface that will be coronal to the healed flap margin (to reduce postsurgical sensitivity).
4. Suture the flap margin so that it rests at or near the crest of the alveolar process (APF-T, APF-C, and APF-SC). The most common error in suturing an apically positioned flap is to suture too tightly, pulling the flap coronally and defeating the purpose of the procedure. Sling-type suturing is usually used for apically positioned flaps.

Special Considerations

Vertical Releasing Incisions

Vertical relaxing incisions may be used when access and visibility are limited. The convex nature of the anatomy on the facial surface stretches the flap during reflection, often resulting in tears and perforations. For that reason, vertical releasing incisions are most commonly used on the

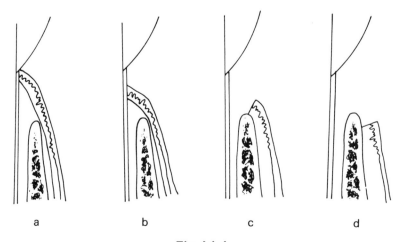

a   b   c   d

Fig. 14-4

facial surface of the jaws. They should be made at line angles to preserve the interdental papillae for suturing and to prevent necrosis of the wound edge (Fig. 14-4A). Under no circumstances should vertical incisions be made over the midfacial (radicular) surface of roots (Fig. 14-4B). Vertical relaxing incisions should not be made indiscriminately, and careful attention must be paid to vital structures, especially on the mandibular lingual and palate.

Palatal Flap

On the palate, the bound masticatory mucosa does not allow the physical movement of the tissue. Any apical displacement of the margin must be accomplished by surgical reduction. The initial incision is begun somewhat apical to the free gingival margin and is aimed at a point slightly apical to the alveolar crest. The exact position of this incision is based on the probing depth, the level of the palatal osseous tissues, and the shape of the palatal vault (the shallower the palatal vault, the closer to the gingival margin the incision needs to be made). This type of incision results in a wedge of tissue (secondary flap) remaining between the outer (primary) flap and the tooth. The removal of this wedge of tissue with curettes or hoes and the position of the initial incision determine the marginal height of the palatal tissues after surgery. If necessary, the gingival margin can be further trimmed with a fresh scalpel blade or sharp scissors.

Special care must be taken when performing a palatal flap because of three anatomic structures:

1. About one third of the time, palatal exostoses are present in the molar region. The presence of these bony nodules creates thin tissue in the region and makes atraumatic flap reflection and proper flap margin placement difficult.
2. The incisive papilla is often in the incision line of a flap procedure in the anterior palate. Surgical removal of this structure at the time of the initial incision seems to have no detrimental effects. In addition, removal of the structure may avoid an excess bulk of tissue between the central incisors.
3. The greater palatine artery and nerve may be damaged if flap reflection is extensive. Generally, this artery and associated nerve run in a bony channel about halfway between the crest of the alveolar and the midpalatal suture. Severing this vessel may lead to extensive bleeding that requires special management.
4. The presence of palatal rugae at or near the flap margin may lead to poor gingival margin contours after surgery. In general, it is preferable to trim these rugae before suturing to obtain an even, thin, confluent flap margin against the teeth.

SUGGESTED READINGS

Caton J, Nyman S. Histometric evaluation of periodontal surgery. I. The modified Widman flap procedures. J Clin Periodontol 1980;7:212–223.

Donnenfeld O, Marks R, Glickman I. The apically repositioned flap: a clinical study. J Periodontol 1964;35:381–387.

Levine HL, Stahl SS. Repair following flap surgery with retention of gingival fibers. J Periodontol 1972;43:99–103.

Ramfjord SP, Nissle R. The modified Widman flap. J Periodontol 1974;45:601–618.

Ramfjord SP. Present status of the modified Widman flap procedure. J Periodontol 1977;48:558–565.

Staffileno H, Levy S, Gargiulo A. Histologic study of cellular mobilization and repair following a periosteal retention operation via split-thickness mucogingival flap surgery. J Periodontol 1966;37:117–131.

Staffileno H. Palatal flap surgery: mucosal flap (split thickness) and its advantages over the mucoperiosteal flaps. J Periodontol 1969;40:547.

Staffileno H. Significant differences and advantages between the full thickness and split thickness flaps. J Periodontol 1974;45:421–425.

Management of Soft Tissue: Mucogingival Procedures

John Rapley

MUCOGINGIVAL CORRECTIVE SURGERY

Indications

Gingival recession (atrophy) is an abnormality of the mucogingival complex. Areas of recession may result from problems with a frenum or the attached gingiva. Exposed root surfaces associated with recession may be unaesthetic or sensitive. The determination and correction of etiologic factors (such as prominent tooth position, frena, tooth brushing technique, restoration margins or contours, and factitious habits) are important for overall treatment success.

Objectives

1. Establish an adequate width and/or thickness of keratinized and attached gingiva.
2. Eliminate tension on the free gingival margin by frena or muscle attachments.
3. Correct areas of gingival recession.
4. Establish new gingival attachment at a more coronal level.

Mucogingival corrective procedures involve pedicle flaps or free soft tissue grafts. Pedicle flap procedures mainly include the laterally positioned flap and the coronally positioned flap. Free soft tissue grafts are the free gingival or subepithelial connective tissue grafts. Materials such as allogeneic freeze-dried skin or barrier membranes have also been used in gingival augmentation procedures.

Techniques

Laterally Positioned Flap

The laterally positioned flap is used to reposition gingiva from an adjacent tooth or edentulous area to a prepared adjacent recipient site. This procedure requires that only one or two teeth need therapy and that sufficient width and thickness of donor tissue are available in adjacent areas. In addition, adequate vestibular depth is necessary for a laterally positioned flap to be performed correctly. When adjacent tooth sites are to be used as donor areas, care must be exercised that the healthy donor gingival tissue is thick, wide, and keratinized, with no underlying bony fenestrations or dehiscences.

Indications

The laterally positioned flap is used to

1. Increase the zone of keratinized attached gingiva.
2. Cover isolated areas of recession where

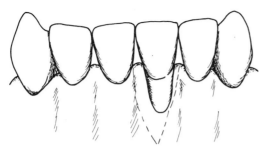

Fig. 15-1

the adjacent proximal gingival height is more coronal.

Either a full- or a partial-thickness flap can be used. Both types of flaps result in satisfactory clinical healing, but studies of root coverage suggest that full-thickness, laterally positioned flaps result in more connective tissue attachment. Partial-thickness flaps may be indicated when protection of the donor area (especially radicular surfaces) against bone loss is desired. Clinical root coverage of about 70% of the original recession area can be routinely expected. Similarly, about 1 mm of recession at the donor site usually occurs.

The surgical technique for the laterally positioned flap is as follows:

1. After local anesthesia, make a V-shaped incision with a suitable scalpel blade (no. 15 or 15c are the most commonly used) and create a beveled wound edge around the recipient site (Figs. 15-1 and 15-2). The wound edge to be sutured must be over bone.

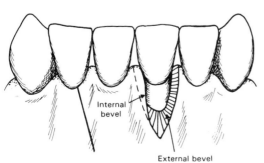

Fig. 15-2

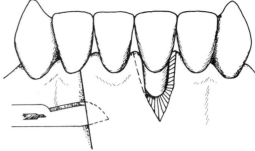

Fig. 15-3

2. Remove the incised tissue with a curet, and root plane the cementum until it is smooth and hard.
3. Make a vertical incision at a distance of at least one and a half times the measurement of the recipient site. This incision should be angled slightly toward the recipient site (Fig. 15-2).
4. Perform a full- or partial-thickness dissection (Fig. 15-3) to free the donor flap tissue from its bed, being careful to maintain its base and blood supply. A useful modification is to perform a partial-thickness dissection in the gingiva and to shift to a full-thickness dissection in the alveolar mucosa. Enough vestibular depth and mobility of the donor pedicle must be present to allow the unstrained, relaxed positioning of the flap at the recipient site.
5. Position the flap at the recipient site to completely cover the defect. If there is tension on the flap as the lip or cheek is extended, further dissection and elevation at the base may be performed (Fig. 15-4).
6. Suture the flap to ensure that the desired coverage of the denuded root surface is maintained (Fig. 15-5). Place interrupted sutures (5–0 suture material is preferred), beginning apically and working coronally. No more than two or three sutures are usually necessary. A sling suture is carried around the tooth and is tied facially to prevent the graft from slipping apically. Particular attention must be paid to the su-

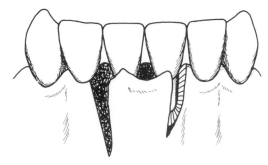

Fig. 15-4

turing of the apical area to immobilize the entire length of the flap to the bed at both the mesial and distal corners.

7. Apply gentle but firm pressure to the flap for 2 to 3 minutes with cotton-free gauze moistened with sterile water or saline solution.

8. Cover the surgical site with an appropriate dressing to protect the flap from displacement. The dressing must not displace the flap or impinge on its base. An improperly placed dressing may impede the blood supply to the coronal part of the flap and result in necrosis and failure.

9. Remove the dressing and sutures after 7 to 10 days. Polish the area and instruct the patient in plaque control. The area should not be probed for at least 3 months.

When properly performed, the laterally positioned flap is a predictable surgical procedure for increasing the zone of

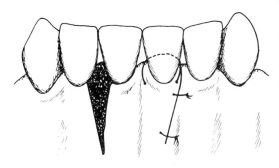

Fig. 15-5

keratinized attached gingiva or repair of gingival clefts when width of keratinized gingiva at the donor site is sufficient.

Double-Papillae Flap

Indications

The double-papillae flap is a modification of the laterally positioned flap. It can be used to repair narrow gingival clefts when there is an adequate amount of healthy interproximal tissue adjacent to the recipient site and minimal keratinized gingiva over the radicular surfaces. Few clinical situations favor this procedure because many recession areas are too wide to allow use of the adjacent papillae. In practice, many clinicians have had limited success with the double-papillae flap.

Free Gingival Graft (Free Soft Tissue Autograft)

Indications

The free soft tissue autograft is an extremely versatile and highly predictable technique. It is used to

1. Increase the zone of keratinized attached gingiva.
2. Eliminate aberrant frena or muscle attachments.
3. Deepen the vestibule.
4. Repair minimal gingival clefts.

Wound healing studies have demonstrated the effectiveness of the technique in the treatment of the first three problems. These same studies, however, indicate that the free soft tissue autograft can also repair narrow clefts but may not adequately bridge deep, wide gingival clefts.

The technique for performing the free soft tissue autograft is as follows:

1. After local anesthesia, use an appropriate scalpel blade to make an internally beveled incision 1 mm coronal

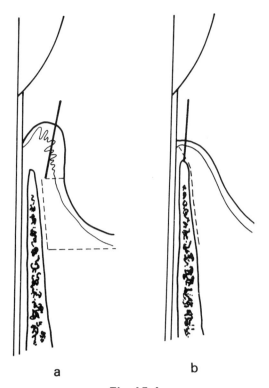

a   b

Fig. 15-6

the sterile surgical blade or suture material.

5. Take the template to the donor site (edentulous ridge or hard palate) and superficially outline with a blade slightly larger than the template. If the palate is used, care must be taken to avoid incorporating rugae in the graft or encroaching on the major palatal blood vessels.

6. Remove the donor tissue with a scalpel blade or one of the special instruments designed to remove thin sections of tissue. The graft should be between 1.0 and 1.5 mm thick and should be wide enough to cover the recipient site. Achieve hemostasis of the donor site wound. A protective surgical stent in combination with hemostatic agents is beneficial in this regard.

to the mucogingival junction. This action may result in resection of the collar of gingival tissue (Fig. 15-6).

2. Sharply dissect the tissue close to the bone, leaving a thin, nonmobile connective tissue bed attached to bone. Extend the incision to include the involved teeth. Prepare the bed by removing excess connective tissue with iris scissors or tissue nippers. All muscle fibers must be removed (Figs. 15-6 and 15-7). Exposure of bone does not jeopardize the results.

3. Optional: Make a periosteal fenestration by exposing a small horizontal strip of bone near the apical border of the recipient site (Fig. 15-7b). The mucosal flap on the lip or cheek side may be sutured to the reflected periosteum apical to the fenestration with small resorbable sutures.

4. Prepare a template of the recipient site by using the sterile wrapper of

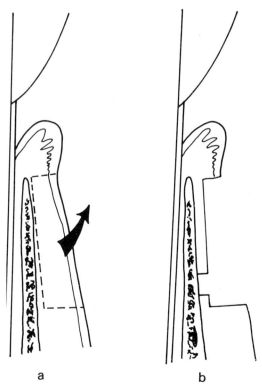

a   b

Fig. 15-7

7. If the donor tissue is removed from the palate, remove some tissue from the inner surface, if necessary, to obtain uniform graft thickness.

8. Rinse the undersurface of the graft and the recipient site with sterile water or saline solution to remove clots and debris. Clot formation will prevent initial nutrition of the graft by diffusion and will result in necrosis of the graft before revascularization can occur.

9. Suture the graft at the coronal margin to ensure immobilization (Figs. 15-8 and 15-9). In addition, vertical external compression sutures may be used for better graft adaptation to an irregular surface.

10. Apply gentle but firm pressure for 2 to 3 minutes with gauze moistened with sterile water or saline solution to assist in initial fibrin clot formation and an effective union between the graft and the recipient site (Fig. 15-10).

11. Carefully apply an appropriate protective dressing to the surgical site. Do not displace the graft while placing the dressing.

12. Remove the dressing and sutures after 7 to 10 days. Polish the area and instruct the patient in plaque control procedures. Inform the patient about the "dead" appearance of the surface

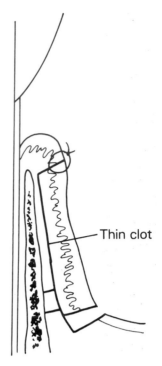

Fig. 15-9

of the graft at the end of the first postoperative week and caution the patient against disturbing the graft until clinical healing is complete. The area should not be probed for at least 3 months.

Healing of the recipient site is usually uneventful. A grayish-white, sloughing epithelial layer is present after 1 week, and the graft is essentially united to the bed in this time frame. Healing of the palatal donor site is usually more of a problem for the patient because the large denuded area is slow to granulate and epithelialize. Dressing retention is difficult on the palate, and many clinicians fabricate an acrylic stent to protect the area during healing.

A progressive coronal shift (up to 1 mm) of the gingival tissue after an adequate band of keratinized attached gingiva has been established is common within the first year. This phenomenon is called creeping attachment and may re-

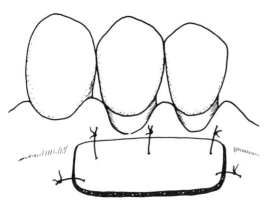

Fig. 15-8

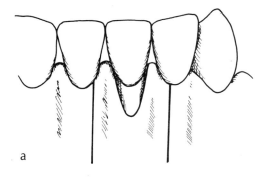

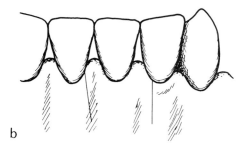

Fig. 15-10

sult in complete or partial coverage of an exposed root surface.

Coronally Positioned Flaps

The coronally positioned flap is another alternative for correcting areas of recession. This procedure is often preceded by a free soft tissue autograft to increase the amount of keratinized tissue available at the local site. This procedure and the laterally positioned flap procedure seem to have similar rates of successful root coverage.

Technique

1. Perform a free soft tissue autograft apical to the area of recession. The graft is allowed to heal for 6 to 8 weeks.
2. After local anesthesia, reflect a full-thickness flap, with vertical incisions at its lateral boundaries (to release the tissue and to allow the flap to be positioned and secured at a more coronal level).

3. Detoxify the roots with curets.
4. Suture the flap in its new coronal position to cover the prepared roots.
5. Apply gentle but firm pressure for 2 to 3 minutes to achieve hemostasis and to minimize the size of the blood clot.
6. Apply an appropriate protective dressing.
7. Remove the dressing and sutures after 7 to 10 days. Polish the area and instruct the patient in home care.

Other Considerations in Root Coverage

Other factors that may influence the results of mucogingival procedures relate primarily to root coverage attempts. The first involves the treatment of endodontically treated teeth. Conflicting reports and clinical impressions abound, but several research reports seem to indicate that root coverage attempts are as successful on endodontically treated teeth as on vital teeth. Another factor influencing the success of root coverage is root preparation. Generally, cementum and dentin exposed to the oral cavity absorb endotoxins and other substances that have an adverse influence on fibroblasts and epithelial cells. As a general rule, aggressive scaling and root planing (and, at times, minimal odontoplasty of the root) are recommended to remove enough root structure to eliminate these toxic substances, as well as to reduce the prominence of the root. Chemical root preparation agents, such as citric acid, may improve the predictability and degree of success but should be used with caution because they can cause postoperative dental sensitivity on areas not covered by root coverage procedures. In addition, most investigators have concluded that patients who smoke have less root coverage with mucogingival procedures because of the long-term effects of smoking on the tissue.

MANAGEMENT OF OTHER SOFT TISSUE PROBLEMS

Aberrant Frena (Frenectomy)

Aberrant frena can be treated by incising the frenum at its insertion, allowing it to retract into the lip or cheek, and allowing healing of that mucosal wound with or without placement of a free soft tissue graft. Occasionally a frenum, especially a maxillary labial or mandibular lingual frenum, is so large that it should be totally excised and the wound sutured. This procedure is termed a frenectomy.

One technique for frenectomy is as follows:

1. After local anesthesia, grasp the frenum with a slightly curved hemostat at its base. Cut the tissue with scissors above the hemostat and then below it, until the hemostat is free (Figs. 15-11a and b).
2. Use scissors to remove any dense fibers that may be observed in the wound (Fig. 15-11c). Extend the lip and check to determine whether there is still pull on the periosteum.
3. Suture the edges of the diamond-shaped wound together (Fig. 15-11d). This will reduce postoperative discomfort and help promote healing.
4. Remove sutures after 7 to 10 days.

Another technique for treating aberrant frena is to perform a free soft tissue autograft in the area where the frenum is causing a problem. This technique not only removes the aberrant frena but also increases the amount of keratinized attached gingiva and therefore helps preclude a return of the aberrant frena.

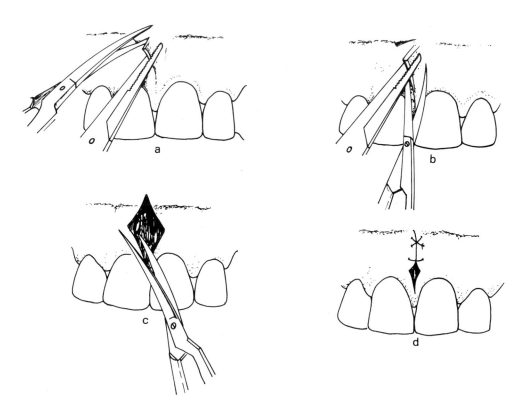

Fig. 15-11

SUBPERIOSTEAL CONNECTIVE TISSUE GRAFTS

The subepithelial connective tissue graft is a successful technique for root coverage; the success is attributed to a double blood supply from both the underlying connective tissue bed and the overlying flap. The technique is indicated for isolated or multiple areas of gingival recession.

The technique for the connective tissue graft is as follows:

1. After local anesthesia, a split-thickness flap with vertical incisions is reflected and should be one-half a tooth wider mesial-distally than the area of recession. The interproximal papillae are left intact, and the flap must be reflected past the mucogingival junction so that it may be coronally positioned.
2. The root is thoroughly debrided, and pronounced convexities may be reduced.
3. The donor tissue is removed from the palate, and the ideal site is palatal to the bicuspids because of its increased thickness. Two parallel horizontal incisions are made in an anterior-posterior direction and are continued toward the palatal bone so that a connective tissue wedge can be removed. The donor site can be sutured with or without the addition of a hemostatic agent. The epithelium may or not be removed from the graft; if left, it is to be placed coronally when the graft is sutured.
4. The graft is placed over the denuded roots and sutured to the recipient tissue bed. The overlying tissue flap is coronally positioned over the graft to cover as much of the graft as possible and then sutured.
5. Gentle pressure is applied to form a fibrin clot, and appropriate dressing is applied to the surgical site.
6. Remove the dressing and sutures after 7 to 10 days. The graft may appear thick during the healing period but may lessen considerably with time. A future gingivoplasty may be indicated to recontour the graft.

SUGGESTED READING

Langer B, Langer L. Subepithelial connective tissue graft technique for root coverage. J Periodontol 1985;56:715–720.

16

Management of Osseous Defects: Osseous Resective Surgery

Arthur R. Vernino

INTRODUCTION TO OSSEOUS SURGERY

An osseous defect is a concavity or deformity in the alveolar bone involving one or more teeth. Osseous surgery is the general term for all procedures designed to modify and reshape defects and deformities in the bone surrounding the teeth.

Diagnosis

A rational approach to osseous surgery must be based on the accurate diagnosis and morphologic classification of existing defects. It is important that the therapist determine the structure of an osseous defect as accurately as possible. It is unfortunate that most of the methods of diagnosing osseous defects record the topography in a single plane in one spatial dimension. Routine probing supplies the linear measurement of probing depth. Radiopaque materials, such as Hirschfeld points and silver points, disclose depth and contour of the pocket with respect to the bony outline (Fig. 16-1).

If local anesthesia is used, one can "sound" (probe both vertically and horizontally through the gingiva with a sharp instrument) to help determine the loca-

tion and number of osseous walls. However, the three-dimensional structure of a defect cannot usually be determined until the defect is visualized at the time of surgery.

Classification

Periodontal pockets in which the base is apical to the crest of the alveolar bone are called infrabony pockets. For this to occur, there must be bone loss apical to the crest of the alveolar bone. The resultant bony defect is referred to as an infrabony defect (infrabony = below the bone). These infrabony defects can be classified according to the number of remaining osseous walls and by their structure.

1. *Three-wall defect.* The three-wall infrabony defect occurs most frequently in the interdental region. The remaining bony walls are the facial, the lingual, and the proximal bone (Fig. 16-2). This defect is also called an intrabony defect (intrabony = within the bone). A three-wall defect may also occur as a trough-like defect on the facial or lingual aspect. Occasionally, a three-wall defect may wrap around the tooth and

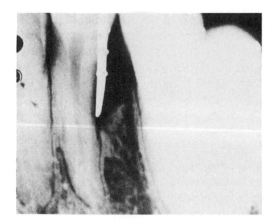

Fig. 16-1

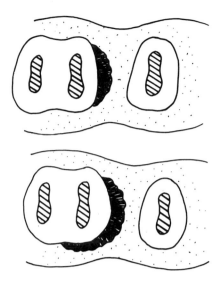

Fig. 16-3

involve two or more contiguous root surfaces (Fig. 16-3). These are referred to as circumferential defects. In addition to designation by the number of remaining walls, the three-wall defect is described as narrow, wide mouth, shallow, or deep, depending on its dimensions. For example, a three-wall defect may be called a "deep and narrow three-wall infrabony defect."

2. *Two-wall defect.* The two-wall defect is the most prevalent osseous defect. It has been referred to as a crater or an interdental crater (Fig. 16-4). The two-wall defect is found interdentally and has a facial and lingual wall. A two-wall defect can also occur when facial and proximal (or lingual and proximal) walls remain (Fig. 16-5).

3. *One-wall defect.* The one-wall defect usually occurs interdentally; if the remaining wall is the proximal wall, the defect is called a hemiseptum. The remaining wall may also be on the facial or lingual side (Fig. 16-6).

4. *Combination defect.* Many osseous lesions occur as some combination of the one, two, or three-wall bony defects (Fig. 16-7). The depth, width, topography, number of remaining osseous walls, and the configuration of the adjacent root surfaces are all important in determining the therapeutic approach.

Objectives

Osseous surgery has four basic objectives:

1. To create contours that permit patients to effectively control plaque.
2. To create contours that will parallel the contours of the gingival tissue after healing.
3. To permit primary wound closure.
4. To expose additional clinical crown for proper construction of restorations (crown lengthening).

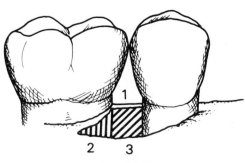

Fig. 16-2

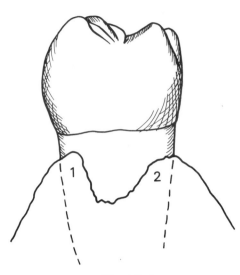

Fig. 16-4

MANAGEMENT OF OSSEOUS DEFECTS

The therapist has five basic choices for resolving osseous defects. The therapist can do the following:

1. Eliminate the defect by removing or recontouring nonsupporting bone (osteoplasty) or by removing tooth supporting bone (ostectomy). Together, this is called osseous resective surgery.
2. Induce or promote regrowth and regeneration of bone. These regenerative techniques most often include bone grafts (Chapter 17).
3. Amputate a root or roots, in cases

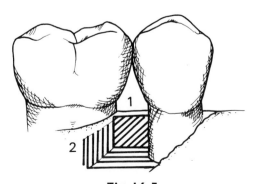

Fig. 16-5

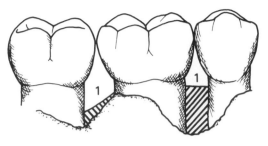

Fig. 16-6

of interradicular involvement, or divide the tooth in half (and remove one half of the tooth) to eliminate the defect. These procedures also involve some osseous resective surgery to adequately correct the bony defect (Chapter 18).
4. Attempt maintenance of the pocket and osseous defect by frequent scaling, root planing, topical antimicrobial therapy, plaque control (nonsurgical antimicrobial therapy, Chapter 12), or combinations of osseous defect therapy (Chapter 19).
5. Extract the tooth.

Of these five basic methods of management of osseous defects, only osseous resective surgery is discussed in this chapter.

Gingival Behavior

Before osseous resective surgery is performed, it is important to understand the normal relationship of gingiva to the tooth and underlying bone. It is also important to understand how gingiva will behave upon healing after periodontal surgery.

In health, the relationship of the gingiva to the tooth is somewhat constant. There will normally be 1 mm of connective tissue attachment to the root and 1 mm of junctional epithelium along the tooth. Finally, there will be approximately a 1-mm space between the gingiva and the tooth called the sulcus. This 1-mm:1-mm:1-mm rela-

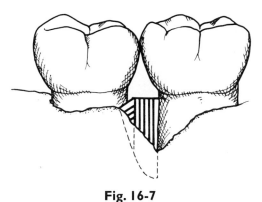

Fig. 16-7

tionship is called the "biologic width" and is easily remembered (Fig. 16-8).

Also observed in health are physiologic contours of the gingiva consisting of facial and lingual scalloping and interdental papillae. The degree of scalloping and papilla height varies in different places in the mouth. There are, however, biological rules that can be used to determine normal (physiologic) contours. Scalloping tends to parallel the cemento-enamel junction. More significant, is the gingival relationship to the convexity of

the root surface and the tooth position in the alveolar bone. The more convex anterior teeth have a greater degree of gingival scalloping than posterior teeth (Fig. 16-9). Gingiva on a very prominent root in the arch has more scalloping than the gingiva on a normally positioned root (Fig. 16-10). Teeth in close proximity to each other have long narrow papillae and therefore greater scalloping than teeth with wide interdental areas. After periodontal surgery, the gingiva will heal according to these anatomic concepts. Gingiva will always be scalloped to some degree, with greater scalloping on prominent convex roots. Posterior teeth that, before surgery, had flat gingival scalloping on a single root trunk will often have a double heavy scalloping on the now prominent two facial roots.

After periodontal surgery, the gingiva will also attempt to reestablish its "biologic width." If the bony contours are parallel to the final healed contours of the gingiva, the equal dimensions of the "biologic width" will be reestablished. If the bony contours are not parallel to the final

BIOLOGIC WIDTH

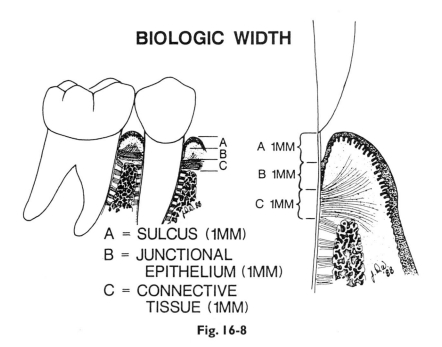

A = SULCUS (1MM)
B = JUNCTIONAL
    EPITHELIUM (1MM)
C = CONNECTIVE
    TISSUE (1MM)

A 1MM
B 1MM
C 1MM

Fig. 16-8

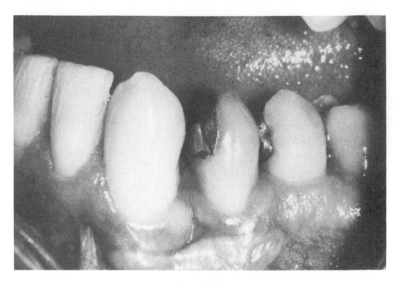

Fig. 16-9

healed gingival contours, one of the dimensions of the "biologic width" will predominate. Although it is possible to achieve longer connective tissue attachment and junctional epithelium, it is unlikely, especially in posterior areas. The sulcus, therefore, is the dimension most apt to increase in length. A deepened sulcus is difficult for the patient to keep clean, and periodontal disease tends to recur at these sites, resulting in recurrent periodontal pocketing.

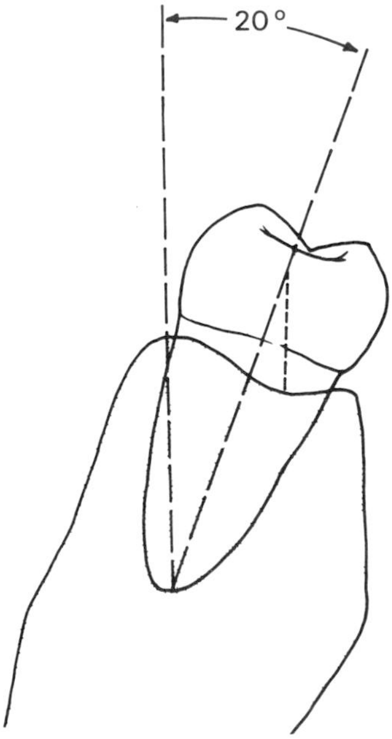

Because of this well-known behavior of gingiva in health and after periodontal surgery, it is often desirable during surgery to obtain physiologic contours in the bone that parallel the anticipated post-surgical gingival form. Osseous resective surgery (osteoplasty or ostectomy) involves techniques to achieve this goal. However, the indications for definitive osseous resective surgery are limited to incipient or moderate osseous defects since the therapist may remove excessive tooth support and lessen the prognosis of the adjacent teeth when the defects are severe. In the severe osseous defect, the therapist must settle for more postoperative probing depth.

Fig. 16-10

OSSEOUS RESECTION: OSTEOPLASTY/OSTECTOMY

Osteoplasty is the removal of nontooth supporting bone to improve physiologic contours. Often, large amounts of bone can be removed without the loss of tooth supporting bone. Ostectomy is the removal of bone that is supporting the tooth (bone containing the fibers of the periodontal ligament).

Indications for Osseous Resection

Osseous resective surgery has limited indications. Use of osteoplasty/ostectomy beyond these indications will sacrifice valuable tooth support, which is necessary for long-term tooth retention. Osseous resection is indicated for the following:

1. Shallow infrabony defects (1 to 2 mm deep).
2. Grade I and selected grade II furcation involvements.
3. Flat or reverse architecture, tori, exostoses, and ledges.
4. Contouring of bone in conjunction with root resection.
5. Achieving primary closure of flaps in conservative new attachment and replaced flap procedures.

Contraindications for Osseous Resection

There are times in periodontal surgery when osseous resection to achieve physiologic osseous contours will remove too much bone and compromise the overall goals of therapy. In these situations, the therapist must compromise and accept greater probing depth after surgery. The therapist must be prepared to adapt the maintenance therapy to this compromise. In the following situations, osseous resection is contraindicated:

1. *Esthetics.* Removal of bone in maxillary anterior areas usually results in an unacceptable esthetic appearance for most patients.
2. *Isolated deep defect.* Too much tooth supporting bone would have to be re-

moved from the adjacent teeth to obtain physiologic contours.
3. *Advanced periodontitis.* Teeth in these patients are already in a compromised situation. Additional removal of tooth supporting bone would be contraindicated.
4. *Local anatomic factors.* Ascending ramus, external oblique ridge, maxillary sinus, and flat palate are some of the anatomic factors that limit achievement of physiologic contours.
5. *High caries index.* Any procedure that results in additional exposure of root surfaces in patients with a high caries index would not be indicated.
6. *Systemic conditions.* Health problems that would limit osseous resective surgery would limit performance of all periodontal surgical procedures.

Technique of Osseous Resection

After adequate local anesthesia, a mucoperiosteal (full-thickness) flap is designed and performed, as discussed in Chapter 14. The apically positioned flap is the technique most applicable when pocket elimination surgery and osseous resection are anticipated. Flap reflection should be adequate for visibility and access to the osseous defects. All granulation tissue should be removed by using sharp curets and other suitable instruments. All calculi should be removed from the teeth and the roots planed.

The first step in osseous resection is to thin the alveolar housing. The facial and lingual surfaces of the bone are reduced to provide a ramping effect into the interproximal areas where the osseous defects occurred and to thin the bone over the facial and lingual surfaces of the teeth. This bone contouring is usually done with large round burs (no. 6 or 8) in a high-speed handpiece and cooled with sterile physiologic saline or sterile water.

The second step is to flatten the interproximal defects by removing the coronal edges. This step is also usually done with rotary instruments. At this point, a reasonable bulk of bone may have already been removed, but none of it was tooth-supporting bone. Consequently, a situation has been established in which the interproximal bone is now apical to the bone on the facial and lingual surfaces of the teeth.

In the third step, this facial and lingual bone is removed with chisels to achieve a physiologic contour similar to that anticipated in the healed gingiva. A back-action chisel will aid in removing bone at the distal line angles of the teeth.

The mucoperiosteal flap is now positioned and sutured to cover the bone and to contact the tooth about 1 mm coronal to the bone. If desired, surgical dressing may be placed over the surgical site. Routine postoperative care for surgical patients is discussed in Chapter 11.

EFFECT OF BONE REMOVAL

Visual Effect

The bone is reduced to the depth of the interproximal defect. The supporting bone is removed primarily on facial and lingual surfaces. This usually amounts to an average of 0.6 mm of bone reduction circumferentially and 1 to 2 mm of bone reduction on the facial and lingual surfaces. Because the facial is a highly visible area, the loss of bone appears to be magnified. Of course, where esthetics will be a problem, osseous resection should not be done.

Effect on Tooth Mobility

Increased tooth mobility can be expected immediately after most periodontal surgical procedures. After adequate healing and tissue maturation, mobility usually returns to presurgical levels. A similar pattern follows osseous resection. After 6 to 12 months of healing, mobility patterns also return to presurgical levels.

Lingual Approach to Osseous Resection

There are advantages to performing the bulk of the osseous removal from the lingual aspect in both the maxillary and mandibular arches.

In the maxillary arch, the osseous defects can be ramped to the palate. Ramping to the palate avoids removing bone from the vulnerable facial furcation areas. This provides a wider area for access to perform the surgery. The palatal approach also provides better access for oral hygiene after surgery and markedly improves the esthetic result.

In the mandibular arch, the teeth have a normal inclination to the lingual, which places the deepest point of most osseous defects in a lingual position (Fig. 16-11). Ramping the osseous defects to the lingual will require less removal of tooth supporting bone which will preserve the bone over an already coronally located facial furcation. The bone on the lingual, however, is often quite thick and will require considerable effort to achieve the desired physiologic contours (Fig. 16-11).

Modified Osseous Resection

Because of the limitations associated with osseous resection, it is often impossible to achieve ideal physiologic contours in treating advanced periodontal disease. When defects are deep, many therapists modify the amount of bone removed to retain tooth supporting bone in areas where they feel it cannot be sacrificed. This leaves reversed or flat contours; this is an admitted compromise but one necessary to achieve maximum retention of functional teeth in a maintainable state of periodontal health.

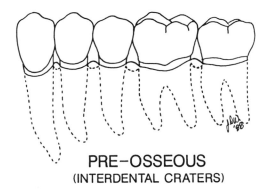

PRE-OSSEOUS
(INTERDENTAL CRATERS)

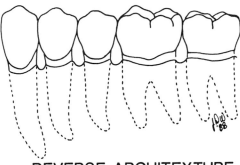

REVERSE ARCHITEXTURE
Fig. 16-11

Advantages of Osseous Resection

1. *Predictability.* By obtaining physiologic osseous contours at the time of surgery, the therapist knows the outcome of the procedure without having to rely on an unpredictable amount of osseous fill or new attachment.

2. *Minimal waiting period.* After a reasonable healing period (8 to 12 weeks), gingival contours will be at their best and restorative procedures can be completed.

3. *Plaque control.* With the periodontal pocket eliminated or reduced to a minimum, the patient has access to root surfaces that had been within the periodontal pocket. The improved access

enables the patient to adequately clean the dentogingival areas for maintaining periodontal health.

Disadvantages of Osseous Resection

1. *Loss of attachment.* By design, the procedure removes bony attachment to achieve the desired result. The loss of attachment may be lessened by use of a lingual approach or modification of the technique.

2. *Esthetics.* Additional clinical crown length is less desirable than teeth with a normal gingival position. Resective techniques should not be used in areas where esthetics are of prime consideration.

Future Considerations

Periodontics is dynamic and changing rapidly. As the profession becomes successful in controlling the pathologic microflora and develops predictable regenerative treatments, the importance of resective surgery will decrease. For today, however, osseous resection provides dentistry with a predictable method of reducing periodontal pockets to a level more maintainable by the patient and the professional.

SUGGESTED READINGS

Johnson R. Principles of periodontal osseous resection. Dent Clin North Am 1976;20: 35–59.

Ochsenbein C. A primer for osseous surgery. Int J Periodontol Rest Dent 1986;6:9–47.

Proceedings of the World Workshop in Clinical Periodontics. Section IV: Resective Procedures. July 23–27, 1989. Princeton, 1989: 1–26.

Selipsky H. Osseous surgery. How much need we compromise? Dent Clin North Am 1976; 20:79–106.

Management of Osseous Defects: Bone Replacement Grafts

Raymond A. Yukna

For many years, researchers and clinicians alike have attempted to regenerate lost osseous architecture by promoting regeneration of bone and its ligamentous attachment to the tooth with various osseous stimulators. Many autogenous, allogeneic, xenogeneic, and alloplastic (synthetic) materials have been tried with varied success. To date, autografts and some allografts offer the best hope for inducing restoration of lost bone and regeneration of a functional attachment apparatus of the periodontium on a predictable basis, but new alloplasts are constantly being developed.

INDICATIONS FOR BONE GRAFTING

Patients Selection

Patient selection is of critical importance when bone replacement graft procedures are being considered. The factors causing the inflammatory periodontal disease must be controlled before reparative procedures are attempted. The patient must demonstrate effective oral hygiene; have no compromising physical problems, mental conditions, or social habits; have a positive attitude toward therapy; and be amenable to a long-term post-therapy maintenance program.

Defect Selection

The structure of the osseous defect to be grafted is as important as patient selection. Realistic expectations of success are directly proportional to the number of vascular osseous walls surrounding the defect and are inversely related to the number of avascular tooth root walls. A narrow (less than 2 mm wide) three-wall defect, confined to a single tooth surface, has great inherent osseous regenerative potential even without the use of bone replacement grafts. A wide (more than 2 mm wide) three-wall defect, confined to one or more surfaces of the tooth root; a two-wall or one-wall defect; or combinations of the foregoing have progressively less inherent osseous regenerative potential. Bone replacement grafts may help regenerate only limited amounts of the lost support. The least predictable situations for new bone formation are furcation defects and supracrestal regeneration of bone.

The basic functions of all osseous

grafting materials are one or more of the following:

1. *Osteoconduction.* The graft acts as a template or trellis to assist in bone formation and deposition.

2. *Osteoinduction.* The graft acts to stimulate or to induce new bone formation by undifferentiated cells.

3. *Osteogenesis.* The cells of the graft actually produce new bone.

TYPES OF BONE REPLACEMENT GRAFTS

Autograft

Autogenous bone grafts are of two general types: free osseous autografts and contiguous autografts.

Free Osseous Autografts

Free osseous autografts contain cortical, cancellous, or a combination of cortical and cancellous bone and can be obtained from extraoral or intraoral sites. Clinical experience suggests that cancellous bone affords greater opportunity for success because of its less dense composition, but it is often more difficult to obtain and then often only in limited amounts. Consequently, most defects are filled with a combination of cortical and cancellous bone, with the higher percentage usually being cortical bone particles.

Studies have consistently shown that cancellous bone and marrow grafts have extremely high regenerative potential because they contain numerous viable pluripotential cells, which may differentiate, proliferate, and actually participate in bone formation (osteogenesis).

Use of extraoral bone marrow has several disadvantages. In most instances, a physician must obtain the material, and the experience is time-consuming, costly, and often traumatic for the patient. Some clinicians have noticed extensive tooth resorption coronal to the crestal area of the graft for as long as 1 year after successful bone fill. Resorption of this type is rarely observed with intraoral autogenous bone. However, because extraoral donor sites, such as the ileum or rib, are rarely used to treat periodontal defects, this section focuses on the use of intraoral bone.

Intraoral Donor Sites

Bone that is removed during osteoplasty or ostectomy is an excellent source of donor material. The size of the chips may vary from fairly large fragments (diameter in millimeters) to very small particles (diameter in microns) depending on how the bone is removed. If rotary instruments are used, the particle size is small (200 to 400 microns). Evidence suggests that the small particles of donor bone may more actively induce regeneration in osseous defects. Small particles offer the advantage (over large fragments) of a greater surface area for resorption and replacement by new host bone.

Osseous Coagulum

A suggested technique uses a large round carbide bur, revolving at 25,000 to 30,000 rpm or more, to reduce bone to small particle size during osteoplasty or ostectomy. This fine donor bone is gathered by placing a large bladed elevator in position to catch the bone particles as they come off the bone surface. A surprising amount of bone can be obtained from cortical bone shavings obtained when performing osteoplasty and ostectomy procedures or reducing the bulk of nonsupporting bone or tori. Hand instruments that are also useful for this purpose are Ochsenbein, Wedelstaedt, or Fedi chisels and Chigo or Sugarman files.

Healing Sockets

Bone may also be obtained from a healing socket 6 to 12 weeks after an extraction. A flap is made over the socket, the cancellous bone and marrow slush is harvested from the socket with rongeurs or large curettes, and the donor material is placed in the periodontal osseous defect. The immature bone and cells appear to offer excellent healing and reparative potential.

Other Sources

Donor bone can also be obtained from maxillary tuberosities, edentulous ridges, or retromolar areas. Usually, a window is made in the outer cortical bone for access to the cancellous areas. Rongeurs, trephines, or large curettes can then be used to harvest the bone. Cancellous bone in the tuberosities once contained hemopoietic marrow, but in the adult the hemopoietic content is minimal. Limited visual and mechanical access, together with the frequent occurrence of an alveolar extension of the maxillary sinus in the tuberosity, severely reduces the availability of graft material in this region.

Contiguous Osseous Autografts (Bone Swaging)

Contiguous osseous autografts, which have been called bone swaging grafts, are seldom used today to eliminate osseous defects. The technique involves the use of a "green stick" fracture of the adjacent alveolar bone, compressing the fractured bone laterally or occlusally into the defect. The difficulty lies in producing a fracture of the alveolar process that is still intact and connected to the main body of bone.

Allografts

An allograft (allogeneic graft) is tissue transplanted between persons of the same species. Although allografts may possess some inductive capacity, they may initiate adverse tissue responses and graft rejection by the host unless specially processed. The most commonly used and safest form of allografts are those processed by freeze-drying (lyophilization).

The bone tissue should be procured under rigidly controlled conditions from carefully selected donor cadavers and must be tested to ensure it is an aseptic donation of tissue that is free of any transmissible pathologic conditions. Considerable research on the use of freeze-dried bone in periodontal osseous defects has been conducted over the past 30 years. By following strict criteria for donor selection and processing, the bone is surgically removed from the body, freeze-dried, ground to an average particle size of 300 to 500 microns, and placed in sterile vacuum-sealed bottles that have an indefinite shelf life. Considerable testing has demonstrated this form of allograft to be nonantigenic. Some freeze-dried bone allograft materials are decalcified with the intent of exposing bone morphogenic protein, thereby theoretically increasing regenerative potential. However, clinical research suggests that the demineralized and nondemineralized forms yield equal results in periodontal defects. The advantage of using allografts over autografts is that there is no need to create an additional surgical wound to procure donor material and still maintain comparable osseous repair potential. Some evidence indicates that combining four parts of freeze-dried bone allograft with one part of tetracycline powder may improve bone repair. Several certified laboratories (bone banks) sell the allograft materials.

Xenografts

Xenografts (xenogeneic) grafts are materials obtained from a different species, usually cows (bovine) or pigs (porcine) for human use.

Particulate bovine natural hydroxylapatite grafts are produced by chemical processing (Bio-Oss) or high-heat processing (OsteoGraf/N) to remove the organic material. This leaves a natural hydroxylapatite skeleton showing the macroporous and microporous structure of human bone, and the particles appear to be resorbed while bone is deposited in juxtaposition to them.

A different form of xenograft is Emdogain, a group of enamel matrix proteins obtained from pigs. This material appears to encourage the formation of acellular cementum that is then followed by associated bone deposition. Clinically detectable results take longer to become evident with this gel-like material than with other grafts, but the material is based on an intriguing biological concept.

Alloplastic Grafts

Alloplastic grafts are synthetic substances, and several hold promise for periodontal use. Currently available synthetic bone replacement graft materials include the following:

1. Porous, resorbable A- and B-tricalcium phosphate (Synthograft, Peri-Oss, Bio-Base).
2. Dense, nonresorbable hydroxyapatite (Calcitite, Osteograf/D, and others).
3. Porous, nonresorbable hydroxyapatite (Interpore).
4. Calcium carbonate (coral) (Biocoral).
5. Polymers (HTR Synthetic Bone).
6. Plaster of Paris (Capset).
7. "Resorbable" hydroxyapatite (Osteogen, Osteograf/LD).
8. Bioactive (silica-based) glasses (Perioglas, Biogran).

Histologic evidence suggests that these substances are essentially biocompatible fillers, with limited evidence of bone or attachment apparatus regeneration. Clinical results indicate that these materials may effectively fill the defect, may encourage bone deposition on their surface, and thus help maintain bone and soft tissue height.

Composite Grafts

Composite grafts are usually combinations of autogenous bone and an allograft, xenograft, or alloplast. Because a form of autogenous bone is the preferred graft material, and at times the amount available is insufficient to meet the therapeutic needs, an expander, in the form of an allograft, xenograft, or alloplast, is used to increase the usable amount of bone replacement graft material. Some evidence indicates that the composite grafts form more new bone than either of their components used independently.

Results with Bone Replacement Grafts

Many clinical studies and limited human histologic evidence suggest that no one type of bone replacement graft material is superior to the others. Moreover, no material is preferable to or yields better results than autogenous bone. However, a limited amount of host bone is often conveniently available in the oral cavity, so allografts, xenografts, or alloplasts may be indicated instead. Evaluation of research reports suggests that all types of bone replacement grafts yield essentially similar clinical results. These results demonstrate fill of the original intrabony defect of about 60% to 70%.

SURGICAL PROCEDURES

The technique for preparation of the osseous defect recipient site is the same regardless of what donor material is used.

1. Make a scalloped, internally bevelled incision around the necks of the teeth to remove the sulcular epithelium and the inner soft tissue wall of the pocket associated with the defect.

Preserve as much gingival tissue as possible to enhance primary closure of the wound.

2. Elevate a full-thickness (mucoperiosteal) flap to expose the defect. Occasionally, one or more vertical relaxing incisions may be needed to provide better access, especially for deep defects.

3. Remove the granulomatous tissue from within and around the osseous defect. The entire inner surface of the bony defect should be exposed and vigorously debrided.

4. Mechanically detoxify the root surface with ultrasonic, sonic, or hand instruments until it is smooth and hard. Chemical conditioning agents may also be used if desired.

5. Intramarrow penetrations with a sharp instrument or a no. 1/2 round bur may be performed. The compact bone that lines the defect is perforated to allow rapid ingress of new blood vessels and bone-forming cells into the defect from the surrounding marrow spaces.

6. Place the bone replacement graft material into the defect in increments, pack gently but firmly, and fill to a level at or only slightly coronal to the existing osseous walls.

7. Replace the flap over the graft and suture. Be sure to approximate the wound edges interproximally to ensure primary flap closure and a circumferential seal against the root surface.

8. Place a suitable periodontal dressing over the surgical area.

9. Provide written and oral postoperative instructions to the patient to minimize post surgical sequelae (Chapter 10). Appropriate prescriptions to control swelling, infection, and pain should be provided.

10. Remove sutures after 7 to 10 days, debride the wound, and deplaque the involved teeth. Redress if necessary.

11. After final dressing removal, instruct the patient in mechanical and chemical plaque control. Biweekly professional plaque debridement for several months after surgery enhances the final results. Do not probe the graft sites for at least 3 months.

An antibiotic regimen is prescribed for the first 10 to 14 days of healing (tetracycline hydrochloride, 250 mg every 6 hours, or its equivalent is preferred). Studies have shown that results are enhanced if therapeutic levels of tetracycline are maintained for plaque and collagenase suppression during the first week or two of healing.

SUGGESTED READINGS

Amler MH. The time sequence of tissue regeneration in human extraction wounds. Oral Surg Oral Med Oral Pathol 1969;27:309–318.

Bowen JA, Mellonig JT, Gray JL, et al. Comparison of decalcified freeze-dried bone allograft and porous particulate hydroxyapatite human periodontal osseous defects. J Periodontol. 1989;60:647–654.

Froum SJ, Ortiz M, Witkin R, et al. Osseous autografts. III. Comparison of osseous coagulum-bone blend implants with open curettage. J Periodontol 1976;47:287–294.

Hiatt WH, Schallhorn RG. Intraoral transplants of cancellous bone and marrow in periodontal lesions. J Periodontol 1973;44:194–208.

Mellonig JT. Periodontal bone graft technique. Int J Periodontol Rest Dent 1990;10:288–299.

Mellonig JT, Prewett AB, Moyer MP. HIV inactivation in a bone allograft. J Periodontol 1992;63:979–983.

Nabers C. Long-term results of autogenous bone grafts. Int J Periodontol Rest Dent 1984;4:51–67.

Passanezi E, Jansen W, Nahas D, et al. Newly forming bone autografts to treat periodontal infrabony defects: clinical and histological events. Int J Periodontol Rest Dent 1989;9:141–152.

Renvert S, Garrett S, Nilveus R, et al. Healing after treatment of periodontal intraosseous defects. VI. Factors influencing the healing response. J Clin Periodontol 1985;12:707–715.

Reynolds M, Bowers G. Fate of demineralized freeze-dried bone allografts in human infrabony defects. J Periodontol 1996;67:150–157.

Robinson RE. Osseous coagulum for bone induction. J Periodontol 1969;40:503–510.

Rosling B, Nyman S, Lindhe J. The effect of systematic plaque control on bone regeneration in infrabony pockets. J Clin Periodontol 1976;3:38–53.

Ross SE, Cohen DW. The fate of a free osseous tissue autograft: a clinical and histologic case report. Periodontics 1968;6:145.

Ross SE, Malamed EH, Amsterdam M. The contiguous autogenous transplant: its rationale, indications and technique. Periodontics 1966;4:246–255.

Sanders JJ, Sepe W, Bowers J, et al. Clinical evaluation of freeze-dried bone allografts in periodontol osseous defects. Part III. J Periodontol 1983;54:1–8.

Soehren SE, Van Swol RL. The healing extraction site: a donor area for periodontal grafting material. J Periodontol 1979;50:128–133.

Yukna RA. Osseous Defect Responses to Hydroxylapatite Grafting Versus Open Flap Debridement. J Clin Periodontol 1989;16:398–402.

Yukna RA. Synthetic bone grafts in periodontics. Periodontology 1993;2000 1:92–99.

Yukna RA, Mayer ET, Miller S. Five year evaluation of durapatite hydroxylapatite ceramic grafts. J Periodontol 1989;60:544–551.

Yukna RA, Yukna CN. A 5-year follow-up of 16 patients treated with coralline calcium carbonate (Biocoralö) bone replacement grafts in infrabony defects. J Clin Periodontol 1998;25:1036–1040.

Zaner DJ, Yukna RA. Particle size of periodontal bone grafting materials. J Periodontol 1984;55:406–409.

Management of Osseous Defects: Furcation Involvement

Arthur R. Vernino

TREATMENT CONSIDERATIONS

Philosophy

Treatment of teeth with furcation involvement complicates periodontal treatment. A furcation involvement may be defined as a pathologic condition that has destroyed the periodontium in the intraradicular area of a multirooted tooth. Treatment of these teeth has varied from conservative (nonsurgical) maintenance to extraction. Recently, the trend has been toward retaining these teeth, especially if they are of strategic importance in the overall treatment plan. Nevertheless, the dentist is cautioned to avoid unnecessary heroics in attempting to salvage seriously involved, multirooted teeth by means of "interesting" techniques. Before attempting extensive therapy, the dentist should ask the following questions:

1. Can a morphologic environment that can be adequately maintained by the patient be established?
2. Will retention of this tooth preserve arch integrity and obviate prosthetic replacement?
3. Will retention permit better prosthetic design?

4. Is the tooth vital to an existing prosthesis?
5. Can the proposed therapeutic effort be considered realistic therapy?
6. Is there a more predicable alternative to retaining this tooth?

Diagnosis

Pathologic conditions in this area are diagnosed by the use of a periodontal probe, a pigtail or cowhorn explorer, a Nabors probe, and radiography. The use of radiography must be related to the clinical examination. For example, radiographic examinations may reveal evidence of a furcation involvement, whereas probing reveals that the soft tissue attachment is still intact, with no entrance into the furcation area. Obviously, the clinical examination is the critical evaluation in this instance.

Maxillary molars, with extensive pocket depths (5 mm or more), on the mesial, distal, or midfacial aspect should automatically be suspected of having furcation involvement. In mandibular molars, extensive midfacial or midlingual pocket formation strongly suggests an intraradicular pathologic process, regardless of the radiographic evidence.

Probing and positive identification of maxillary furcation involvement can be especially difficult. Occasionally, local anesthesia must be used to permit adequate diagnosis. The mesial entry in the furca is best accomplished from the palatal aspect. The distal entry may be accomplished from either the palatal or the facial aspect. Although careful presurgical diagnosis can minimize the possibility of an unexpected furcation problem, final, positive evidence is often found only at the time of surgery.

Classification

Classification of furcation abnormality can be divided into four grades:

1. Grade I (incipient defects).
2. Grade II (moderate involvement).
3. Grade III.
4. Grade IV.

The classification may be defined in greater detail as follows.

Grade I

A soft tissue lesion extending to the furcation level but with minimal osseous destruction. The probe will just enter the furcation area (less than 1 mm). Radiography of these incipient lesions reveals little, if any, evidence of a pathologic condition (Fig. 18-1).

Grade II

A soft tissue lesion combined with bone loss that permits a probe or explorer to enter the furcation from one aspect but not to pass completely through the furcation. Grade II is further subdivided as follows:

Degree I. Greater than 1 mm and less than 3 mm of horizontal bone loss in the furcation. The probe or explorer enters

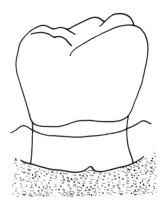

Fig. 18-1

the furcation more than 1 mm and less than 3 mm.

Degree II. Horizontal loss of bone of 3 mm or greater, but no through-and-through involvement. The probe or explorer enters the furcation more than 3 mm but does not go through and through (Fig. 18-2).

Grade III

A lesion with extensive osseous destruction that permits through-and-through communication but the furcation is still covered by soft tissue (Fig. 18-3).

Grade IV

A through-and-through furcation involvement that is clinically exposed and open. There is complete visualization through the furcation (Fig. 18-4).

Prognosis

The prognosis of teeth with a furcation involvement depends on the following factors:

1. Extent of horizontal and vertical bone destruction in the intraradicular space.
2. Number of roots, their structure, and furcal roof structure.
3. Structure of the intraradicular space (e.g., width and depth).

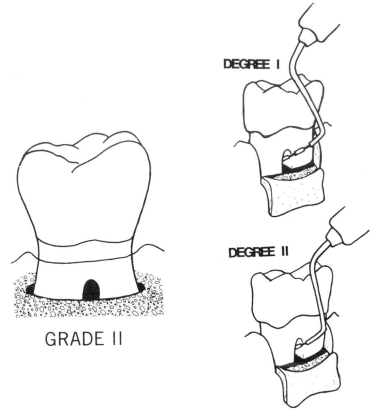

Fig. 18-2

4. Health status of the periodontal ligament (determined by tooth mobility, percussive response, and so forth).
5. Access for surgical correction.
6. Access for plaque control by the patient after surgical correction.
7. Pulpal status and prospects for successful endodontics therapy and root removal procedures.
8. Ability to control occlusal factors.
9. History of caries.

When the foregoing factors are equal, mandibular first molars generally have the best prognosis, followed by mandibular second molars and maxillary first molars. The prognosis of maxillary premolars is considered poor, even with only moderate furcation involvement. The anatomic features of premolar teeth do not lend these teeth to satisfactory plaque control or to root amputation.

The possibility of new attachment in the furcation area, with or without osseous grafting, is not a highly predictable.

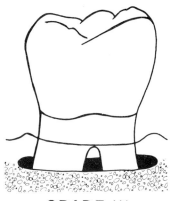

GRADE III

Fig. 18-3

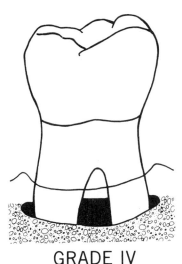

GRADE IV

Fig. 18-4

Some evidence suggests that guided tissue-regenerative procedures may be more successful for treating furcation involvements.

Pulpal-Periodontal Relationships

The relationship between pulpal disease and periodontal disease has been increasingly appreciated. It is apparent that there are many direct communications between pulpal tissues and the periodontal ligament. Dentists cannot consider these areas as separate and unrelated environments. Therefore, in diagnostic terms, a pulpal evaluation should be a part of every periodontal examination.

Pulpal-periodontal interaction is especially important in intraradicular areas. Because of the potential accessory foramina in the furcation areas, grade II and grade III furcation lesions are sometimes associated with pulpal disease. It has been demonstrated that the intraradicular periodontal apparatus is especially sensitive to excessive occlusal stress. Thus, the combination of pulpal disease, periodontal traumatism, and inflammatory periodontitis might reasonably be expected to produce extensive destruction in the furcation area.

The potential for pulpal-periodontal interrelationships provides continual diagnostic challenges to the therapist. The clinician must be highly suspicious of pulpal disease, especially when the following conditions exist:

1. Periodontal pockets near or leading to the furcation area or apex.
2. Sinus tract of uncertain origin.
3. Discolored teeth.
4. Chronic drainage from the sulcus.
5. History of acute or chronic pulpal insult (for example, periodontal trauma, extensive restorative dentistry).
6. Prolonged hypersensitivity.
7. Evidence of slow or inadequate healing of periodontal lesions.

THERAPY

Grade I Involvement

Treatment for incipient furcation lesions is essentially the same as that for an uncomplicated soft tissue pocket. If the width of attached gingiva is adequate (see Chapters 1 and 15), gingivoplasty or odontoplasty may be used, together with thorough debridement and root preparation. The surgery is accomplished to permit access to the furcation for both the therapist and patient.

1. Careful attention should be given to the character of the cervical crown area. Inadequate class IV restorations, cervical caries, and poor crown contours may be predisposing factors that should be corrected.
2. Projections of enamel into the furcation area may influence the spread of gingival inflammation. This anomaly occurs on the buccal aspect of about 25% of all molars. Although the importance of such projections is not clear, the therapist should be aware of them. Removal of the enamel projections by

odontoplasty may be indicated, especially if new attachment is anticipated. On the other hand, if the furcation is left permanently exposed, removal of these anomalies may cause unnecessary tooth sensitivity.

Grade II Involvement

The prognosis and treatment approach are related to the severity of the grade II furcation involvement.

Grade II, Degree I

The prognosis for maintaining a furcation with this severity of involvement is good. Therapy will vary from conservative (nonsurgical) root preparation to surgical access of the furcal area for osseous surgery. Furcation plasty may be necessary for maintenance of oral hygiene by the patient.

Grade II, Degree II

The prognosis for maintaining a furca with degree II severity of involvement is less favorable than a degree I involved tooth. Therapy will include, in addition to the procedures for the degree I furcation, more aggressive approaches such as guided tissue regeneration, root resection, or hemisection.

Grade III and IV Involvement

There are several categories of therapy for grade III and grade IV furcation involvement. These involve the following:

1. Increasing the furcation opening to facilitate plaque control.
2. Eliminating the furcation by various root removal procedures.
3. Extracting the tooth.

Attempts to reestablish total furcation integrity (new bone, periodontal attachment apparatus, and dentogingival rela-tionship) by bone grafting continue to be an unpredictable form of treatment.

Furcation Plasty

Enlargement of an existing class III furcation defect may facilitate plaque control and permit retention of the tooth. Enlargement may be at the expense of the tooth structure, the bone, or both. This approach, however, is generally limited to mandibular molars. Occasionally, a trifurcation area can be opened widely, but adequate plaque removal is difficult. Even after successful treatment of the class III furcation involvement, caries in the furcation area is a constant threat. Caries control is essential for success in the treatment of all furcation involved teeth. The use of the various topical fluorides is recommended.

Root Resection

Root amputation is a predictable procedure for grade III trifurcation involved teeth. The root with the greatest overall bone loss is the logical candidate for amputation. If there is no marked difference, then the disto-buccal root is the root most likely chosen for removal. The mesio-buccal root is the most desirable for retention because of favorable root size and position in alveolar bone (Fig. 18-5; RT = root trunk, PAL = palatal). Several points should be considered before root resection is attempted.

1. Review root and furcation anatomy on extracted molars.
2. Check for and correct occlusion. The occlusal table should be narrowed, and lateral occlusal forces should be removed (Fig. 18-6).
3. Establish the need for splinting.
4. Thoroughly evaluate the strategic importance of teeth indicated for root resection.
5. Locate and avoid the maxillary sinus.

PAL 24%

DB 17%   **MB 25%**

RT 32%

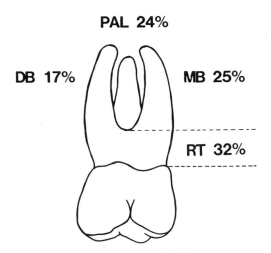

MAX 1ST MOLAR

Fig. 18-5

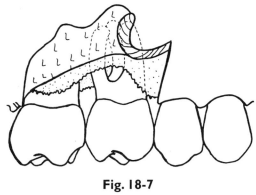

Fig. 18-7

Technique

1. Elevate a mucoperiosteal (full-thickness) flap to expose the defect (Fig. 18-7). Relaxing incisions may be required for adequate access and tissue placement.

2. Make the initial cut on the root, with an appropriate bur, apical to the cementoenamel junction, beginning in the furcation area. Amputation should be at the expense of the root rather than of the crown (Fig. 18-8).

3. Remove the severed root, with appropriate instruments.

4. Contour the resected root stump. The root surface must be tapered and gently curved to permit complete access by the patient for plaque control (Fig. 18-9).

5. Suture the flap (Fig. 18-10) and cover it with a suitable periodontal dressing.

6. Remove sutures in 1 week and recheck the contour.

7. Polish the stump with a fluoride-containing polishing agent.

8. Teach the patient techniques for proper plaque control.

9. Initiate endodontic therapy before or soon after (within two weeks) root amputation.

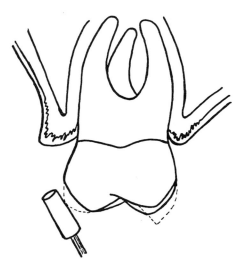

Fig. 18-6

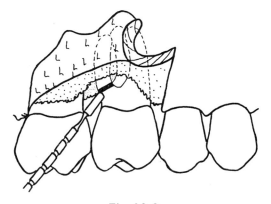

Fig. 18-8

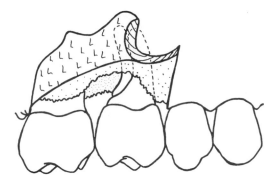

Fig. 18-9

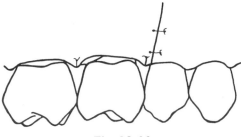

Fig. 18-10

Hemisection

Hemisection involves the removal of one half of the tooth. The same technique is used as was described for root resection. This procedure is most often performed on the mandibular molars, and the retained root can often serve as a suitable abutment for fixed prosthesis or fixed splinting.

Guided Tissue Regeneration

Guided tissue-regenerative procedures show some promise for successfully re-establishing the periodontium in the grade II and grade III involved teeth. The procedure has shown predictability for connective tissue attachment in grade II furcation involvements; predictability for bone regeneration has been lower. The guided tissue procedures have not shown reliability in managing the grade III furcations.

SUGGESTED READINGS

Bower R. Furcation morphology relative to periodontal treatment: furcation entrance architecture. J Periodontol 1979;50:23–37.

Gher M, Vernino A. Root morphology: clinical significance in pathogenesis and treatment of periodontal disease. J Am Dent Assoc 1980;101:627–633.

Herman D, Gher M, Dunlap R, Pelleu G. The potential attachment area of the maxillary 1st molars. J Periodontol 1983;54:431–434.

Kerns D, Greenwell H, Wittwer J, et al. Root trunk dimensions of 5 different tooth types. Int J Periodontics Restorative Dent 1999;19:83–91.

Management of Osseous Defects: Additional Techniques and Summary

John Rapley

FLAP CURETTAGE/DEBRIDEMENT

Several reports have suggested that thorough surgical debridement of osseous defects and adjacent pathologic root surfaces may result in some bony fill of the defects. Full-thickness (mucoperiosteal) flaps (replaced flap or modified Widman flap) coupled with osseous defect debridement for osseous regeneration appear to work best in narrow three-wall defects. Results achieved in other types of defects are less favorable. Thorough and frequent professional and personal plaque control after surgery is critical to maximizing the bony repair. Almost every clinical research evaluation that has compared flap curettage with bone replacement grafts has demonstrated better clinical results when graft material was used as part of the treatment of the defect.

GUIDED TISSUE REGENERATION

Extensive animal and clinical research has established the use of the concept of guided tissue regeneration for treatment of some periodontal defects. Most intrabony defects, grade II furcations, and some dehiscences have been shown to respond well to this type of therapy.

Guided tissue regeneration is based on the following principles:

1. Create a biologically acceptable wound repair area by debridement of the osseous defect and/or furcation and root detoxification (mechanical and chemical).
2. Insert a barrier or membrane between the external tissues (gingival connective tissue and epithelium) and the internal tissues (bone, periodontal ligament, root surface).
3. Create and maintain a space between the barrier and the tooth that will heal with bone, cementum, and periodontal ligament. This space must be maintained for 4 to 8 weeks.
4. Position the flap to cover the barrier and suture it to stabilize the wound.
5. Monitor the patient closely during the 6-week post-surgical period.
6. Nonresorbable barriers must be surgically removed at about 6 weeks. Resorbable barriers do not need to be removed.

Although an expanded polytetrafluoroethylene (e-PTFE or Teflon) nonresorbable barrier has been the main commercially available product to date, several other nonresorbable and resorbable types are becoming commercially available. Results with all of them are generally favorable, but at times the use of a barrier by itself or in combination with bone replacement grafts has not shown an advantage over the bone replacement grafts or flap curettage. Histologic new attachment achieved with use of guided tissue-regeneration barriers alone often does not include new bone formation. Patient and defect selection are important when the clinician is considering the extra time and expense involved in using guided tissue regeneration for periodontal defects.

SELECTIVE EXTRACTION

Selective extraction (strategic extraction) of some periodontally involved teeth can significantly improve the prognosis of adjacent teeth. For example, in Figure 19-1, severe periodontal involve-ment of this vital first premolar has also resulted in bone loss of the adjacent teeth. The tooth exhibits grade III mobility, and its prognosis is poor. If it is extracted, the socket will fill approximately to the highest level of the alveolar crest on the adjacent teeth, as shown in Figure 19-1. Consequently, the prognosis for the adjacent teeth is improved. Selective extraction can be a predictable method of case management.

MINOR TOOTH MOVEMENT

Orthodontic tooth movement can create favorable alterations of gingival form and osseous structure. These changes often modify the extent or eliminate the need for pocket elimination or pocket reduction surgery. Teeth can be moved into a vertical bony defect to narrow the lesion and improve the chances for success with regenerative techniques. Teeth can also be moved away from the osseous defect (such as in molar-uprighting techniques), thereby leveling the bone and modifying or eliminating the bony defects. Similarly, forced eruption can be

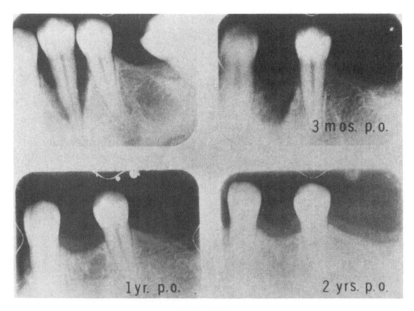

Fig. 19-1

used to modify the osseous topography. Some corrective osseous surgery is frequently needed after the forced eruption to finalize the hard and soft tissue contours. In all cases, inflammation must be controlled before orthodontic therapy begins.

SUMMARY OF TREATMENT OF OSSEOUS DEFECTS

The prognosis for successful resolution of infrabony pockets is influenced by the following:

1. Number of remaining osseous walls.
2. Size of the osseous defect.
3. Number of root surfaces involved.
4. Extent of bony destruction.
5. Presence or absence of furcation involvement.
6. Ability to effectively detoxify and debride the defect and tooth.

As a general rule, the greater the number of osseous walls and the narrower the defect, the better the prognosis for new attachment (provided there is no furcation involvement). The type of therapy chosen for the defects found at the time of surgery depends on the osseous structure and location of the defects, as well as the clinician's experience, knowledge, and skill. Osseous resection, flap curettage, and bone replacement grafts have all been used for each type of bony defect. Preference for one technique over the others for a given clinical situation is often determined by success in transferring information from the literature or lectures to clinical reality.

Some Guidelines for Treating Various Osseous Defects

1. Broad interproximal ledges: consider osteoplasty.
2. Abrupt interproximal irregularities of bone: consider osteoplasty.
3. Exostoses that interfere with pocket

reduction or proper flap closure: consider osteoplasty.
4. Three-wall defect.
   a. Narrow: consider the following:
      i. Bone replacement graft.
      ii. Flap curettage.
   b. Broad defect: consider the following:
      i. Bone graft replacement.
      ii. Guided tissue regeneration.
5. Two-wall defect.
   a. Shallow crater: consider the following:
      i. Osteoplasty or ostectomy (Fig. 19-2).
      ii. Flap curettage.
   b. Deep crater: consider the following:
      i. Bone replacement graft.
      ii. Flap curettage.
      iii. Guided tissue regeneration.
      iv. Combined procedures, including osteoplasty or ostectomy, defect debridement, and/or bone replacement graft, and/or guided tissue regeneration.
6. One-wall defect.
   a. Shallow: consider the following:
      i. Osteoplasty/ostectomy (if adjacent teeth are not jeopardized).
      ii. Bone replacement graft.
      iii. Orthodontic extrusion.
   b. Deep: consider the following:
      i. Bone replacement graft.
      ii. Guided tissue regeneration.
      iii. Combined procedures.

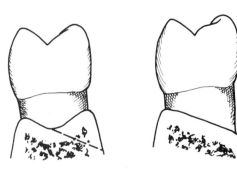

Fig. 19-2

7. Combination defects: consider combination procedures.
8. Grade I furcation involvement: consider the following:
   a. Scaling and root planing.
   b. Gingivectomy or gingivoplasty.
   c. Osteoplasty/ostectomy plus odontoplasty.
   d. Apically positioned flap.
9. Grade II furcation involvement: consider the following:
   a. Osteoplasty/ostectomy and odontoplasty.
   b. Root resection or hemisection.
   c. Bone replacement graft.
   d. Guided tissue regeneration.
   e. Combination procedures.
   f. Extraction depending on severity of furcation involvement.
10. Grade III and grade IV furcation: consider the following:
   a. Root resection or hemisection.
   b. Osteoplasty or ostectomy with odontoplasty (tunneling) and apically positioned flap to open defect through and through for plaque control.
   c. Extraction.

Suggested Readings

Anderegg CR, Martin SJ, Gray JL, et al. Clinical evaluation of the use of decalcified freeze-dried bone allograft with guided tissue regeneration in the treatment of molar furcation invasions. J Periodontol 1991;62: 264–268.

Cortellini P, Pino Prato G, Baldi C, Clauser C. Guided tissue regeneration with different materials. Int J Periodontics Restor Dent 1990;10:137–151.

DeVore CH, Beck FM, Horton JE. Retained "hopeless" teeth: effects on the proximal periodontium of adjacent teeth. J Periodontol 1988;59:647–651.

Gottlow J, Nyman S, Lindhe J, et al. New attachment formation in the human periodontium by guided tissue regeneration. Case reports. J Clin Periodontol 1986;13: 604–616.

Kozlovsky A, Tal H, Lieberman M. Forced eruption combined with gingival fiberotomy. A technique for clinical crown lengthening. J Clin Periodontol 1988;15:534–538.

Machtei EE, et al: Proximal bone loss adjacent to periodontally "hopeless" teeth with and without extraction. J Periodontol 1989;60: 512–515.

Polson AM, Heijl LC. Osseous repair in infrabony periodontal defects. J Clin Periodontol 1978;5:13–23.

Saadoun AP. Periodontal and restorative considerations in strategic extractions. Compend Cont Educ Dent 1981;2:48.

Schallhorn RG, McClain PK. Combined osseous composite grafting, root conditioning, and guided tissue regeneration. Int J Periodontics Restor Dent 1988;8:9–32.

VanVenrooy JR, Yukna RA. Orthodontic extrusion of single-rooted teeth affected with advanced periodontal disease. Am J Orthod Dent Orthoped. 1985;87:67.

Vernino A, Wang H, Rapley J, et al. The use of biodegradable polylactic acid barrier materials on the tratment of Grade II periodontal furcation defects in humans—Part II: A multicenter investigative surgical study. Int J Periodontics Restorative Dent 1999;19:57-65.

Dental Implants

Donald Callan

INTRODUCTION

Dental implants have become a predictable treatment alternative for the replacement of missing teeth in partially or completely edentulous patients. Many dental practitioners have incorporated dental implants into their practices. Most dentists already possess the necessary skills and abilities, which can be maximized to include some aspect of implant therapy into their practice.

The surgical placement of dental implants with or without augmentation procedures requires additional commitment and training beyond the experience received in the undergraduate dental experience. The dentist must have a good understanding of bone physiology, soft tissue physiology, wound healing, occlusion, anatomy, implant designs, advanced prosthetic designs, pharmacology, and advanced surgical skills.

PATIENT SELECTION AND CONSIDERATIONS

The selection of the appropriate patient for dental implants must be determined by evaluating a variety of oral, systemic, and economic factors. Not every edentulous or semi-edentulous area is a site for a dental implant. Dental implants, like any other implants, are merely artificial replacements for lost or traumatized nat-

ural structures; therefore, they cannot be better or last longer than what was given as original equipment.

The past and present state of oral repair is of paramount importance with regard to a favorable long-range prognosis. If the patient lost his or her teeth because of decay or periodontal disease, an accurate pretreatment index of their ability to care for dental implants must be achieved. If a patient's mouth is in a poor state of repair and in need of periodontal and endodontic therapy and clean-outs of decay and temporization, education must be a primary goal. Implant maintenance is presented Chapter 21.

The quantity and quality of the horizontal and vertical bone structure, the proximity of the adjacent vital structures (such as the maxillary sinus, inferior alveolar canal, and the mental foramen) will help in planning for implant therapy. The presence or absence of keratinized gingival tissues, unfavorable muscle attachment, decreased vertical dimension and freeway space, along with class II or class III maxillomandibular relationships, could also influence the treatment plan. The presence of hard or soft tissue abnormality, in addition to the presence of intraoral plates, screws, or wires in the area of anticipated implant placement, must be eliminated before surgery.

The desires and expectations of the patient should be verbalized and documented. If these desires and expectations are realistic and obtainable, the treatment plan process can proceed. The treatment objective is to provide the patient a positive result. The goal in implant dentistry is to restore the patient's mouth to a condition that the patient can and will maintain. The following indications should be met to obtain this goal.

IMPLANT INDICATIONS (PATIENT NEEDS)

1. Restore function.
2. Improve esthetics.
3. Decrease gag reflex.
4. Preservation of teeth.
5. Preservation of bone.
6. Improve speech problems.
7. Improve psychological state.

After the dental evaluation, a medical evaluation is needed. The medical history will determine the degree of presurgical work-up required. Because patient selection influences the success rate, the patient must be carefully screened for potential medical, dental, and psychological contraindications. The purpose of a medical evaluation is to determine whether a patient is a candidate for dental implants and what alterations in the treatment plan may be required to account for existing medical conditions. As a general rule, patients who have undergone primary or secondary radiation of the head and neck region, those who have received chemotherapy, those with brittle diabetes, and those with connective tissue disorders (erythema multiforme, pemphigus, pemphigoid, lupus erythematosus) have a poor risk or should not have implant reconstruction surgery. In addition, the category of patients who have undergone or are currently receiving active psychiatric therapy are also poor implant candidates. If a patient has undergone other implant procedures, such as total hip, total knee, prosthetic valves, or artificial vascular graft procedures, a thorough consultation with the vascular or orthopedic surgeon is indicated. If in doubt, consult with the physician.

IMPLANT CLASSIFICATIONS

Generally speaking, the design of the implants would fit into four major classifications:

1. Subperiosteal (over the bone).
2. Transosseous (staple) (through the bone).
3. Epithelial (mucosal) (soft tissue).
4. Endosseous (into the bone).
   a. Ramus frame.
   b. Endostabilizer.
   c. Blade.
   d. Sinus ("S").
   e. Basket.
   f. Root form (most used today)

IMPLANT MATERIAL

The implant system or grafting material should be biocompatible to the host at the hard and soft tissue interface. Without biocompatibility, the host tissue has a potential for damage and rejection. Numerous articles have documented the biocompatibility of titanium for the use of implants. Titanium and titanium alloy appear to be the materials of choice, although other materials show biocompatibility. In recent years, inorganic bioactive coatings have been applied to metal implants.

Hydroxylapatite (HA) appears to be used most often and can bond directly to bone. Compared with implants coated with a non-HA material, those coated with HA have a faster rate of bone formation, 5 to 8 times more interfacial strength, biointegration as early as 8 weeks, and more bone to the implant surface. Greater bone density and less fibrous tissue encapsulation of HA-coated implants have also been reported. The dental implant is anchored mechanically (osseointegration) or by bone attachment (biointegration). Biointegration is seen with HA-coated implants. Implants coated with a non-HA material are osseointegrated.

The HA-coated implants have the following advantages:

1. Biointegration (bone bonding).
2. Greater bone-implant surface.
3. Stronger (implant/bone interface).
4. No metal ion release from the implant.
5. Faster integration.
6. Applicable to all implant methods.
7. Bridging of bone deficiencies.
8. Increased success with type IV bone.

Integration involves more than biocompatibility of the dental implant material. Fit of the dental implant is extremely important. Although the implant may be biocompatible, its surface must be acceptable to the host tissue. Steam sterilization causes deposition of organic substances on implants, thereby rendering the surfaces less than clean and directly affecting wetting profiles. Glow discharge treatment appears to be the best approach to clean and sterilized dental im-

plants. It is best not to re-sterilize implants. If in doubt, contact the implant manufacturer for instructions.

Although charts list the surface area for tooth roots and implants, a direct one-to-one correlation cannot be made. The information listed below is intended for reference purposes only. There are no hard and fast rules for the surface area of an implant required to replace a given tooth. Common sense dictates that the total surface area of the implants being used comes as close to the surface area of the teeth being replaced as possible. The surface areas shown in the tables do not include any factor for surface roughness of the implant. Surface area of a rough (TPS = titanium plasma–sprayed) coating may be six times the area of a similar smooth implant. All factors must be considered when determining the load bearing area of an implant.

Implant factors to consider for implant selection include the following:

1. Size (length, diameter).
2. Cylinder vs. thread type.
3. Neck design (micro-leakage).

Approximate Surface Area Root Form Implants (mm^2)

Length (mm)	3.25D Cylinder	3.25D Threaded	3.8D Cylinder	3.8D Threaded	4.5D Threaded
8	90	118	107	140	164
10	110	149	131	175	206
12	130	180	155	211	248
14	150	210	178	247	291
16	170	241	202	283	333
18	190	271	226	319	376

Approximate Surface Area of Natural Dentition (mm^2)

Tooth	Central	Lateral Cuspid	First Bicuspid	Second Bicuspid	First Molar	Second Molar
Maxilla 204	179	273	234	220	443	431
Mandible 154	168	268	180	207	431	426

Data obtained from Jepsen A. Root surface measurement and a method for X-ray determination of root surface area. Acta Odontol Scand. 1963;21:35.

4. Surface activity (HA/Non-HA).
5. Mechanical limits.
6. Hard tissue compatibility (implant material).
7. Soft tissue compatibility (smooth neck).

PROSTHETICS

The long-term success of an implant depends on treatment planning, proper selection, fabrication, occlusion, and hygiene maintenance of the prosthetic device. The choice may be narrowed by the preference of the patient and hygiene history, as well as the anatomy of available bone, soft tissue quality, and existing dentition. The team members are encouraged to refer to current published literature for current prosthetic principles. *The case selection for presurgical treatment planning must start with the vision of the final result.* The case type and the retainment must be considered before the start of treatment. A more detailed discussion will follow within this chapter.

CASE TYPES

Single unit.
Three-unit bridge.
Multiple units.
Full replacement.
Bar/denture.
Partial denture.

RETAINMENT

Fixed prosthesis (prosthesis cemented to abutment).
Fixed-removable prosthesis (screw-retained prosthesis).
Patient-removable prosthesis (bar-over-denture).

IMPLANT SITE PREPARATION

Endosseous implant design and the protocols for dental implant surgery have now advanced to a point at which it is rarely the implant or the surgery that is at fault when an implant fails. Instead, other culprits are frequently found on examination of a failed implant: inadequate hard or soft tissue, poor oral hygiene, substandard restorative procedures, implant neck design, or failure to follow the well-established surgical protocols. Clinical experience routinely demonstrates that even the best-designed implants placed with the most meticulous surgical technique are at risk if they are surrounded by inadequate or poor bone or an insufficient amount of attached gingival tissue. The human body's ability to repair both hard and soft tissue is a natural biological phenomenon. Regeneration, however, is another matter. This is certainly the case when a tooth is lost. The absence of a tooth is only the most visible aspect of loss. Because the function of the alveolar bone of the maxillary and mandibular arches is to support teeth, when teeth are removed, this bone recedes, resorbs and is lost. Likewise, attached gingival tissue recedes around the extraction site and may be lost altogether. The dental implant is our human-made answer to tooth root regeneration. Replacement bone materials and soft tissue grafts are our weapons against loss of alveolar bone and gingival tissue. They enable us to recreate the soft and hard tissue environment that natural teeth would normally enjoy.

For soft tissue grafting, free gingival autografts have typically been the material of choice. Chapter 15 discusses several mucogingival procedures that can enhance the success of dental implants.

By anticipating that any extraction site may someday be an implant site, clinicians might consider osseous grafting the extraction site at the time of extraction to preserve the site for future restoration with implants or removable prosthesis. Even though implants are not to be placed after bone grafting, other advantages are created: better support for a partial or full denture or the restoration of normal shape to the arches for a better tissue-clinical crown relationship for conventional dentistry. Bone grafting of the extraction socket to maintain the alveolar process is now considered the standard of care.

Just as bone maintenance measures are advisable as soon as possible after tooth loss, soft tissue grafting is best performed early in the course of implant treatment. Soft tissue grafting may be performed at the time of the implant surgery, but it is recommended that the clinician wait for the second-stage surgery (implant uncovering) to enable the implant site to heal before undertaking a second procedure at the site. If a mucogingival defect develops after the second-stage surgery, the procedure can also be used with good results. Indeed, successful acellular dermal allografts may be performed even after the implants have been restored. Long delays are not recommended because of possible recession and bone loss, which can cause a loss of support for the implant and possible implant loss (Fig. 20-1).

ADVANTAGES OF BONE GRAFTING FOR IMPLANT PLACEMENT

Improved quality and quantity of bone for support of the implant.
Improved implant placement location.
Control of biological and mechanical limits (distribution of forces).
Longer implants.
Larger implants.
Better esthetics.
Multiple implants.
Proper angle placement.
Greater predictability.
Ease of placement.
Maximizing of restorative options.

With all the advantages of bone grafting, the question is when, where, and what material to use for grafting. The sequence of tissue grafting is as follows.

Grafting Sequence

1. Hard tissue before placement of implants.
2. Soft tissue after placement of implants.

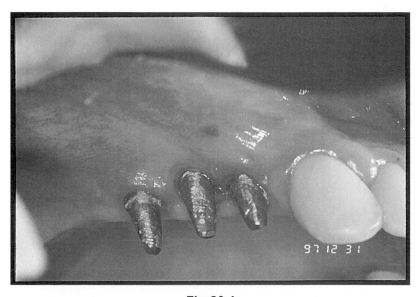

Fig. 20-1

It is best to bone graft before implant placement to prevent or correct the existing defects.

BONE GRAFTING APPLICATIONS

Extraction sockets (Fig. 20-2).
Osseous defects (Fig. 20-3).
Ridge enlargement (Fig. 20-4).
Sinus lifts (Fig. 20-5).
Implants repair (caution!) (Fig. 20-6).

IMPLANT PLACEMENT

Surgical Guides

Many designs of surgical guides have been developed. It is best to have a surgical guide with teeth forms that have defined cemento-enamel junctions. The guide is used by the surgeon as a positional guide for implant placement so that ideal mesio-distal, bucco-lingual, and long-axis orientation of the implant can be determined. A proper design is also important for the best emergence profile and proper axial directed loading forces. The surgical guide (template) may also be also used to determine the need for grafting for better implant placement. If a lack of available bone or anatomical structures prevents ideal placement, secondary sites may be chosen as predetermined in the alternate treatment plan. Guided by the surgical guide, if the required number, location or axial orientation of the implants cannot be achieved successfully as dictated by the treatment plan, the surgeon may elect to place no implants. To fabricate the surgical guide, the implant laboratory may assist the surgical and the restorative dentists as well as providing suggestions. It is best to start with a wax-up of the ideal end result (Fig. 20-7). From this wax-up, the surgical guide is fabricated in a hard clear acrylic material (Fig. 20-8). Holes are then placed in the center of each tooth that is to be supported by the dental implant. The surgical guide is then delivered to the surgical dentist. The guide gives a dry run of the case.

PRESURGICAL CHECKLIST

1. Radiographs/computerized images.
2. Mounted study cast.
3. Surgical guides.

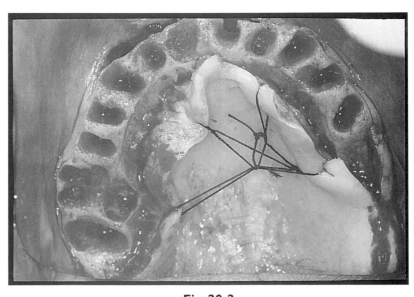

Fig. 20-2

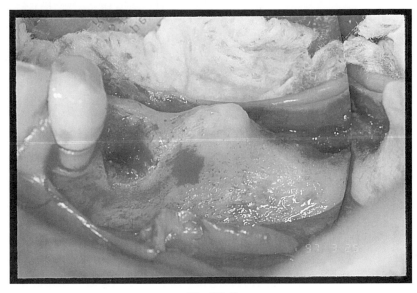

Fig. 20-3

4. Medical clearance/health history review.
5. Signed consent form.
6. Agreement among all team members (treatment plan).
7. Alternate treatment plans.
8. Financial arrangements.
9. Medications.
10. Pre- and postoperative instructions.
11. Implants ordered and received.
12. Communication with the patient about the procedure.

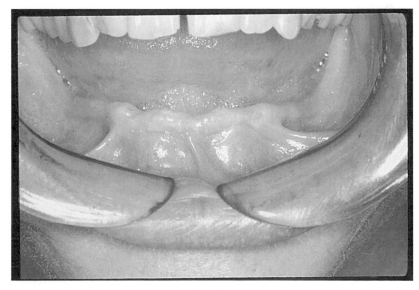

Fig. 20-4

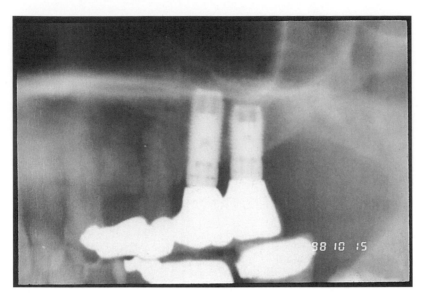

Fig. 20-5

13. Follow-up appointment for suture removal.

IMPLANT SURGICAL PROCEDURE

As in any surgery, it is important the implant procedure be performed under aseptic conditions. The surgical procedure is completed in two phases: 1) implant placement and 2) implant uncovering. Both phases can be performed in the office under local anesthesia, with or without sedation. For implant placement, make a mesiodistal incision along the alveolar crest through the mucoperios-

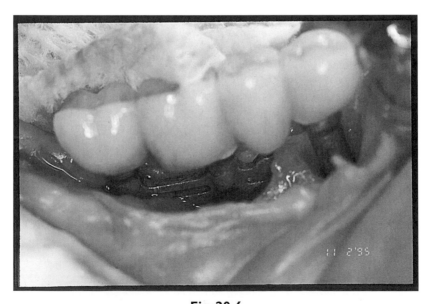

Fig. 20-6

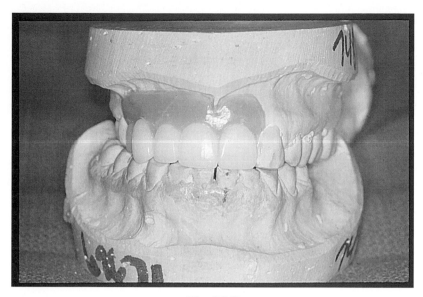

Fig. 20-7

teum and attached gingiva to the bone. The incision should be long enough to permit adequate reflection without tearing the tissue and to provide a broad field of view. (Vertical incisions may be used if necessary.) Using a periosteal elevator, carefully lift the periosteum to expose enough of the alveolar bone as necessary to provide an adequate surgical working area (Fig. 20-9).

Place retraction sutures as needed. Remove spinous ridges or other bone irregularities using the rosette bur or a rongeurs forceps to create as flat a bone plateau as possible. Keep bone removal to a minimum. Insufficient bone width and

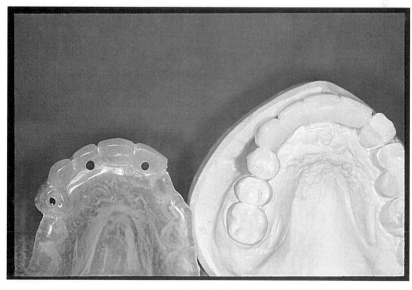

Fig. 20-8

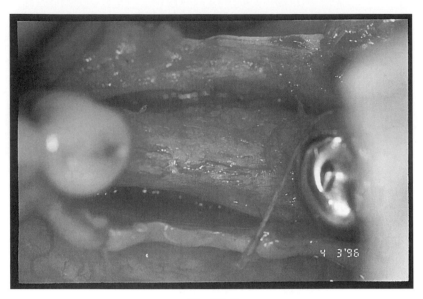

Fig. 20-9

abnormal defects or contours not previously detected may now contraindicate placement of the implant. Ridge width should allow at least 1 mm of bone to remain buccal and lingual to the implant after placement. Maintain proper spacing as previously determined (Fig. 20-10).

The surgical guide may be placed over the surgical site to verify proper location placement (Fig. 20-11).

Bone cutting procedures must be performed with a low-speed, high-torque, internally irrigated handpiece. This instrument minimizes excessive heat generation and preserves the vitality of the bone that is in contact with the implant. Place the implants, and suture the full mucoperiosteal flaps sutured together with 4–0 plain gut followed with 4–0 monocryl. Provide written postoperative instructions to the patient.

The technique of implant placement varies depending on the system being used. The surgical dentist must follow the guidelines as set forth by the manufacturer. If the guidelines are not followed, the success of the case may be decreased. The final decision is the responsibility of the surgical dentist.

POSTOPERATIVE CARE

Instruct the patient to follow a postoperative regimen, including cold packs for the initial 24 hours. An antibiotic of choice may be prescribed. Sutures may be removed after 10 days. When a prosthetic appliance is to be worn during the healing phase, the prosthesis is relieved and relined with a soft liner to prevent premature loading and micromovement of the implants. Patients are called to evaluate soft tissue health, to review the condition of the reline materials, and to confirm that the implants are not being loaded by the prosthesis.

SUMMARY OF POSTOPERATIVE CARE

Educate patients on postoperative care (written instructions).
Review with patient the healing time required on the basis of the procedure.
Be available for postoperative care.
Prescribe the needed postoperative medications.
Schedule postoperative visits for suture removal and evaluation.

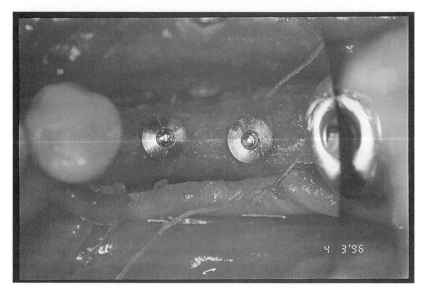

Fig. 20-10

Figures 20-12, 20-13, and 20-14 are photographs of a completed case that followed the proper protocol.

PROSTHETIC FACTORS, DETERMINED BEFORE SURGERY

Occlusion (location) (nut-cracker effect).
Position and inclination.
Surface area (length, thread, cylinder, diameter).
Spacing to distribute occlusal load.
Occlusal table.
Opposing occlusion.
Muscle mass.
Progressive loading.
Spacing (rim to rim) determined by tooth being replaced.
Type of restoration (screw or cement retained).
Parafunctional habits.
Amount of bone loss (crown root ratio).
Arch form.
Bone quality.
Implant surface material.
Tooth being replaced (diameter).
Length of edentulous span.

Replacing roots of teeth.
Self-cleansing.
Open embrasures.
Good accessibility for maintenance.
Patient's ability to maintain.
Esthetics.
Functionality.

RESTORATIVE OPTIONS

Fixed crown and bridge (cement-retained prosthesis).
Fixed-removable crown and bridge (screw-retained prosthesis).
Bar overdenture.
Attachment-retained overdenture (O-ring and ball abutments).
Fixed-removable denture (screw-retained prosthesis).
Milled bar overdenture.

Fixed Crown and Bridge (Cement-Retained Prosthesis)

Fixed implant restorations are similar to conventional crown and bridge restorations. The restoration is cemented to a prepared abutment, which is either threaded or cemented into the implant.

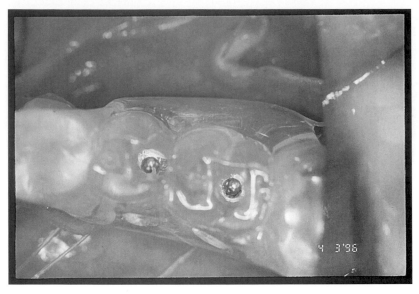

Fig. 20-11

The use of provisional cement may provide retrievableness.

Fixed-Removable Crown and Bridge (Screw-Retained Prosthesis)

Fixed-removable restorations are retained by a coping screw that enters through the occlusal or cingulum of the restoration.

The coping screw passes through the crown and threads either into an abutment or directly into the implant. The restoration is removed by the dentist.

Bar Overdenture

A bar overdenture is a conventional acrylic denture retained by attachments

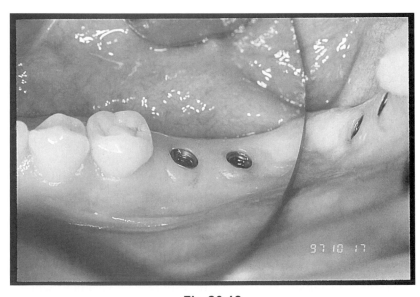

Fig. 20-12

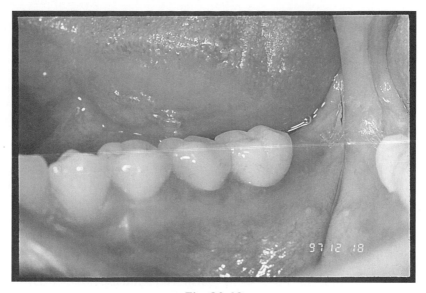

Fig. 20-13

(e.g., clips, O-rings) to an implant-supported cast bar. The denture can be supported by tissue and implant (resilient) or by implants only (rigid). Intraoral considerations, patient manual dexterity, and attachment selection determine the type of bar overdenture. Design of the bar is determined by the number, length, and location of the implants and the quality and quantity of the supporting bone.

Attachment-Retained Overdenture (O-Ring and Ball Abutments)

An attachment-retained overdenture is an implant- and tissue-supported con-

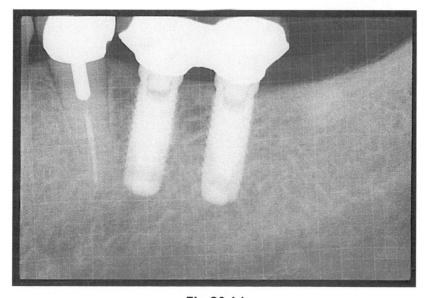

Fig. 20-14

ventional overdenture retained by attachments, which are threaded directly into the implants.

Fixed-Removable Denture (Screw-Retained Prosthesis)

A fixed-removable denture incorporates more conventional denture procedures with a screw-retained bridge. Denture teeth are processed to a metal framework, which is attached directly to the implants or to the abutments.

Milled-Bar Overdenture

A milled bar overdenture is a precision-milled, attachment-retained, double-bar restoration. The cast and milled, implant-supported, primary bar supports a removable prosthesis, which is processed to a secondary (telescoping) cast framework. Stability and retention of the prosthesis are gained through the precision fit and use of attachments. This is an excellent prosthesis for a severely resorbed maxillary reconstruction.

DENTAL IMPLANT TEAM

After the medical and dental information has been obtained and evaluated, the case planning can start. The treatment plan for each patient is different. Considering the expense and knowledge required to provide dental implants or regenerative therapy for the patient, the team approach has merit. The team approach means more than a division of labor. It implies that each member not only is knowledgeable in his or her own right but also understands the needs and problems of his or her counterpart.

Team Members

Restorative dentist and staff.
Surgeon and staff.

Patient and family.
Laboratory.
Manufacturer.
Physician.

All team members should help to determine the problems as well as the solutions. The knowledge of each member will differ. The abundance or lack of knowledge must be shared with all members. The lack of knowledge may be assumed by another team member. Whether it be the full-service or the team approach or not, we must not lose sight of the goal of implant dentistry: to provide the best possible care to our patients. The best results are achieved when all team members are in close communication and carry out prudent planning.

Restorative Dentist and Dental Hygienist

The restorative dentist normally gathers the diagnostic information and coordinates the treatment plan with the patient, surgical dentist, and the laboratory technician. The restorative dentist monitors the prosthetic needs of the patient through the surgical, healing, and restorative phases. Ideally, the restorative dentist works in conjunction with the laboratory technician and surgical dentist to develop the surgical guide to maximize esthetics and to optimize occlusion. The surgical guide is then supplied to the surgical dentist to aid in optimum placement of implants. Excellent oral hygiene maintenance by the patient is important to the long-term success of dental implants. The dental hygienist will play a crucial role in this success by educating and motivating the patient towards excellent oral hygiene. As part of the team, the dental hygienist can also identify and educate potential implant patients during routine hygiene visits.

Surgical Dentist

The surgical dentist gathers additional information and evaluates all diagnostic information provided by the restorative dentist and laboratory technician. If necessary, the surgical dentist may request more extensive radiographic or medical information before patient consultation. This information is then presented to the potential implant patient during the consultation appointment.

Patient and Family

The desires and expectations of the patient should be verbalized and documented. If these desires and expectations are realistic and obtainable, the planning process can proceed. The patient needs to know what to realistically expect from the implant treatment. A satisfied patient is an invaluable resource for future referrals.

Dental Laboratory Technician

The dental laboratory technician brings prosthetic insight to the implant case before surgery. By evaluating the case through a complete work-up, including an esthetic wax-up, the laboratory technician addresses potential esthetic and functional concerns. Other functions include the design and fabrication of provisional and final prosthesis, radiographic and surgical guides, and abutment selection alternatives. Consulting the laboratory technician before surgical procedures gives the restorative dentist a more accurate financial analysis of the final restoration. It is recommended that this be done before the patient is quoted a fee.

Manufacturer

The role of the manufacturer is to support all members of the implant team through product development, manufacturing, and education. Strict manufacturing protocols are followed to assure compliance with Food and Drug Administration standards and with quality assurance requirements. The manufacturer may assist the restorative dentist in the selection and use of prosthetic components to maximize esthetics and function. The dental laboratory technician and restorative dentist can look to the manufacturer for suggestions on case design and proper use of laboratory components. The hygienist may receive support from the manufacturer through the development of effective hygiene instruments and maintenance products, such as specially designed implant scalers and the patient education brochures.

Physician

The physician should be willing to communicate with the dentist and have a reasonable knowledge of dental implants. The physician should provide support and understand the dentist's needs and be available for advice and consults.

Final Consultation

Now that all factors have been gathered, a final patient consultation for the treatment plan presentation can be appointed. During this appointment with the patient, All information must be reviewed to prevent misunderstandings later.

SUGGESTED READINGS

Albertsson T. Direct bone anchorage of dental implants. J Prosthet Dent 1983;50:255–261.

Albertsson T, Dahl E, Enborn L, et al. Osseointegrated oral implants: A Swedish multicenter study of 8139 consecutively inserted Nobelpharma implants. J Periodontol 1988; 59:287–296.

Amier MH. The time sequence of tissue regeneration in human extraction wounds. Oral Surg Oral Med Oral Pathol Oral Rdiol Endod 1969;27:309–318.

Block M, Kent J, Kay J. Evaluation of hydroxylapatite-coated titanium dental implants in dogs. J Oral Maxillofac Surg 1987;45: 601–607.

Callan DP. Guided tissue regeneration without a stage 2 surgical procedure. Int J Periodontol Rest Dent 1993;13:173–179.

Callan DP, O'Mahony A, Cobb CM. Loss of crestal bone around dental implants: a retrospective study. Implant Dent 1998;7:258–266.

Carlsson L, Rostlund T, Albertsson BMP, et al. Implant fixation improved by close fit. Cylindrical implant-bone interface studied in rabbits. Acta Orthop Scand 1988;59:272–275.

Eriksson L, Albertsson T. Temperature threshold levels for heat induced bone injury: a vital microscopic study in the rabbit. J Prosthet Dent 1983;50:101–107.

Eriksson L, Albertsson T, Grane B, et al. Thermal injury to bone: a vital microscopic description of heat effects. Int J Oral Surg 1982;11:115–121.

Hansson HA, Albertsson T, Branemark PI. Structural aspects of the interface between tissue and titanium implants. J Prosthet Dent 1983;50:108–113.

Jansen JA, Van de Walden J, Wolke J, et al. Histologic evaluation of osseous adaptation to titanium and hydroxylapatite-coated titanium implants. J Biomed Mat Res 1991; 25:973–989.

Mombelli A, VanOsten MAC, Schurch E, et al. The microbiota associated with successful or failing osseointegrated titanium implants. Oral Microbiol Immumol 1987;2: 145–151.

Implant Maintenance

John Rapley

Periodontal maintenance has long been viewed as an essential part of total periodontal therapy and is considered a major factor in the success of periodontal therapy. Long-term studies have demonstrated that regular periodontal maintenance can maintain the periodontal attachment. Similarly, the importance of long-term implant maintenance cannot be underestimated.

A basic understanding of implant maintenance entails knowledge about the peri-implant attachment apparatus, its susceptibility to disease and reinfection, and specific microbiology. Clinical measures of implant health, evaluated at each maintenance appointment, consist of probing, radiographs, tissue health evaluation, and mobility. Clinical instruments and materials for patient home care and therapist's debridement may differ from those used for periodontal maintenance and need to be understood.

PERI-IMPLANT ATTACHMENT APPARATUS AND DISEASE SUSCEPTIBILITY

Numerous authors have found a similar epithelial attachment in the peri-implant tissues. This epithelial attachment is also mediated by hemidesmosomes, while the connective tissue component is different. Instead of the connective tissue fibers inserting perpendicular as found in the periodontal attachment, a peri-implant connective tissue cuff surrounds the implant. This cuff, which has a parallel-fiber orientation, has no insertion to the implant. This difference is significant in that it may result in an altered susceptibility to plaque-induced disease. Research tends to illustrate the increased susceptibility of the peri-implant tissue to plaque-induced disease, which may be related to the lack of a connective tissue attachment or the absence of a periodontal ligament.

Reinfection

The phenomenon of reinfection from diseased sites to nondiseased sites has been shown to occur in patients with periodontal disorders, and the same has been seen in partially edentulous patients with implants. This possibility of reinfection from diseased periodontal sites to implant sites necessitates completion of needed periodontal therapy before implant placement and should be an integral part of treatment planning. Therefore, concurrent periodontal and implant maintenance is vital in partially edentulous patients with implants.

Microbiology

Implant and periodontal microbiology are similar in that a stable healthy implant has a similar microflora as a healthy tooth (mainly gram-positive, nonmotile, aerobic, organisms, mainly cocci). The ailing implant has microflora similar to that found in a periodontally involved tooth (gram-negative, motile, anaerobic, organisms, with a high percentage of spirochetes). The pathogens in periodontitis, such as *Prevotella intermedia* and *Porphyromonas gingivalis,* are the same pathogens seen in peri-implantitis. Implant plaque formation is identical, with comparable time frames and succession, to that seen in peri-implant disease: the progression is from cocci to filamentous forms and then to pathogens with spirochetes. There is also a positive correlation with increased plaque and inflammation and with the amount of plaque and peri-implant probing depth. Therefore, the importance of the prevention of plaque accumulation is similar in both periodontal and peri-implant tissues. Tests using microbial monitoring may be indicators or predictors of implant health in the future.

CLINICAL MEASURES

Clinical measures are evaluated at both periodontal and implant maintenance appointments. Measures include probing depth, bleeding on probing, radiographs, tissue health, and mobility.

Probing

Implant probing is somewhat controversial; some therapists feel that it may be an invasive procedure because the probe penetrates into the connective/bone zone as a result of the lack of an inserting connective tissue attachment. This wounds the tissue or seeds bacteria into the tissue. Others believe it is a valuable measure if the change of probing depth is evaluated and monitored. The probe reading is influenced by many variables, such as force of probing, angulation of the probe, tissue health, probe diameter, type of probe, and implant access. It must be emphasized that there is no clear numerical value of a "healthy probing depth" as is associated with the dentate individual. Additional factors influence the peri-implant probing depth, including the thickness of the tissue, position of the implant, and amount of countersinking.

Several studies have correlated bleeding on probing to disease activity in the dentate patient; it may also be of value in patients with implants. The bleeding status may provide knowledge of the health of the tissue but may be related to probing force and tissue woundability.

Radiographs

The most viable measure for monitoring implant health is still the dental radiograph, used by most therapists. An accurate radiograph is exposed at 65- to 70-kilovolt peaks with a long cone paralleling technique and adequate exposure time to distinguish any vents or implant fixture landmarks. Two periapical radiographs at 6 to 12 degrees of variation on the horizontal plane may enhance the evaluation of the interproximal bone. A disposable grid overlay on the radiographs may aid in the assessment of implant bone levels.

Radiographic inaccuracies can result from magnification error or a nonparallel technique. Image magnification on periapicals ranges from 2 to 5%, and magnification on a panoramic radiograph may be as high as 15 to 25% depending on the manufacturer. Even with the best technique, a parallel image-to-film may not be possible because of implant angulation or anatomic limitations for film placement (as in resorbed maxilla or mandibles).

It is recommended that radiographs be taken at the following times:

1. Day of second-stage implant uncovering as a baseline radiograph.
2. One year after prosthetic loading to

evaluate the bone loss resulting from physiologic adaptation.

3. Every year or as needed during maintenance.

Tissue Health

During maintenance, the peri-implant tissues are evaluated for changes in color, contour, and consistency. Some studies report no correlation of disease with the presence or absence of keratinized tissue adjacent to the implant. Others feel that mobile connective tissue associated with nonkeratinized tissue adversely affects the epithelial seal. Augmentation of keratinized tissue would be indicated if patient discomfort during normal oral hygiene procedures results in unhealthy tissue. The overall conclusion is that the type of peri-implant tissue has a minimal influence on implant health in the presence of good oral hygiene.

Mobility/Occlusion

Mobility of an implant fixture is an unfavorable finding; mobile implants must be removed. However, it is difficult to determine slight mobility. Occlusion should be evaluated at each maintenance appointment and discrepancies adjusted as detected. Untreated overload can lead to rapid and substantial peri-implant bone loss. It is also recommended that the prosthesis be periodically removed to assess the individual mobility of each fixture.

Monitoring of Gingival Crevicular Fluid

Various investigators have explored the monitoring of enzymes in the gingival crevicular fluid to assess the status of an implant. Enzymes that have been investigated include neutral protease, arylsulfatase, elastase, myeloperoxidase, β-glucuronidase, and aspartate aminotransferase.

Patient's Home Care

Several home care aids for patients with implants are beneficial in plaque removal:

1. The primary aid is the soft toothbrush, which includes the manual and the powered counter-rotational toothbrush. Patients may find the smaller head toothbrushes superior in accessing the lingual and palatal aspects of the prosthesis.
2. Interproximal plaque can be removed by using normal floss, yarn, nylon "floss," or other products that can be threaded beneath the prosthesis and around the abutments.
3. Gauze can be used to debride the distal aspects of implants, especially under cantilever areas.
4. Antimicrobial mouthrinses, such as chlorhexidine, can decrease supragingival plaque formation.
5. Water irrigation systems, adjusted at low power, may aid in removing food debris beneath and around the prosthesis.
6. The interdental brushes with a Teflon-coated wire core are effective for areas with poor or minimal access.

These home care aids do not alter the implant abutment surface and are safe for the patient to use. However, oral hygiene may be more difficult or uncomfortable for patients with implants because of poor access.

Therapist Instrumentation

Recommended instruments for debridement include plastic, nylon, or special alloy scaler-type instruments that do not cause any adverse surface alterations of the implant material. Many of the instruments available have the inherent problem of lacking a working surface "edge" to effectively and easily remove calculus. A rubber cup with or without flour of pumice is also a useful adjunct and may actually improve the abutment surface.

Instruments not recommended for use include metal hand scalers, ultrasonic scalers, and sonic scalers because of the danger of significant alteration of the implant surface. Some sonic scalers are available with hard plastic tips, which may be safe. There is still some debate over the air-powder abrasive because it may remove the protective oxide layer and increase corrosion.

Adjunctive Therapy

Evidence suggests that subgingival irrigation can be a benefit in the treatment of peri-implant inflammation. The use of various local drug delivery systems into the peri-implant space may be a useful option in the treatment of peri-implant inflammation.

SUGGESTED READINGS

Bauman G, Mill M, Rapley J, et al. Plaque-induced inflammation around implants. Int J Oral Maxillofac Implants 1992;7:330–337.

Bauman G, Rapley J, Hallmon W, et al. The peri-implant sulcus. Int J Oral Maxillofac Implants 1993;8:273–280.

Becker W, Becker B, Newman M, et al. Clinical and microbiological findings that may contribute to dental implant failure. Int J Oral Maxillofac Implants 1990;5:31–38.

Berglund T, Lindhe J, Marinello C, et al. Soft tissue reaction to de novo plaque formation in implant and teeth. An experimental study in the dog. Clin Oral Implant Res 1992;3:1–8.

Leukholm U. Osseointegrated implants in clinical practice. J Oral Implantol 1986;12:357–364.

Lindhe J, Berglund T, Ericsson L, et al. Experimental breakdown of peri-implant and periodontal tissues. A study in the beagle dog. Clin Oral Implant Res 1993;3:9–16.

Listgarten M, Lang N, Schroeder H, et al. Periodontal tissues and their counterparts around endosseous implants. Clin Oral Implant Res 1991;2:1–19.

Mombelli A, Lang N. Antimicrobial treatment of peri-implant infections. Clin Oral Implant Res 1992;3:162–168.

Quirymen M, Listgarten M. The distribution of bacterial morphotypes around natural teeth and titanium implant ad modum Branemark. Clin Oral Implant Res 1990;1:8–13.

Rapley J, Swan R, Hallmon W, et al. The surface characteristics produced by various oral hygiene instruments and materials on titanium implant abutments. Int J Oral Maxillofac Implants 1990;5:47–52.

Schou S, Holmstrup P, Hjorting-Hansen E, et al. Plaque-induced marginal tissue reactions of osseointegrated oral implants: a review of the literature. Clin Oral Implant Res 1992;3:149–161

Periodontal Emergencies

Joseph J. Lawrence and Peter F. Fedi, Jr.

A periodontal emergency is any circumstance, or a combination of circumstances, that adversely affects the periodontium and requires immediate attention. This definition encompasses a wide variety of conditions that involve the periodontium; however, this chapter will be limited to the emergencies most often encountered.

PERICORONITIS

Cause

Pericoronitis is probably the most common periodontal emergency, and the partially erupted or impacted mandibular third molar is the site most frequently involved. The overlying gingival flap is an excellent harbor for the accumulation of debris and an ideal breeding ground for bacteria. Additional insult to the pericoronal flap is often produced by trauma from an opposing tooth.

Signs and Symptoms

The clinical picture is a red, swollen, possibly suppurating lesion that is extremely painful to the touch. Swelling of the cheek at the angle of the jaw, early necrotizing ulcerative gingivitis, partial trismus, lymphadenopathy, and radiating pains to the ear are common findings. The patient may also have systemic complications, such as fever, leukocytosis, and general malaise.

Treatment

The treatment of pericoronitis consists of irrigation of the undersurface of the flap and the surrounding area with warm saline solution or antimicrobial rinses. A 10-mL syringe with a blunt 10-gauge needle, bent at an 80-degree angle, is an excellent irrigating instrument. An ultrasonic or sonic instrument can also be used effectively in this region. It may be necessary to extract the opposing third molar at the first visit if it impinges on the pericoronal flap. The patient is instructed to rinse with warm salt water every 2 hours, and antibiotics are administered if systemic complications are present. Once the acute symptoms have subsided, a careful evaluation is made to determine whether the tooth should be retained and whether further periodontal therapy is indicated to alter the environment.

ABSCESS FORMATION

Gingival Abscess

A gingival abscess is a localized (usually superficial), painful, rapidly expanding lesion that appears suddenly in the marginal gingiva or interdental papilla. The lesion consists of a purulent focus in connective tissue. It is initiated by the forceful embedding of a foreign body (e.g., a toothbrush bristle or popcorn husk) into the gingiva or gingival sulcus. A gingival abscess may occur in tissue entirely free from periodontal disease.

Treatment

Treatment consists of drainage to relieve the acute symptoms and removal of the foreign body. If the lesion has become fluctuant, topical anesthesia is first applied to the gingival margin and the gingival sulcus is gently opened with a curet to permit evacuation of pus. The sulcus is gently instrumented, and copious amounts of warm saline are used to flush the area. The patient is advised to rinse with warm salt water every 2 hours. Once the irritant is removed and drainage is established, the tissues usually return to normal with no further treatment.

Periodontal Abscess

A periodontal abscess is a localized, purulent inflammatory process involving the deeper periodontal structures. Abscess formation is usually associated with infrabony pockets, deep tortuous pockets, and furcation involvement. Conditions that force material into deep pockets, prevent free drainage, or occlude the orifice of a pocket may result in abscess formation. The latter may occur when patients become conscientious about plaque control and improve the tissue health in the marginal area without treatment of the deeper problem.

Periodontal abscesses may be acute or chronic. Acute lesions often subside and persist in the chronic state, while chronic lesions may suddenly become acute.

Signs and Symptoms

The following are clinical signs of an acute abscess:

1. Severe pain.
2. Swelling of the soft tissues.
3. Tenderness to percussion.
4. Extrusion of the involved tooth.
5. Mobility of the involved tooth.

Periodontal destruction in an acute periodontal abscess may be rapid and extensive, and treatment should be instituted promptly.

Treatment

Treatment of the periodontal abscess is performed in two stages.

The first stage involves management of the acute symptoms by drainage. Whenever possible, drainage is established through the lumen of the pocket. If this cannot be done, as is often the case when there is a furcation involvement or a tortuous pocket, drainage is obtained externally by making a "stab" wound through the pointed lesion. The patient is advised to rinse with warm salt water every 2 hours, and antibiotics are prescribed if systemic complications are present. It may often be necessary to adjust the occlusion of the involved tooth or teeth.

The second stage of treatment is directed toward elimination of the pocket as soon as the acute symptoms have subsided and before the chronic stage is reached.

Treatment consists of careful elevation of a mucoperiosteal flap. All granulomatous tissue is removed and the root surface is lightly planed. Emphasis is placed on gentle manipulation of the soft tissue. The flap is replaced in its original position (replaced flap) and sutured. A periodontal dressing may be used for 7 to 10 days.

Clinical experience has demonstrated a marked propensity for healing and repair after acute periodontal destruction. For this reason, teeth affected by an acute periodontal abscess should be carefully evaluated before extraction is recommended, and periodontal surgery, if indicated, should be instituted.

Acute Periapical Abscess

It is sometimes necessary to differentiate between a periodontal and periapical abscess. A nonvital pulp usually indicates a periapical abscess, and the tooth should be treated endodontically or extracted. A clinically responsive vital pulp is not always assurance that the problem is still not pulpal. Radiography is of some assistance in differential diagnosis, but clinical findings, such as extensive caries, tooth vitality testing, pocket formation, and continuity between the abscess and the gingival margin, are of greater practical significance.

Various investigators have confirmed pulpal pathosis and infection in periodontally involved teeth. Thus, the probability exists that periodontitis can result in death of the pulp. Studies have has also shown that, as a result of pulpal disease, tissue destruction may proceed from the apical region toward the gingival margin. This process is termed *retrograde periodontitis,* to differentiate it from marginal periodontitis, in which the disease spreads from the gingival margin to the apex of the tooth. Whether the periodontal pocket is a result of retrograde or marginal periodontitis, or a combination of both, is academic. In all cases, treatment should consist of combined endodontic-periodontal therapy or extraction of the tooth.

CHEMICAL AND PHYSICAL INJURIES

Injuries caused by toothbrush trauma, chemical burns, cheek and tongue biting, factitious habits, and periodontal dressings sometimes occur. Emergencies of this type are painful but otherwise of little consequence. Healing usually occurs uneventfully in 10 days to 2 weeks. Treatment is chiefly of the symptoms, and patient discomfort is controlled through the use of topical anesthetics or warm saline rinses.

NECROTIZING ULCERATIVE GINGIVITIS

History

Necrotizing ulcerative gingivitis is an emergency of special importance. As long ago as 400 B.C., Greek soldiers were plagued by what appears to have been necrotizing ulcerative gingivitis. In the 1890s, Plaut and Vincent were the first to associate specific organisms with the disease process; thus, the term *Vincent's infection* has been associated with the disease for many years. The disease has also been called Vincent's stomatitis, Plaut-Vincent's disease, Plaut-Vincent's stomatitis, trench mouth, and many other names. Because the trend in dental and medical terminology is to dispense with the use of eponyms, the descriptive term *necrotizing ulcerative gingivitis* is preferred.

Incidence

An increase in necrotizing ulcerative gingivitis among college students after final examinations and periods of stress has been reported. The condition has also been related to cigarette smoking, increased consumption of alcohol, low socioeconomic status, poor nutrition, age, general debilitation, and climate. In effect, any factor that increases emotional stress, lowers patient resistance, or inhibits plaque control can contribute to the initiation of necrotizing ulcerative gingivitis.

Contagion

For many years, necrotizing ulcerative gingivitis was considered a communicable disease contracted from eating utensils, personal contact, and so forth. Numerous studies have failed to establish any pattern of transmission among affected patients. Some hardy investigators have even injected fusospirochetal microorganisms into their own mouths and have not contracted the disease. The 1966 World Workshop in Periodontics concluded, on the basis of existing evidence, that necrotizing ulcerative gingivitis was not a communicable disease.

Cause

The cause of necrotizing ulcerative gingivitis can be divided into predisposing and exciting (causative) factors.

1. *Predisposing factors.* Local factors include calculus, gingival flaps over molar teeth, caries, overhanging margins of restorations, improper tooth contacts, malpositioned teeth, and food impaction. Systemic predisposing factors include emotional and nonspecific stress, anxiety, heavy alcohol intake, cigarette smoking, fatigue, malnutrition, mouth breathing, AIDS, gross neglect, pre-existing gingivitis, and general debilitation.
2. *Exciting (causative) factors.* The exciting or causative factors are microorganisms. As in most forms of gingivitis, the primary etiologic factor is bacterial plaque. The acute disease develops from a host-parasite imbalance as a result of an overwhelming increase in the number of bacteria or lowered patient resistance. Organisms that have been associated with necrotizing ulcerative gingivitis are the following:
   a. *Bacillus fusiformis.*
   b. *Borrelia vincentii.*
   c. Alpha hemolytic streptococci.
   d. *Bacteroides melaninogenicus.*
   e. Other unidentified vibrios, spirochetes, and streptococci.

It is interesting to note that the number of spirochetes is proportional to the amount of inflammation and the amount of necrosis present. Current research has shown organisms penetrating the tissue in the lesions of necrotizing ulcerative gingivitis. Even though a specific organism has not been conclusively demonstrated to produce necrotizing ulcerative gingivitis, it has been established that microorganisms are the exciting causative agents of the disease. The dramatic response to antibiotics, both topical and systemic, is valid evidence of the role of bacteria in the cause of necrotizing ulcerative gingivitis. Once antibiotic administration is stopped, the disease usually recurs unless the predisposing factors have been eliminated.

Diagnosis

Necrotizing ulcerative gingivitis can be diagnosed on the basis of clinical findings alone. The onset of the disease is sudden, and patients report severe pain about the teeth or gums. Usually, they cannot determine any one particular area that hurts but say, "My entire mouth hurts" or "All of my teeth hurt." The pain is more intense at the sites of ulceration. The second most prominent symptom is bleeding gums. Bleeding is often spontaneous, and patients may observe blood on their pillows or notice the taste of blood when they awaken. Patients may also experience marked pain and bleeding while brushing their teeth or when eating. Alcoholic beverages, hot or cold liquids, or spicy foods may be intolerable.

The most characteristic and pathognomonic finding of necrotizing ulcerative gingivitis is ulceration and cratering of the interdental papillae (Fig. 22-1). Frequently, the papillae are reduced to punched-out masses of necrotic tissue covered by a gray-white pseudomembrane. Acute pain and bleeding result from the slightest pressure on the area. Ulcerated areas spread by contiguity and by contact. The mucosa of the lips, the jaws, and the palate may be affected, and ulcerated areas may be found on the tongue. The fetid odor of necrosis is usually present, but this distinctive odor is not pathognomonic of necrotizing ulcera-

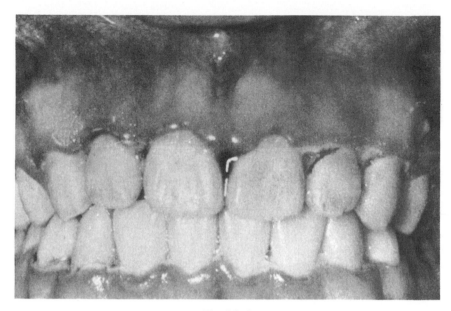

Fig. 22-1

tive gingivitis in that the odor may be present in any site of tissue necrosis. There may or may not be many systemic findings. Fever, headache, general malaise, loss of appetite, and regional lymphadenopathy may be present. The constitutional symptoms seem to parallel the severity of the disease and are usually more pronounced in younger patients.

Differential Diagnosis

Several diseases produce lesions similar to those of necrotizing ulcerative gingivitis. Lesions most commonly mistaken for necrotizing ulcerative gingivitis include the following:

1. Acute gingivitis.
2. Primary herpetic gingivostomatitis.
3. Recurrent aphthous stomatitis.
4. Desquamative gingivitis.
5. Infectious mononucleosis.
6. Acute leukemia.
7. Agranulocytosis.
8. Secondary stage of syphilis.

Only necrotizing ulcerative gingivitis, however, produces ulceration and cra-

tering of the interdental papillae. It should be emphasized that necrotizing ulcerative gingivitis can occur in conjunction with any number of systemic debilitating diseases.

1. *Acute gingivitis (Fig. 22-2).* An intense generalized or even localized acute gingivitis can mimic any of the signs and symptoms of necrotizing ulcerative gingivitis. In gingivitis, pain is not as severe or as persistent, and spontaneous bleeding is rare. In many patients with acute gingivitis, the interproximal areas and gingival margins are filled with food, plaque, and materia alba. Once this debris is removed and the interproximal areas can be examined, the lack of necrosis and crater formation will verify the diagnosis of nonulcerative gingivitis.
2. *Primary acute herpetic gingivostomatitis (Fig. 22-3).* This disease is characterized by small ulcers with elevated, halo-like margins. The lesions are yellowish and cheesy in appearance and bleed less readily on pressure than do the lesions

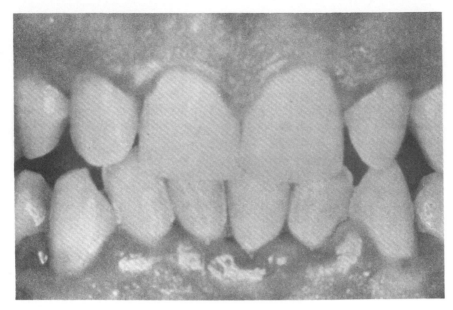

Fig. 22-2

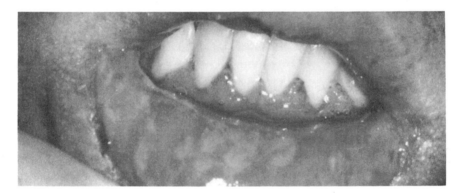

Fig. 22-3

of necrotizing ulcerative gingivitis. The lips, tongue, buccal mucosa, palate, gingiva, pharynx, and tonsils may be involved. The disease is accompanied by generalized soreness, which interferes with eating or drinking. The typical interdental crater of necrotizing ulcerative gingivitis is lacking. Patients usually display severe systemic symptoms with typical herpetic lesions, extraorally and intraorally. Diagnosis is based on clinical findings and patient history. Acute herpetic gingivostomatitis usually lasts 7 to 10 days. Treatment consists of palliative measures. The patient is placed on a regimen of warm water rinses, soft diet, and forced fluids. Plaque and superficial calculus are removed to reduce gingival inflammation. If the patient experiences pain when eating, a 0.05% solution of dyclonine hydrochloride or viscous Xylocaine may be prescribed for use before meals. The solution is swished in the mouth for about 2 minutes and then expectorated. Local anesthesia is produced and lasts up to 1 hour. Dyclonine hy-

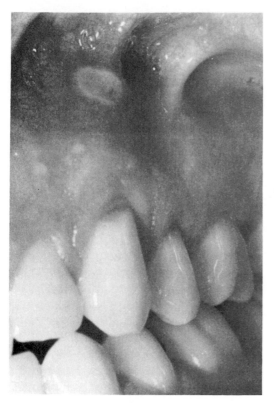

Fig. 22-4

drochloride can be used several times daily, without fear of toxicity.

3. *Recurrent aphthous stomatitis (canker sores) (Fig. 22-4).* This condition is characterized by single or multiple epithelial erosions, which can occur on the buccal mucosa, lateral margin of the tongue, floor of the mouth, soft palate, and pharynx. The ulcers are covered by a gray-white membrane with an erythematous margin and minimal adjacent erythema. The condition is extremely painful, and one or more oral lesions may be present. Common precipitating factors include mucosal trauma, psychic stress, and endocrine imbalance. In patients who continuously develop with this condition, a recommended treatment is tetracycline hydrochloride, oral suspension. One teaspoon containing 250 mg is

swished around the mouth for 2 minutes and then swallowed. This is done four times a day until the lesions are gone. The mouth rinse is followed by a topical application of a steroid. The treatment should begin as soon as the prodromal signs are recognized. This treatment is not recommended for persons who experience only the occasional aphthae or those who should not take tetracyclines.

4. *Chronic desquamative gingivitis.* This gingival condition is probably a clinical syndrome rather than a disease entity. The cause is not known; however, the condition is probably an oral manifestation of a bullous dermatologic disease, such as benign mucous membrane pemphigoid or lichen planus. Desquamative gingivitis is most commonly observed in women (40 to 55 years of age) and can occur in mild, moderate, and severe forms. In the mildest form, there is diffuse, painless erythema of the gingiva. In the moderate to severe form, scattered red and gray areas involve the marginal and attached gingiva. The gingiva can usually be rubbed off with finger massage or blown off with an air syringe (Nikolsky's sign), leaving a bleeding surface. The papillae do not undergo necrosis; therefore, there is no interdental cratering. Patients report a burning sensation, thermal sensitivity, and pain when brushing the teeth. The mild form of this condition may be painless, but the severe form is extremely painful. Diagnosis is based on clinical findings and biopsy. Local treatment consists of gentle prophylaxis, plaque control, and elimination of all forms of local irritants. In the most severe cases, topical or systemic corticosteroid therapy is used to supplement local therapy. Topical hormones are often effective supplements to local therapy: for female patients, a cream containing 1.25 mg/g of conjugated es-

trogen, and for male patients, methyltestosterone ointment, 2 mg/g. Some therapists have successfully eliminated the condition by gingivectomy.

5. *Infectious mononucleosis.* This benign infectious disease is usually seen in children and young adults. The symptoms include a sudden onset of fever, nausea, headache, vomiting, malaise, loss of appetite, swelling, and tenderness of the lymph nodes. The patient often first reports a sore mouth and throat. There may be diffuse erythema of the mucosa and petechiae. The marginal gingiva and interdental papillae are swollen and inflamed and bleed spontaneously or upon gentle pressure. There is no ulceration or interdental crater formation, but secondary development of necrotizing ulcerative gingivitis affords a diagnostic challenge. Diagnosis is based on hematologic and immunologic findings.

6. *Leukemia (Fig. 22-5).* Oral manifestations occur with great frequency in patients with leukemia, particularly acute and subacute monocytic leukemia. Clinical changes may vary from diffuse cyanotic discoloration of the entire gingival mucosa to a tumorous gingival enlargement. The enlargement may be localized or generalized, diffuse or marginal, but in all cases it is associated with local irritants, such as plaque, calculus, faulty restorations, and trauma. The clinical signs of necrotizing ulcerative gingivitis are often superimposed upon leukemic gingival enlargement. When local treatment of necrotizing ulcerative gingivitis fails, a complete blood count, urinalysis, and bone marrow studies are essential to rule out the presence of leukemia and other blood dyscrasias.

7. *Agranulocytosis (malignant neutropenia).* This condition is manifested orally as ulceration and necrosis of the gingiva, which resembles necrotizing ulcerative gingivitis. The ulcers are covered by a gray or gray-black membrane, but less inflammation associated with the lesions of agranulocytosis than with the lesions of necrotizing ulcerative gingivitis. Lesions are also observed in the oral mu-

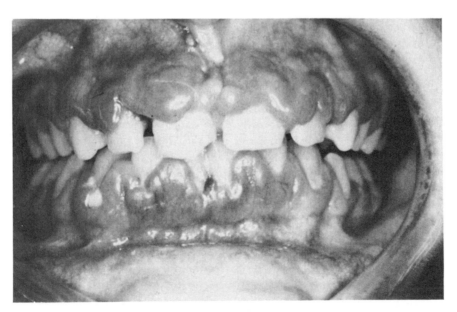

Fig. 22-5

cosa, tonsils, and pharynx. The most common cause is a reaction to a wide variety of drugs. Diagnosis is based on blood studies and bone marrow biopsy.

8. *Secondary syphilis (mucous patch)*. The oral lesions of syphilis are usually on the tongue, the gingiva, or the buccal mucosa. They are usually ovoid or irregularly shaped and are surrounded by an erythematous zone. The mucous patch rarely affects the marginal gingiva, and the overlying gray-white plaque is not detachable. The lesions are usually painless but are highly infectious. Diagnosis is made by positive results on serologic analysis and dark-field examination of an affected lymph node.

Treatment

The dentist should attempt to do the following:

1. Control the acute bacterial phase.
2. Educate the patient in plaque control.
3. Eliminate the predisposing factors, both local and systemic.

Early and vigorous local treatment during the acute phase will produce rapid and dramatic results in most cases. Drugs should never be considered a substitute for scaling and debridement. Antibiotics should be used only when systemic complications are evidenced.

The basic steps in treatment are as follows.

First Visit

1. Remove as much calculus, plaque, and debris as possible. Do this as soon as possible and as gently as possible. Ultrasonic or sonic instrumentation are the methods of choice because they provide irrigation and debridement.
2. Instruct the patient in plaque control. Begin patient education and motivation. Have the patient hold the soft

toothbrush under warm water to soften the bristles further and then instruct the patient in the proper use of the brush. Be sure to advise the patient to discard the old toothbrush and to use a new brush.

3. Antibiotics may be administered systemically if there is evidence of elevated temperature, lymphadenopathy, and general malaise. Most cases do not require antibiotics. Mild analgesics may be prescribed for pain.
4. Instruct the patient in specific home care procedures. It is advisable to give the patient a photocopied sheet of specific instructions to be followed at home.

Recommended Home Care Instructions

1. Rinse the mouth vigorously with warm saline solution (1 teaspoon of table salt dissolved in one 8-ounce glass of warm water) every 2 hours.
2. Follow a soft, bland diet of milk, eggnog, broth, and so forth. Dietary supplements (Nutrament, Metrecal, Carnation Instant Breakfasts) are especially useful during this period.
3. Drink plenty of water.
4. Avoid foods that are hard, fried, coarse, spicy, or starchy.
5. Eliminate or reduce smoking and drinking of alcoholic beverages.
6. Rest as much as possible.
7. After eating, rinse the mouth with the warm saline solution.
8. Brush the teeth in the manner prescribed.
9. Return to the dental office after 24 hours.

Second Visit

1. Check oral hygiene and review plaque control procedures.
2. Continue the removal of calculus, plaque, and debris.
3. Polish the teeth.

4. Have the patient return after 24 to 48 hours.

Third Visit

1. Check oral hygiene and review plaque control procedures, if indicated.
2. Continue the elimination of all irritants, which includes all calculus, overhanging margins, and open contacts.
3. If the tissues have not responded dramatically by the third visit (48 to 72 hours), evaluate for systemic factors (e.g., leukemia, infectious mononucleosis, HIV). Refer for medical consultation, if necessary.
4. If improvement is apparent, make an appointment for reevaluation in 7 to 10 days; otherwise, continue to see the patient every 24 to 48 hours.

Fourth Visit

1. Check plaque control.
2. Check for calculus and other irritants. Remove if present.
3. Evaluate for further periodontal treatment.

Necrotizing ulcerative gingivitis responds rapidly and dramatically to local therapy and effective plaque control. As a result, some patients and clinicians become somewhat complacent about the severity of the disease. It is important to remember, and to caution the patient accordingly, that unless the treatment is continued to completion, necrotizing ulcerative gingivitis is likely to recur. Likewise, uncontrolled necrotizing ulcerative gingivitis can result in localized osteonecrosis and extensive soft tissue destruction. Ludwig's angina has been observed in necrotizing ulcerative gingivitis cases among patients with infectious mononucleosis, acute leukemia, uncontrolled diabetes, and HIV infection. For this reason, if necrotizing ulcerative gingivitis has not responded dramatically to local treatment by 72 hours, the patient should be referred for medical consultation.

HYPERSENSITIVITY

Hypersensitivity is often a management problem for both the patient and the dentist. This is true despite the wide variety of medicaments and desensitizing paraphernalia available.

Cause

Hypersensitivity of exposed dentin can occur when dentinal tubules are exposed by caries, fracture, periodontal disease, or periodontal instrumentation. Trauma from occlusion is also a frequent cause of hypersensitivity. Under such circumstances, thermal stimuli (hot or cold foods) and tactile stimuli (toothbrushes and dental instruments) can incite a painful response. It is most discouraging to the patient, and futile for the dentist, to insist on vigorous plaque control when the procedures are painful.

Treatment

Hypersensitivity can be controlled by eliminating the etiologic factors and by using desensitizing agents. Several patient-applied and dentist-applied preparations are available, all of which have some degree of success. One of the first treatments to be considered, especially after surgical procedures, should be occlusal adjustment. Even a slightly heavy occlusal contact can make a tooth or teeth in a recently treated area very sensitive. Refinement of the occlusal contacts often renders immediate relief.

Patient-applied commercial products can be very effective. Strontium chloride and potassium nitrate–containing toothpastes may be used as medicaments, applied for 1 to 2 minutes after regular plaque control procedures. Relief should be achieved within 1 week.

Dentist-applied medicaments include ophthalmic suspensions of prednisolone acetate, sodium fluoride solution, stannous fluoride gels and solutions, sodium fluoride-glycerin-kaolin paste, and dibasic calcium phosphate. Each of these are applied after the sensitive area is polished with a suitable polishing agent. The medicament is then applied with a cotton pledget or porte polisher. Several applications may be needed for complete relief. Local anesthesia may be required before the medicaments can be applied. Refractory cases may need root canal therapy if the tooth is to be retained.

PRIMARY PERIODONTAL TRAUMATISM

Definition

In primary periodontal traumatism, tissue injury (trauma from occlusion) is produced in an otherwise normal periodontium by excessive occlusal force (traumatogenic occlusion). In secondary periodontal traumatism, relatively normal occlusal forces produce injury in a weakened periodontium. In combined periodontal traumatism, excessive occlusal forces produce an injury in a weakened periodontium (in the presence of inflammation). On microscopic examination, the periodontal ligament may demonstrate necrosis, hemorrhage, thrombosis of blood vessels, and dissolution of principal fibers; bone loss and widening of the periodontal ligament space also occur. It should be reemphasized that excessive occlusal stress does not initiate gingivitis and pocket formation.

Signs and Symptoms

Traumatogenic occlusion may result in the following:

1. Pain on chewing.
2. Tenderness to percussion.
3. Sensitivity to temperature change.
4. Tooth mobility.

The symptoms of traumatogenic occlusion are usually localized and are often associated with the recent insertion of a restoration or dental appliance, parafunctional habits, or a recent injury to the jaw or teeth. If the tooth is vital, it is frequently hypersensitive to electrical stimuli.

If excessive occlusal forces are of long duration, the tooth or teeth become mobile, but usually there is little or no pain when chewing and little response to percussion. The traumatized tooth frequently migrates. The patient reports increasing thermal sensitivity and occasionally a dull, aching sensation. Diagnosis can often be made by placing the index finger over the mobile tooth and having the patient glide into working and nonworking excursions. The tooth will move in and out of alignment as the excursions are accomplished (fremitus).

Treatment

Treatment of primary periodontal traumatism consists of eliminating the etiologic factor or factors; this may entail selective grinding of the teeth or removal of the irritating appliance. When the cause was a severe blow, it may be necessary to splint the teeth until the acute symptoms have subsided. Bite guards have been used effectively to manage this problem. Once the traumatogenic force is eliminated, the potential for complete reversibility of the lesion is good. In most cases, root sensitivity will disappear after adjustment of the occlusion. Desensitizing solution is often applied to immediately relieve the sensitivity and to encourage plaque control.

TEMPOROMANDIBULAR JOINT PAIN DYSFUNCTION SYNDROME

Cause

Injury to the temporomandibular joint (TMJ) and the muscles related to the function of the joint may result from an extrinsic source, such as a traumatic blow, or from an intrinsic source, such as a muscle spasm. It is not within the scope of this chapter to discuss the multitude of signs, symptoms, etiologic factors, and therapies proposed for TMJ dysfunctions; however, it is important that all dentists have a basic understanding of this extremely painful and demoralizing condition. It is generally, but not universally, agreed that the cause of the dysfunction pain is a combination of psychic tension and occlusal disharmony. These factors together result in hyperactivity and pain in the masticatory muscles and dysfunction of the jaw. No evidence shows organic changes of the joint, except for degenerative arthritis; consequently, the sequelae are similar to those that occur in any joint complex after long-standing functional disorder.

Symptoms

The clinical syndrome is associated with five symptoms, which may vary from patient to patient:

1. Pain in the region of the TMJ, ear, face, and neck.
2. Cracking or popping noises associated with TMJ movement.
3. Limitation or deviation of mandibular movement (muscle spasm).
4. Subluxation or dislocation of the mandible.
5. Difficulty in mastication of food.

Treatment

Many forms of therapy have been proposed for this problem, and some success has been reported with most methods. Studies continue to indicate that psychological factors play a major role in the onset of most TMJ problems. Consequently, many clinicians are adopting techniques that do not result in irreversible alterations of teeth, muscle, or joint structures, yet afford successful treatment. The following approach is recommended as one concerted but effective method of management of TMJ pain dysfunction syndrome.

1. Talk and listen to the patient. Diagnose the problem. Always take a positive approach to patient management. Assure the patient that the problem can be corrected.
2. Make an impression for a bite guard as soon as possible. The bite guard can be used both as a diagnostic instrument as well as for active therapy.
3. When extensive trismus is present, prescribe a tranquilizer until the trismus subsides. Diazepam (5-mg tablets) is specific for this problem and is the drug of choice if one is needed. It is administered by asking the patient to take one tablet in the morning and one tablet in the evening.
4. Instruct the patient to do the following:
   a. Limit mandibular movements.
   b. Eat a soft diet, avoid incising foods, chew bilaterally.
   c. Avoid yawning. This can be accomplished by clasping the hands on the back of the neck and pulling forward with the arms when the urge to yawn arises. This forces inspiration and usually prevents yawning.
   d. Apply warm, moist heat as often as possible (four to six times daily).
   e. Avoid teeth clenching, pipe smoking, fingernail biting, and so forth.
   f. Relax by walking, jogging, playing tennis, and taking hot showers, hot baths, and sauna baths.
   g. Sleep on one's back.
5. Insert and adjust the bite guard as quickly as possible.
6. Instruct the patient to wear the bite guard 24 hours daily, removing it only to accomplish plaque control.
7. Once the acute symptoms have subsided, ask the patient to continue to wear the bite guard during sleep or during periods of stress.

SUGGESTED READINGS

Cuenin MF, Scheidt MJ, O'Neal RB, et al. An in vivo study of dentin sensitivity: the relation of dentin sensitivity and the patency of dentin tubules. J Periodontol 1991; 62(11):668–673.

Horning GM, Cohen ME. Necrotizing ulcerative gingivitis, periodontitis, and stomatitis: clinical staging and predisposing factors. J Periodontol 1995 Nov;66(11): 990–998.

McLeod DE, Lainson PA, Spivey JD. Tooth loss due to periodontal abscess: a retrospective study. J Periodontol 1997;68(10): 963–966.

Stevens AW Jr, Cogen RB, Cohen-Cole S, Freeman A. Demographic and clinical data associated with acute necrotizing ulcerative gingivitis in a dental school population (ANUG-demographic and clinical data). J Clin Periodontol 1984;11(8): 487–493.

Truelove EL, Sommers EE, LeResche L, et al. Clinical diagnostic criteria for TMD. New classification permits multiple diagnoses. J Am Dent Assoc 1992;123(4):47–54.

Periodontal Maintenance Therapy (Recall)

William J. Killoy

S cientific evidence clearly shows that periodontal treatment can be successful in most patients. One of the major elements of successful periodontal treatment is an effective periodontal maintenance program. In fact, most clinicians feel that periodontal therapy, regardless of the therapeutic procedure, will fail without proper maintenance. Thorough periodontal maintenance is the key to success in periodontal therapy.

RATIONALE FOR A PERIODONTAL MAINTENANCE PROGRAM

During the past two decades, many studies from the University of Michigan, the University of Gothenburg (in Sweden), the University of Minnesota, the University of Nebraska, and a private practice setting in Arizona were performed to evaluate the effectiveness of a variety of surgical and nonsurgical techniques. Of interest, the investigators found no major differences among the various techniques, but they did observe that the deciding factor between success or failure was the frequency and thoroughness of the maintenance therapy provided by the practitioner. These studies noted that the periodontal health of patients who were recalled every 2 weeks to every 3 months and received professional prophylaxis, scaling, and oral hygiene reinforcement could be stabilized. The maximum recall interval for stabilizing periodontal health appeared to be every 3 months. There are occasional exceptions to extending this 3-month interval.

RECALL INTERVAL

The interval between recall appointments must be tailored to each patient's needs. The following are some of the recall sequences used.

One-Week Interval

1. *Immediate post-surgery:* to minimize the effects of plaque in wound healing.
2. *Infection control phase of therapy:* for periodontal disease control.
3. *Acute conditions:* The 1-week interval is most appropriate in the acute therapy phase.

Two-Week Interval

1. Used to minimize the disease process in patients with inadequate oral hygiene.
2. May not be practical for an extended period because of the cost and time involved.

Three-Month Interval

1. The most common recall after active periodontal therapy.
2. Depending on the patient's level of oral hygiene and disease activity, the interval can be increased or decreased.

ELEMENTS OF A PERIODONTAL MAINTENANCE PROGRAM

The maintenance appointment has three distinct parts or phases. First is the examination phase, second is a decision phase, and third is the actual treatment. The treatment phase can be divided into routine and personalized.

All phases of periodontal maintenance are demanding procedures. To do them thoroughly and properly (which is what the patient has the right to expect) takes time. Although it is not possible to project how long maintenance procedures will take in a specific situation, some well-managed and respected periodontal practices assign 60 minutes for the average maintenance appointment. The following can be done in this time frame: seating the patient, history review, clinical examination, plaque evaluation, and routine maintenance therapy. However, the time involved must be adjusted to the patient's personal needs.

During each appointment, a significant amount of time may be spent being courteous and interested in the patient. This time is necessary and well spent because personal attention increases patient rapport and will help to build and maintain a successful practice. Figure 23-1 is an example of a form that provides an excellent method of recording data collected at the maintenance visit. The form also allows recording of the treatment rendered and future recommendations.

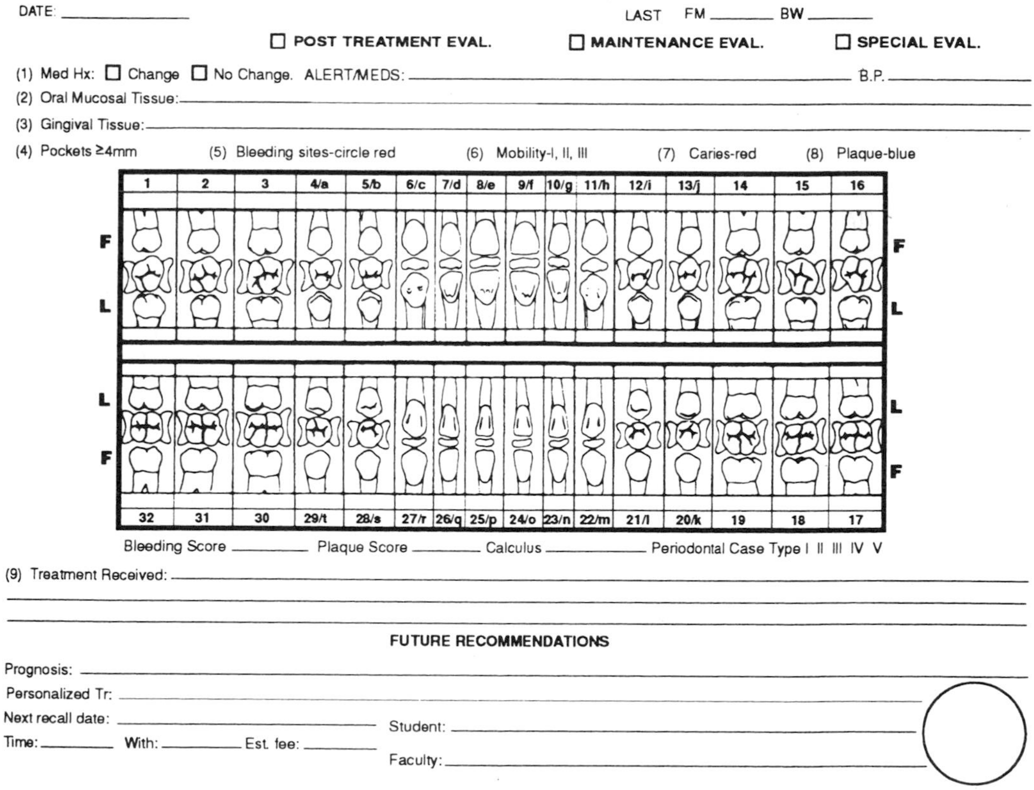

DATE: _____

LAST   FM _____   BW _____

☐ POST TREATMENT EVAL.   ☐ MAINTENANCE EVAL.   ☐ SPECIAL EVAL.

(1) Med Hx: ☐ Change ☐ No Change. ALERT/MEDS: _____ B.P. _____

(2) Oral Mucosal Tissue: _____

(3) Gingival Tissue: _____

(4) Pockets ≥4mm   (5) Bleeding sites-circle red   (6) Mobility-I, II, III   (7) Caries-red   (8) Plaque-blue

Bleeding Score _____ Plaque Score _____ Calculus _____ Periodontal Case Type I II III IV V

(9) Treatment Received: _____

FUTURE RECOMMENDATIONS

Prognosis: _____

Personalized Tr: _____

Next recall date: _____   Student: _____

Time: _____ With: _____ Est. fee: _____   Faculty: _____

Fig. 23-1

Examination Phase

Before treatment or re-treatment of any patient, review of the medical history is mandatory. Patients may have had significant changes in their medical status between appointments. Some of these medical problems can be life-threatening under the stress of a routine dental appointment. Systemic risk factors, such as smoking and diabetes, should also be assessed.

It is also advisable to review the nature of the dental treatment the patient has previously received and the prognosis assigned to the dentition and individual teeth.

Next, the current dental and periodontal status of the patient must be determined. An examination sequence that permits a thorough evaluation of the patient should be followed. The following sequence is one that has proven reliable for many practitioners:

1. *Tissue examination.* This is done before any plaque indicator (red or other-colored dye) is applied to the teeth and gingiva. Observe tissue color, contour, and consistency. Record only the observations that vary from normal limits.
2. *Probing depths.* Probe all areas and record 4-mm depths on the dental chart.
3. *Bleeding and/or suppuration sites.* After probing a small segment of the mouth (4 to 6 teeth), look for bleeding (and suppuration) sites. These bleeding sites should be recorded by circling the probing depth in red. If bleeding occurs at a site with an unrecorded depth of less than 4 mm, simply circle the space where a recording would have been made. Even shallow sulci can be infected and show bleeding upon gentle probing. Identification and treatment of these areas ensure maintenance of periodontal health. By comparing bleeding sites from visit to visit, fluctuating problems can be observed, as well as persistent and serious problem areas. Bleeding is a sign of existing disease and must be addressed in therapy. Areas that continually bleed are major problems, are more likely to break down, and demand immediate, active, and aggressive treatment. Sites that bleed only occasionally also need immediate attention but may not be as serious a problem. Sites that seldom if ever bleed are apt to be stable indefinitely.
4. *Tooth mobility.* Measure tooth movement by applying force on the tooth, faciolingually. Two dental instrument handles can be used. Mobility should be recorded according to the criteria in Chapter 6.
5. *Furcations.* Determine and record health status of each furcation. The more severe the furcation involvement, the more difficult the treatment and worse the prognosis. Because furcation involvement seldom disappear, previous records are important.
6. *Caries.* At all recall appointments, as well as at the initial examination, examine for caries. Record the findings in the dental record. Be particularly aware of root caries and caries beneath crowns.
7. *Radiographs.* Routine bite-wing radiographs should not be taken more than once a year. Vertical bite-wing radiographs will provide a better picture of the alveolar bone and are preferred over standard bite-wings in periodontics. Full-mouth radiographs should be taken whenever required, but seldom more frequently than every 3 years. A guide to radiographs would be the following:
   a. Initial examination: Full-mouth radiographs and four posterior vertical bite-wings (these may or may not be supplemented with a pantographic radiograph).
   b. First year: Four vertical posterior bite-wings.
   c. Second year: Anterior and posterior vertical bite-wings.

d. Third year: Four vertical posterior bite-wings.

e. Fourth year: Full-mouth radiographs and four posterior vertical bite-wings.

8. *Plaque evaluation.* After performing the entire clinical examination, complete a plaque evaluation. The sequencing is important because the dyes usually used in plaque detection will color the teeth and especially the soft tissue, thereby making a clinical examination of the tissue color and tone difficult. All sites with plaque present can be recorded on an oral hygiene chart and the plaque index calculated. The oral hygiene chart will show areas that patients have difficulty in cleaning. The plaque index can be used to demonstrate, to patients, how well they are performing plaque control procedures.

Decision Phase

On the basis of the findings, the clinician must decide what routine maintenance treatment should be provided and whether special or personalized treatment is necessary. Decisions to reactivate the patient may also be required. A decision regarding when the patient should return for future maintenance must also be made. A decision matrix specified for guiding maintenance treatment and adjusting the maintenance interval is provided in Table 23-1.

Treatment Phase

Routine Maintenance Therapy

1. *Oral hygiene instructions.* At each visit, oral hygiene instruction is tailored to the individual needs of each patient. Some patients will always need reinforcement and encouragement. Refer to Chapter 7 for a discussion of plaque control.

2. *Polishing.* Almost all the plaque and stain can be removed with a polishing cup charged with a polishing agent. The air-powder abrasive instruments effectively remove plaque and stain by spraying a solution or paste of water and sodium bicarbonate crystals on the clinical crowns of teeth. The abrasive action of this instrument appears to be helpful in the rapid removal of plaque and stain from supragingival surface. As with any instrument, if used improperly, an excessive amount of cementum and dentin may be removed from the exposed root surfaces.

3. *Scaling.* All interproximal and subgingival areas must be thoroughly debrided. Areas of deepened pockets will require actual root detoxification (root planing). Refer to Chapter 8 for a discussion of root preparation.

4. *Adjuncts to maintenance therapy.*

a. Irrigation: Chlorhexidine has been shown to be an effective antiseptic with the ability to bind to hard and soft tissue releasing the active component for up to 12 hours. Subgingival irrigation of pockets will help in the suppression of periodontopathic microorganisms. Irrigation can be delivered during the scaling in the coolant/irrigation of modern ultrasonic instruments or can be performed after the scaling procedure with irrigating devices.

b. Antimicrobial application: A 1.64% stannous fluoride solution has been shown to significantly decrease the percentages of spirochetes and motile rods in periodontal pockets for an extended period. Placing stannous fluoride subgingivally by means of an irrigation syringe has the potential of reducing microorganisms that may have been left behind, after scaling and root detoxification procedures. If used in addition to chlorhexidine, the stan-

Table 23-1   Decision Matrix for Periodontal Maintenance Therapy

MM PD	PD Changes	Bleeding Status	Treatment	Recall Interval
0–3	Constant	None	1. Routine (polish, light scale)	Same or lengthen (3–12 months)
0–3	Constant	Bleeds	1. Routine	Shorten if bleeding is repetitive in area (1–3 months)
			2. Root plane	
			3. Review oral hygiene	
3–5	Constant	None	1. Routine	Same or lengthen (3–6 months)
3–5	Constant or Increases	Bleeds	1. Routine	Shorten (1/2–3 months)
			2. Root plane with anesthesia	
			3. Review oral hygiene	
			4. Advise patient	
5+	Constant	None	1. Routine	Same (3–4 months)
			2. Irrigation	
			3. Advise patient	
5+	Constant or Increases ≤1 mm	Bleeds	1. Routine	Shorten (1–3 months)
			2. Root plane with anesthesia, and/or tetracycline fiber	
			3. Local delivery of an antimicrobial agent	
			4. Review oral hygiene	
			5. Advise patient	
5+	Increase >1 mm	Bleeds	1. Routine	Shorten (1–3 months)
			2. Root plane with anesthesia, and/or chemical curettage	
			3. Local delivery of an antimicrobial agent	
			4. Review oral hygiene	
			5. Surgery	
			6. Systemic Antibiotics	

MM = millimeter; PD= probing depth.

nous fluoride application should always follow the chlorhexidine irrigation.

c. Topical fluorides: Topical fluorides are applied by brushing or in trays to control dental caries and the supragingival microorganisms.

Personalized Maintenance Treatment

1. *Controlled local delivery of antimicrobial agents.*
   a. Tetracycline fibers (Actisite): A nondegradable polymer fiber 25% saturated with tetracycline hydrochloride has been in use for many years.
   b. Chlorhexidine chip (PerioChip): A biodegradable gelatin chip containing 2.5 mg of chlorhexidine gluco-

nate has been approved for the treatment of periodontitis.
   c. Doxycycline polymer (Atridox): A biodegradable gel polymer containing doxycycline hyclate is being studied and is expected to be approved soon

Research is continuing on other products that will deliver antimicrobial agents subgingivally in a biodegradable matrix.

For local delivery systems of these agents, the future is now. When placed subgingivally, these fibers, chips, and polymers have demonstrated efficiency in reducing probing depths, stabilizing attachment levels, and reducing bleeding on probing. These local delivery systems provide another option to re-treatment of the non-maintainable local pocket. For a more thorough discussion of local delivery systems, see Chapter 12.

2. *Periodontal surgery.* Site-specific surgical therapy is occasionally needed as part of the maintenance phase of treatment. The clinician should not be reluctant to recommend a surgical procedure that is clearly needed in those nonmaintainable areas to extend the life of the dentition.

3. *Systemic antibiotic therapy.* A small percentage of patients do not respond to thorough periodontal therapy and are considered refractory. Assuming the treatment has been thorough up to this point, systemic antibiotic therapy may be indicated in these patients to bring the disease under control. A variety of antibiotics have been used to successfully treat these refractory patients. These have included tetracyclines, metronidazole, amoxicillin, amoxicillin–clavulanate potassium, and combinations of amoxicillin or Augmentin with metronidazole. To best determine the proper antibiotic to use culture and sensitivity testing is recommended. Universities in Atlanta, Los Angeles, and Philadelphia offer this microbiological testing.

THE EFFECT OF AN EXCELLENT MAINTENANCE PROGRAM ON TOTAL DENTAL HEALTH

The 6-year data from the studies performed in Sweden showed that following active periodontal therapy and a thorough maintenance program performed every 2 to 3 months stabilized periodontal disease in an adult population. The effect of this maintenance program on caries reduction was also very impressive. The group of patients on the two- to three-mount regular maintenance program had 61 times less caries experience than the control group, which received traditional dental care.

There is no doubt that the maintenance aspect of therapy is a valuable and effective service for dental patients. Maintenance deserves the highest priority in the daily practice of dentistry.

SUGGESTED READINGS

Axelsson P, Lindhe J. Effect of controlled oral hygiene procedures on caries and periodontal disease in adults. Results after 6 years. J Clin Periodontol 1981;8:239–248.

Axelsson P, Lindhe J. The significance of maintenance care in the treatment of periodontal disease. J Clin Periodontol 1981;8:281–294.

Becker W, Becker B, Berg L. Periodontal treatment with and without maintenance: a retrospective study in 44 patients. J Periodontol 1984;55:505–509.

Becker B, Becker W, Caffesse R, et al. Three modalities of periodontal therapy: five years final result [Abstract]. J Dent Res 1990;69(Spec Issue).

Becker W, Becker BE, Ochsenbein C, et al. A longitudinal study comparing scaling, osseous surgery and modified Widman procedures. Results after one year. J Periodontol 1988;59:351–365.

Garrett S, Johnson L, Drisko CH, et al. Two multicenter studies evaluating locally delivered doxycycline hyclate, placebo control, oral hygiene, and scaling and root planing in the treatment of periodontitis. J Periodontol 1999;70:490–503.

Goodson JM, Cugini MA, Kent RL, et al. Multicenter evaluation of tetracycline fiber therapy. I. Experimental design, methods, and baseline data. J Periodontol Res 1991;26:361–370.

Goodson JM, Cugini MA, Kent RL, et al. Multicenter evaluation of tetracycline fiber therapy. II. Clinical response. J Periodontol Res 1991;26:371–379.

Goodson JM, Haffajee A, Socransky SS. Periodontal therapy by local delivery of tetracycline. J Clin Periodontol 1979;6:83–92.

Hill RW, Ramfjord SP, Morrison EC, et al. Four types of periodontal treatment compared over two years. J Periodontol 1981;52:655–662.

Hirshfeld L, Wasserman B. A long term survey of tooth loss in 600 treated periodontal patients. J Periodontol 1978;49:225–237.

Jeffcoat MK, Bray KS, Ciancio SG, et al. Adjunctive use of a subgingival controlled-release chlorhexidine chip (PerioChip) reduces probing pocket depth and improves attachment level compared with scaling and root planing alone. J Periodontol 1998;69: 989–997.

Kaldahl WB, Kalkwarf KL, Patil KD, et al. Long-term evaluation of periodontal therapy. I. Response to 4 therapeutic modalities. J Periodontol 1996;67:93–102.

Kaldahl WB, Kalkwarf KL, Patil KD, et al. Long-term evaluation of periodontal therapy. II. Incidence of sites breaking-down. J Periodontol 1996;67:103–108.

Killoy W, Cobb C. Controlled local delivery of tetracycline in the treatment of periodontitis. Compend Cont Ed Dent 1992;13:1150–1160.

Killoy WJ, Polson AM. Controlled local delivery of antimicrobials in the treatment of periodontitis. Dent Clin North Am 1998;42: 263–283.

Knowles J, Burgett F, Morrison E, et al. Comparison of results following three modalities of periodontal therapy related to tooth type and initial pocket depth. J Clin Periodontol 1980;7:32–47.

Lang N, Joss A, Orsanic T, et al. Bleeding on probing. A predictor for the progression of periodontal disease. J Clin Periodontol 1986;13:590–596.

Lindhe J, Westfelt E, Nyman S, et al. Long-term effect of surgical/nonsurgical treatment of periodontal disease. J Clin Periodontol 1984;11:448–458.

Mazza JE, Newman MG, Sims TN. Clinical and antimicrobial effect of stannous fluoride on periodontitis. J Clin Periodontol 1981;8: 203–212.

Newman MG, Kornman KS, Doherty FM. A 6-month multicenter evaluation of adjunctive tetracycline fiber therapy used in conjunction with scaling and root planing in maintenance patient: clinical results. J Periodontol 1994;65:685–691.

Pihlstrom BL, McHugh RB, Oliphant TH, et al. Comparison of surgical and nonsurgical treatment of periodontal disease. A review of current studies and additional results after 6½ years. J Clin Periodontol 1983;10: 524–541.

Schallhorn R, Snider L. Periodontal maintenance therapy. J Am Dent Assoc 1981;103: 227.

Soskolne W, Heasman P, Stabholz A, et al. Sustained local delivery of chlorhexidine in the treatment of periodontitis: a multicenter study. J Periodontol 1997;68:32–38.

Wilson T, Glover M, Schoen J, et al. Compliance with maintenance therapy in a private periodontal practice. J Periodontol 1984; 55:468–473.

Mucocutaneous Diseases of the Periodontium

Terry Rees

The tissues of the oral cavity are susceptible to many autoimmune or immunologically mediated diseases that affect the skin and mucous membranes. Several of these disorders may affect the periodontal soft tissues as part of their overall oral manifestations. The conditions often present similar clinical features, and careful diagnosis is required. The following conditions are discussed in this chapter:

Lichen planus.
Chronic ulcerative stomatitis.
Cicatricial pemphigoid (benign mucous membrane pemphigoid).
Pemphigus vulgaris.
Lupus erythematosus.
Erythema multiforme.

LICHEN PLANUS

Lichen planus is a chronic inflammatory condition of unknown cause. It affects 1 to 2% of the population, and lesions may occur on skin or oral mucosa alone or in combination. A relationship with emotional and environmental stress has been suggested, but study results are inconclusive to date. A vulvovaginal-gingival syndrome has been described, and women with oral lichen planus should probably be referred for gynecologic ex-

amination. Skin lesions usually manifest as violaceous, pruritic papules that are generally transient, disappearing spontaneously within 1 to 2 years of onset. In contrast, oral lesions may persist for many years, and their clinical appearance may change. Lesions are more common in women, and they generally affect individuals older than 50 years of age.

Oral lesions may manifest as asymptomatic papular, reticular, or plaque-like white lesions, but they also occur in painful atrophic, ulcerative, or bullous forms. Reticular lesions occur most frequently, and bullous lesions are the least common (Fig. 24-1). For the purpose of this discussion, the atrophic, ulcerative, and bullous forms are grouped under the term *erosive lichen planus*.

Lichen planus can affect any surface of the oral cavity, although buccal mucosal lesions are most common. Erosive lesions, however, may frequently affect the gingiva and give the clinical appearance of desquamative gingivitis (sloughing of the gingival tissue surface) (Fig. 24-2). Histologic examination of lichen planus reveals thickening of the epithelium (acanthosis with hyperorthokeratosis), a saw-toothed configuration of epithelial rete ridges, and liquefaction degeneration of the epithelial basal cell layer. The degeneration of the epithelial basal cells accounts for the tendency of the surface lesional tissue to slough when traumatized. Underlying connective tissue features a dense band of lymphocytic inflammatory cells immediately subjacent to the basement membrane. If dysplastic changes are found, these areas should be carefully monitored and re-biopsied in event of any significant changes in appearance. Direct immunofluorescence of a portion of the biopsy specimen may help establish the diagnosis by identifying the presence of fibrinogen in a linear pattern in the basal membrane zone or the presence of immuno-positive cytoid bodies in underlying connective tissues.

Several studies have suggested a possible relationship between oral lichen planus and chronic hepatitis, especially that induced by the hepatitis C virus. Some data suggest, however, that this relationship may be induced by a lichenoid reaction to interferon and other drugs used to treat chronic hepatitis. In general, drug-induced hypersensitivity reactions will manifest with clinical, histologic, and immunofluorescence features consistent with idiopathic lichen planus. These reactions commonly occur with antihypertensive medications and nonsteroidal anti-inflammatory agents. In recent years, several studies and case reports have described an association between dental restorations, especially silver amalgam, and localized lichenoid reactions in tissue directly contacting the restoration to which the patient is hypersensitive (Fig. 24-3A and B). There are also reports of lichenoid reactions to flavoring agents, such as cinnamic aldehyde, used in many toothpastes, mouthrinses, soft drinks, candies, and chewing gums.

The painless forms of lichen planus usually do not require treatment. Proper management of erosive lichen planus requires a careful diagnosis, elimination of drugs or other agents that may be causing a lichenoid reaction, control of local irritants, and application of topical or systemic corticosteroid therapy. Other therapies have been reported as sometimes successful, but not with the consistency of corticosteroids. Therapeutic goals are directed toward elimination of erosive lesions and control of the painless forms of the disease. Lesions tend to recur, and long-term patient recall is necessary for this reason. Recall is also needed to monitor affected patients for any tissue changes suggestive of possible malignant transformation.

CHRONIC ULCERATIVE STOMATITIS

Chronic ulcerative stomatitis is a newly described autoimmune disease of the oral mucosa that may induce desquamative gingivitis closely resembling erosive lichen planus or oral lupus erythematosus in its clinical and histologic manifestations (Fig. 24-4A and B). Diagnosis is generally based on specific direct and indirect immunofluorescence tests. Chronic ulcerative stomatitis should be suspected in patients who do not respond to routine therapy for lichen planus. Such patients should be referred to a dermatologist or oral medicine expert for diagnostic confirmation and treatment. Treatment may include topical corticosteroid, systemic corticosteroid, or antimalarial therapy.

BENIGN MUCOUS MEMBRANE PEMPHIGOID (CICATRICIAL PEMPHIGOID)

Cicatricial pemphigoid is the term preferred by dermatopathologists for a distinct chronic vesiculobullous disorder of the elderly that usually affects mucous membrane. Oral pathologists tend to prefer the term *benign mucous membrane pemphigoid* for the same condition. The condition is autoimmune in origin, and oral lesions are almost invariably present. On occasion, concomitant lesions may affect the conjunctiva of the eye, the skin, genitalia, rectum, nares, larynx, or esophagus. Although oral lesions rarely heal with scarring, conjunctival scarring (symblepharon) can lead to loss of vision. For this reason, early ophthalmologic evaluation is an essential component in management of this disease.

Lesions may occur on any mouth tissues. The gingiva is the most common target site, with involvement in approximately 97% of reported oral cases. Gingival lesions often feature blistering and loss of the epithelial surface in response to trauma (Nikolsky's sign). This leaves raw, painful erythematous gingival surfaces (Fig. 24-5). Blistering and ulceration may affect other mucosal tissues as well.

Histologic examination of cicatricial pemphigoid reveals a separation of the surface epithelium from underlying connective tissue by a split just beneath the epithelial basal cell layer. Direct immunofluorescence reveals the presence of IgG and complement in a linear pattern at the basal membrane zone of the tissue.

Treatment depends on the severity and responsiveness of the oral lesions. Topical or intralesional corticosteroid therapy should be applied, but systemic intervention is often necessary. Corticosteroids are most commonly used for systemic therapy, but dapsone has also been used with some success. Meticulous oral hygiene is very important in managing oral cicatricial pemphigoid, but patients often have difficulty with oral physiotherapy because of gingival discomfort. Frequent, gentle interoffice debridement and scaling is often necessary to help promote patient comfort. The dentist is the health care provider best qualified to evaluate progress in management of the oral condition.

Bullous pemphigoid is a related condition that usually affects skin as the primary site, although oral mucosal lesions may occur. Oral lesions are very similar in appearance to cicatricial pemphigoid clinically, histologically, and by direct immunofluorescence. Diagnosis is usually based on skin manifestations and by the presence of circulating immunoglobulins (indirect immunofluorescence) in approximately 70% of affected patients. Systemic therapy is usually required.

PEMPHIGUS VULGARIS

The term *pemphigus* refers to a group of autoimmune vesiculobullous diseases that affect mucosa and skin. Pemphigus vulgaris is the most common and severe form of the disorder. It can occur at any age but it is more common in adults between the fourth and sixth decades. Skin lesions manifest as large bullae that rupture and leave eroded, weeping wounds. These wounds may significantly alter the patient's fluid and electrolyte balance and may become secondarily infected. Pemphigus vulgaris is fatal in 5 to 15% of affected patients.

Oral lesions are common, and they often precede skin manifestations. Early diagnosis and treatment of oral lesions may enable afflicted patients to avoid the more serious effects of the disease. Oral lesions are similar to those occurring on the skin. Blisters develop and burst quickly, leaving painful eroded areas with irregular borders (Fig. 24-6). Gingival desquamative lesions are common and are sometimes the only manifestation of the disease (Fig. 24-7).

Histologic examination of pemphigus vulgaris reveals separation of the cells of the epithelium (acantholysis) and blistering within the epithelium above the basal cell layer. Direct immunofluorescence reveals a distinct pattern of IgG and complement located between the cells of the epithelium. In this and other autoimmune mucocutaneous diseases, immunofluorescence findings may be positive even in clinically normal mucosa.

Systemic corticosteroid therapy is frequently used to treat pemphigus vulgaris, although favorable results have also been reported with a variety of other immuno-suppressive agents. Again, maintenance of meticulous oral hygiene is important for patient comfort.

Pemphigus vulgaris–like lesions have been associated with such medications as captopril and penicillamine; an association between pemphigus vulgaris and underlying cancer has been identified in some cases. Paraneoplastic pemphigus lesions may be present exclusively in the oral cavity because of the presence of a variety of underlying benign or malignant neoplasms (Fig. 24-8).

LUPUS ERYTHEMATOSUS

Lupus erythematosus is an autoimmune disease that may involve the skin, the mucosa, and multiple body systems. It occurs more commonly in women and in black persons. The discoid form of the disease exclusively involves skin and mucosa. Mouth lesions are common. In systemic lupus erythematosus, various organ systems may be involved and oral lesions are present in 25 to 40% of affected patients. Typical oral lesions in either form of lupus erythematosus are characterized by a central erythematous erosion or ulceration surrounded by radiating keratotic striae (Fig. 24-9). The gingiva may appear erythematous, and lupus erythematosus can easily be clinically misdiagnosed as one of the desquamative diseases described previously (Fig. 24-10).

Diagnosis is based on clinical, histologic, and immunologic data. Microscopic features include hyperkeratosis, atrophy of rete ridges, and liquefaction degeneration of the basal layer of epithelium. A band-like lymphocytic inflammatory infiltrate is evident in superficial connective tissue. These features are similar in some respects to lichen planus, and a lichen planus/lupus erythematosus overlap condition has been described, in which exact diagnosis is difficult.

Direct immunofluorescence discloses granular deposits of IgG, complement, and fibrinogen in the basement membrane zone, thus displaying features that might be confused with cicatricial pemphigoid.

Because of the similarities in the oral features of lupus erythematosus, lichen planus, and cicatricial pemphigoid, treatment must occasionally be empiric. Oral and skin lupus erythematosus may respond to topical or systemic corticosteroid therapy, but results are unpredictable. Antimalarial drugs sometimes yield satisfactory therapeutic results, as do immunosuppressive or cytotoxic drugs.

ERYTHEMA MULTIFORME

Erythema multiforme is an acute, inflammatory, mucocutaneous disorder that may manifest with distinct, "target" lesions of skin, with or without mucosal involvement. A target skin lesion appears as a central dusky-red zone surrounded by a raised, circumferential, erythematous zone. The oral cavity may be involved and dentists often encounter patients with oral lesions in the absence of skin manifestations. Mouth lesions appear as bullae that burst rapidly and leave erythematous erosions and ulcerations that develop a grayish pseudomembrane, creating a "parboiled" appearance. Hemorrhagic crusting of the lips is common. In the major form of erythema multiforme (Stevens-Johnson syndrome), lesions may also occur on the genitalia and conjunctiva, and multiorgan involvement may be present.

The condition is believed to represent a hypersensitivity reaction to an antigen that may or may not be identifiable. Sulfonamide drugs have been implicated, as have many additional drugs, including antibiotics and anticoagulants. Occasionally erythema multiforme is preceded by bacterial or viral infections, and recent outbreaks of herpes simplex virus lesions have been described preceding the development of erythema multiforme.

Clinically, patients with erythema multiforme may experience prodromal symptoms such as fever, headache, and general malaise. Once lesions begin to occur, full development may take 10 days to several months. Spontaneous remission may occur 2 to 3 weeks after onset but may also take many months.

The histopathologic and immunofluorescence features of erythema multiforme are not specific, and diagnosis is often based on clinical features. Erythema multiforme can be differentiated from the other bullous diseases by its acute onset, by the presence of target skin lesions, and, occasionally, by the presence of slight fever. When lesions are confined to the oral cavity, however, the clinical features may be similar to those encountered in primary herpetic gingivostomatitis (Fig. 24-11A and B). Once the diagnosis is established, treatment usually includes administration of systemic corticosteroid therapy and elimination of any drug associated with disease onset.

SUMMARY

Mucocutaneous diseases are relatively uncommon, yet they occur with sufficient frequency to suggest that all dentists and dental hygienists will encounter them in clinical practice. Many of these diseases produce gingival and other soft tissue lesions that require careful differential diagnosis and knowledgeable management. Primary management responsibility may rest in the hands of a physician or an oral medicine specialist, but all dental health care providers share in the responsibility for successful management of these troublesome disorders.

SUGGESTED READINGS

Axell T, Rundquist L. Oral lichen planus: a demographic study. Comm Dent Oral Epidemiol 1987;15:52–56.

Barnett ML. Pemphigus vulgaris presenting as a gingival lesion. J Periodontol 1987;59:611–614.

Daniels TE, Quadra-White C. Direct immunofluorescence in oral mucosal disease: a diagnostic analysis of 130 cases. Oral Surg Oral Med Oral Pathol Oral Radiol Endod 1981;51:38–47.

Eisen D. The vulvovaginal syndrome of lichen planus. The clinical characteristics of 22 patients. Arch Dermatol 1994;130:1379–1382.

Holmstrup P, Thorn JJ, Rindum J, et al. Malignant development of lichen planus-affected oral mucosa. J Oral Pathol 1988;17:219–225.

Lamey PJ, Rees TD, Binnie WH, et al. Mucous membrane pemphigoid. Treatment experience at two institutions. Oral Surg Oral Med Oral Pathol Oral Radiol Endod 1992;74:50–53.

Lamey PJ, Rees TD, Binnie WH, et al. Oral presentation of pemphigus vulgaris and its response to systemic steroid therapy. Oral Surg Oral Med Oral Pathol Oral Radiol Endod 1992;74:54–57.

Lemak MA, Duvic M, Bean SF. Oral acyclovir for the prevention of herpes-associated erythema multiforme. J Am Acad Dermatol 1986;15:50–54.

Lewis JE, Beutner EH, Rostami R, et al. Chronic ulcerative stomatitis with stratified epithelium-specific antinuclear antibodies. Int J Dermatol 1996;35:272–275.

Plemons JM. Position paper of the American Academy of Periodontology. Vesiculobullous diseases of the oral cavity. Chicago: American Academy of Periodontology, 1999. (In press).

Rees TD. Drugs and oral disorders. Periodontology 1998;18:21–36.

Rees TD. Phenothiazine: another possible etiologic agent in erythema multiforme. Report of a case. J Periodontol 1985;56:480–483.

Robinson JC, Lozada-Nur F, Frieden I. Oral pemphigus vulgaris. Oral Surg Oral Med Oral Pathol Oral Radiol Endod 1997;84:349–355.

Rojo-Moreno JL, Bagan JV, Rojo-Moreno J, et al. Psychologic factors and oral lichen planus. Oral Surg Oral Med Oral Pathol Oral Radiol Endod 1998;86:687–691.

Schiodt M. Oral discoid lupus erythematosus. II. Skin lesions and systemic oral lupus erythematosus in sixty-six patients with six-year follow-up. Oral Surg Oral Med Oral Pathol Oral Radiol Endod 1984;57: 177–180.

Silverman S, Gorsky M, Lozada-Nur F. Oral mucous membrane pemphigoid. Oral Surg Oral Med Oral Pathol Oral Radiol Endod 1986;61:233–237.

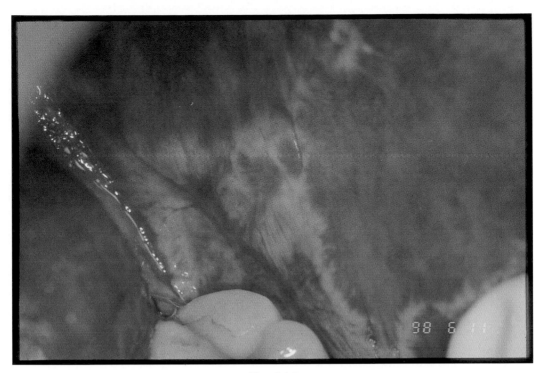

Fig. 24-1

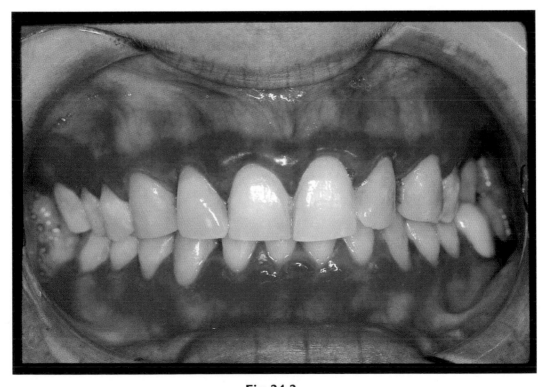

Fig. 24-2

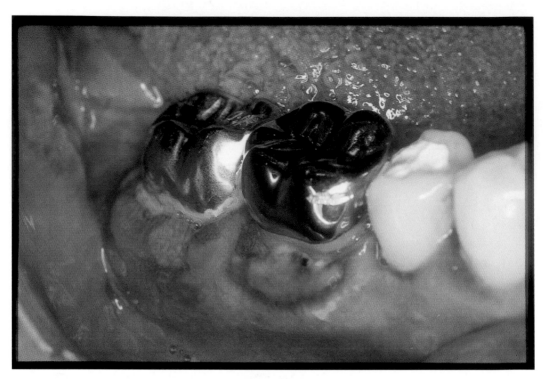

Fig. 24-3A

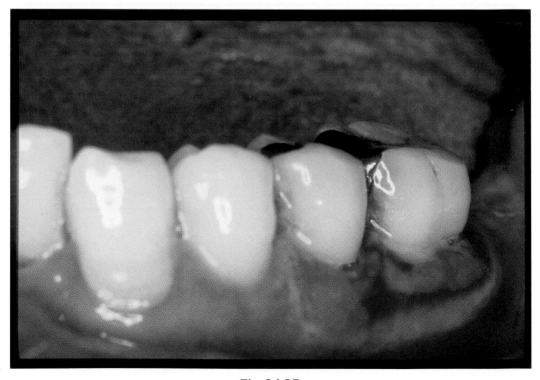

Fig. 24-3B

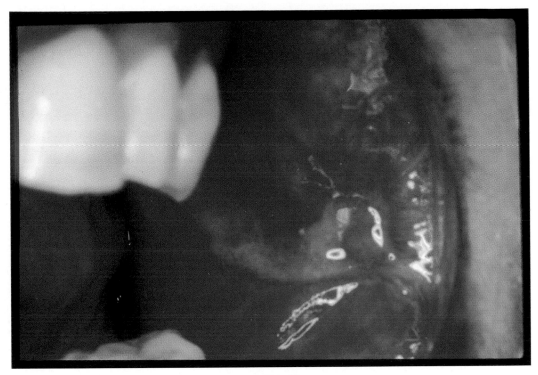

Fig. 24-4A

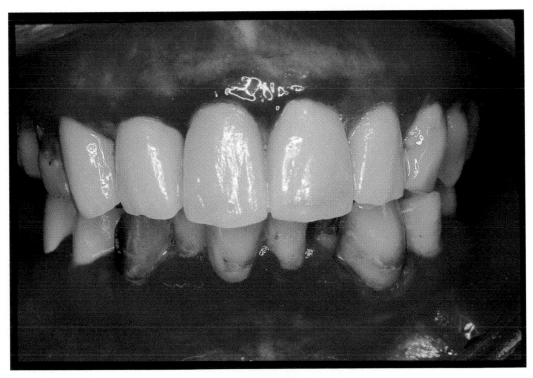

Fig. 24-4B

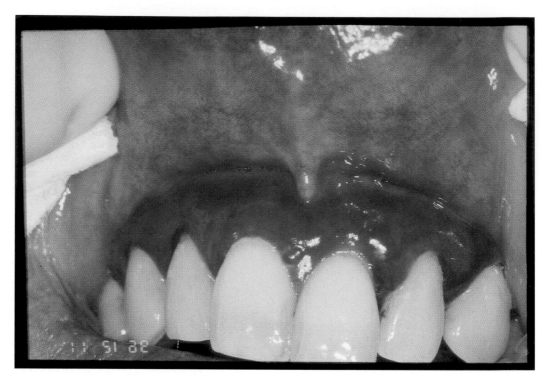

Fig. 24-5

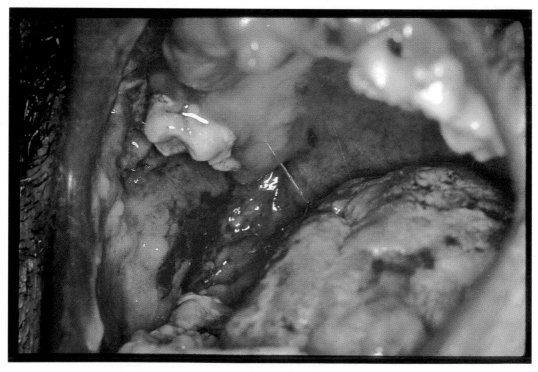

Fig. 24-6

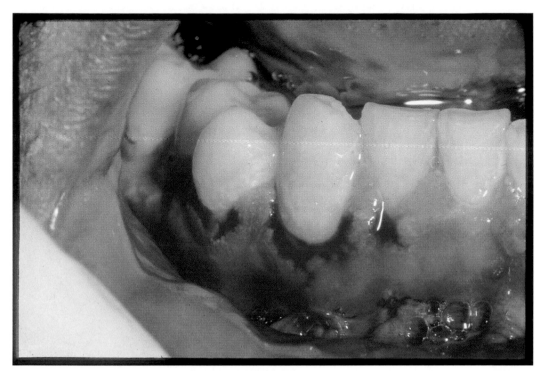

Fig. 24-7

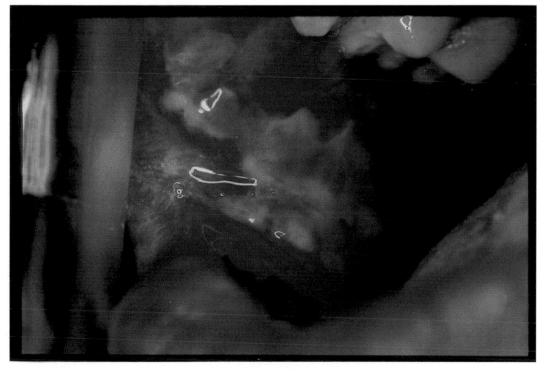

Fig. 24-8

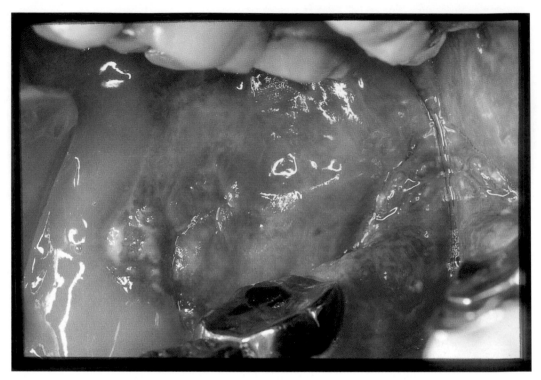

Fig. 24-9

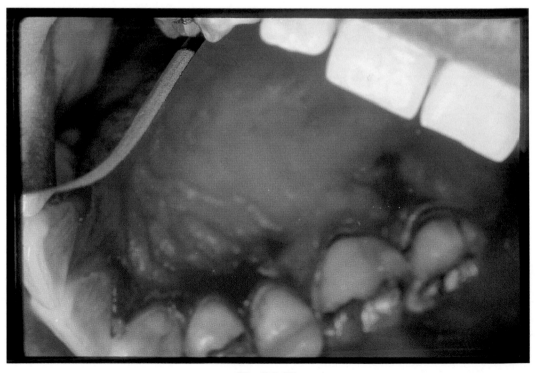

Fig. 24-10

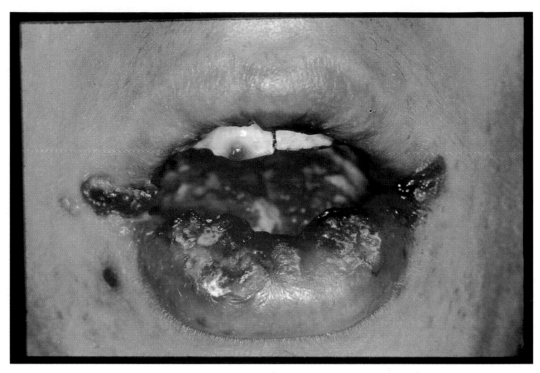

Fig. 24-11A

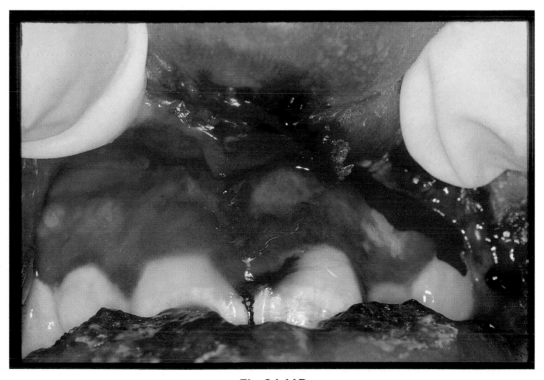

Fig. 24-11B

Instrument Sharpening

Sherry Burns

FACTORS FOR CONSIDERATION

Dental clinicians recognize the many benefits of using properly sharpened instruments in providing high-quality periodontal therapy. Sharp cutting edges will ease the work, improve the quality of the technique, expedite instrumentation, and increase patient and practitioner satisfaction.

Three main factors must be carefully considered: the specific features of instrument design, methods to assess a sharp cutting edge, and the characteristics of the sharpening stones.

INSTRUMENT DESIGN

The terminal shank is the specific segment that extends between the blade and the first angle (or bend) in the shank located closest to the blade. In Figure 25-1, the terminal shanks of the various instruments are identified between the dotted lines. The key feature of each individual scaler and curet is the terminal shank, which determines the position and angulation of the blade in relationship to the handle. To effectively use any instrument, the clinician must be fully aware of the length, strength, and angulation of the terminal shank. In sharpening procedures and instrumentation techniques, the terminal shank provides a visual cue for the practitioner to assess correct angulation of the blade.

Each instrument in the Gracey Periodontal Finishing Curet Series is distinguished by the unique length and angle of the terminal shank. To effectively adapt the lower cutting edge of any Gracey curet, the clinician only has to focus on the alignment of the terminal shank in relation to the tooth surface. When the terminal shank is held parallel to the surface being instrumented, the 60- to 70-degree offset blade automatically places the lower cutting edge in the correct position for instrumentation.

The practitioner must carefully observe the contours of the Gracey blade from many different perspectives. When one is looking down on the face, the blade may appear to have a long, continuous curvature from the heel to the toe (Fig. 25-2, view #1). However, this perceived curvature may be an optical illusion.

When the same blade is examined from a different vantage point, the cutting edge forms a straight line from the heel to the toe (Fig. 25-2, view #2). The cutting edge of a posterior Gracey curet appears to have a greater curvature in the heel one-third of the blade as it turns off the terminal shank, and then a straight edge in the middle one-third to the toe one-third of the blade (Fig. 25-2, view #1).

The blade, shank designs, and dimensions of any instrument may vary among

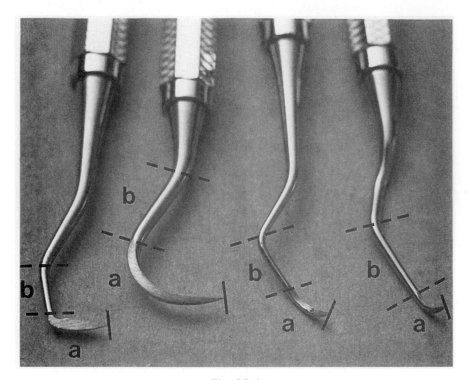

Fig. 25-1

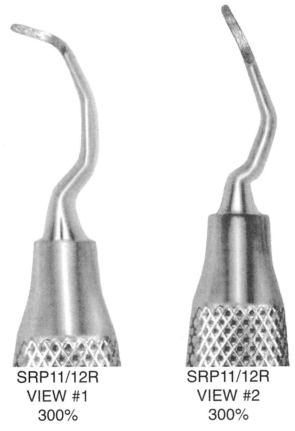

SRP11/12R
VIEW #1
300%

SRP11/12R
VIEW #2
300%

Fig. 25-2

different manufacturers. It is essential to scrutinize the blade contours of each new instrument and to form a mental image of the original dimensions so they may be retained during the sharpening process.

METHODS TO ASSESS SHARPNESS

Minute particles of metal are torn away from the cutting edge when the instrument is repeatedly pulled over rough calculus deposits and hard tooth surfaces. The sharp cutting edge takes on a rounded shape, resulting in a dull, ineffective blade (Fig. 25-3).

Effectiveness of Instrumentation

As the dulling process begins to occur, the clinician loses the ability to "feel" the sharp edge "grabbing" onto a surface. The tactile sensation becomes one of sliding over the surface or deposit. The practi-

tioner's automatic response is to work harder by applying more lateral pressure against the surface. The patient may exhibit some discomfort or may perceive this increased pressure to be due to a rough or heavy-handed operator. The clinician will become more fatigued and frustrated because the procedure will require more time to complete while more energy is expended.

Plastic Test Stick

The quality of the cutting edge can be assessed during instrumentation procedures and checked during the sharpening process by using a plastic test stick. The technique is simple. Hold the instrument with a modified pen grasp and place the cutting edge against the side of the test stick at the same angle used for scaling deposits. Establish a fulcrum with the fourth finger placed on the opposite side of the test stick at approximately the

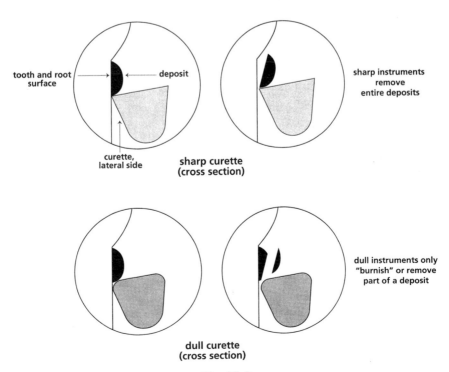

tooth and root surface → ← deposit

sharp instruments remove entire deposits

curette, lateral side

sharp curette (cross section)

dull curette (cross section)

dull instruments only "burnish" or remove part of a deposit

Fig. 25-3

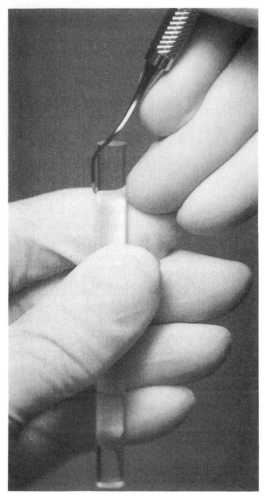

Fig. 25-4

same level as the blade (Fig. 25-4). Apply firm lateral pressure. If the edge is sharp, it will "bite" into the plastic and resist any attempts to "shave" the surface of the stick. If the edge has been worn down and becomes dulled, it will glide over the surface just as it will over a deposit.

CHARACTERISTICS OF SHARPENING STONES

Sharpening stones are composed of a mass of tiny crystals that are harder than the metal of the instrument blades. The size, shape, and hardness of these crystals determine the grit of a stone, which is generally classified as coarse, medium, fine, or ultra-fine. Coarse stones have large crystals or particles that will abrade or grind away more metal at a faster rate. Finer grits have smaller particles that will abrade metal at a slower rate and are recommended for regular, routine sharpening of dental instruments.

Although many sharpening devices are commercially available, including power sharpeners, a keen edge can be restored on scalers and curets with a few relatively inexpensive hand-held stones.

The hard Arkansas stone is a natural stone with a fine grit, and is preferred by many clinicians for sharpening periodontal scalers and curets. It is composed of a hard, compact silica crystal called novaculite that is said to impart a polishing effect to the blade as the crystals abrade away the metal. In the past, the use of a lubricant such as premium-grade honing oil or water has been recommended with use of an Arkansas stone for sharpening dental instruments. The lubricant does not act as a coolant but rather serves as a vehicle to float the metal particles as they are ground away from the blade and prevent these shavings from becoming embedded in the natural pores of the stone. Over time, the pores may become clogged with metal and lose some of the abrasive quality.

The India oilstone, also very popular for grinding away metal from the blades of dental instruments, is an artificial stone composed of aluminum oxide crystals with a medium grit. During the manufacturing process, the India oilstone is impregnated with oil.

Other types of artificial stones widely used by practitioners are ceramic stones, which are hard, dense, and available in a fine or medium grit. The medium-grit ceramic stones are excellent for routine sharpening of dental instruments. The fine-grit ceramic stones are made of small crystals and grind away metal at a much slower rate. These stones do not require lubrication with oil; they can be used wet or can be used dry.

After each use, thoroughly clean the surface of the stone, scrubbing with a stiff brush, soap, and water, or ultrasonically clean to remove the metal residue. The stone should then be properly sterilized.

The selection of an appropriate stone may be dictated by the time and place for use. The ideal sharpening situation is to regularly set aside time and perform the task on sterilized instruments in a prepared, well-lighted work area. After sharpening the presterilized instruments, thoroughly remove any debris from the instruments and the stones, clean them thoroughly, and resterilize before use. Contrary to previous beliefs, research studies have documented the fact that steam autoclaving will not dull the cutting edges of stainless steel instruments.

During root detoxification procedures, the cutting edges may become inefficient because of dullness. To eliminate the need for chairside sharpening and possible puncture wounds with a contaminated instrument, procedural instrument set-ups may be expanded to include several sets of the curets most often preferred by the clinician.

When it is absolutely necessary to sharpen contaminated instruments during an appointment, careful consideration must be given to appropriate infection control procedures for the safety of both the practitioner and the patient. It may be advantageous to reduce the contaminated debris by cautiously wiping off the blade to be sharpened and then submersing the instrument in a disinfectant. A sterile sharpening stone should be included in the procedural set-ups for root detoxification. These stones may be used without a lubricant to reduce contamination of the stone and the instruments.

Current concepts actually preclude the use of oil as a lubricant during sharpening procedures. Complete sterilization may be prevented if any oil residue remains on the instrument blade or the stone. The oil is water insoluble and may insulate and protect microorganisms from sterilization. In addition, the release of the oil vapors during heat sterilization may damage the mechanisms of the automatic sterilizers over time.

Dr. Ester Wilkins, in the 7th edition of her textbook, suggests the use of a dry stone for sharpening procedures to eliminate contamination problems caused by using oil and tap water as lubricants. According to Wilkins, an additional advantage of using a dry stone is to reduce the possibility of nicks in the blade, which may be caused by metal particles floating in the lubricant on the surface of the stone.

SIMPLIFIED STRATEGY FOR SHARPENING

Many acceptable techniques are available for sharpening scalers and curets with hand-held stones. However, the simplified approach explained here eliminates the confusion caused by the use of complicated geometric concepts and terms and the traditional reference to "degrees of angulation." The practitioner is afforded the option of using the more familiar context of "telling time" according to positions of the hands on the face of a clock. This "timely" strategy is a modified approach to the widely recognized "stationary instrument–moving stone" technique.

Basic Principles

The basic orientation for sharpening and testing all instruments is the 12:00 high noon position on the face of a clock. The directions, as stated, are for dominant right-hand operators. The positions on the hands of the clock are reversed for dominant left-hand operators.

Directions for Grasping the Instrument

1. In your nondominant hand, hold the instrument upright (top at 12:00 high noon), positioning the blade to be sharpened at the bottom.
2. Turn the toe (or tip) of the blade to be sharpened toward you.
3. Brace your elbow on the table top with the forearm and wrist upright, keeping the top of the instrument positioned at 12:00 noon. Bring your arm straight upward so the toe of the blade to be sharpened is approximately at your eye level.
4. Hold the entire handle with a secure palm grasp. You may flex your wrist slightly in a backward and upward position to swing the blade at the bottom out and away from your wrist (Fig. 25-5).
5. Brace the top shank with your index finger or thumb. It is essential to firmly stabilize the opposite end of the instrument to counterbalance the pressure of grinding the stone against the blade at the bottom (Fig. 25-5).

Directions for Holding the Stone

1. Grasp the lower half of the stone in your dominant hand (Fig. 25-6).
2. Hold the top of the stone at 12:00. Place your thumb on the edge toward you and your fingers on the edge away from you. Confine your grasp to the lower half of the stone. Tilt the top of the stone toward 1:00.
3. Do not stabilize your dominant hand or arm or rest it on the table.
4. Move the dominant arm smoothly and freely by activating the shoulder muscles. Bend the arm only at the elbow and keep the wrist rigid.
5. Generate a fluid, rhythmic, up-and-down vertical motion of the stone.
6. Keep the stone moving in one plane. Avoid turning or rotating the wrist.

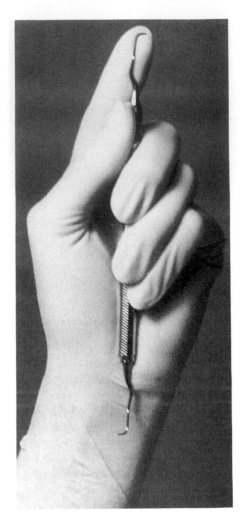

Fig. 25-5

Grasping only the lower half of the stone will minimize the natural tendency of the arm and hand to move in a "rolling" or "rotating" up-and-down motion, which may cause the stone to roll over the actual cutting edge itself.

DIRECTIONS FOR SHARPENING ALL SICKLE SCALERS AND UNIVERSAL CURETS

1. Hold the instrument in a vertical position, with the blade to be sharpened at the bottom and the tip (or toe) pointed toward you.

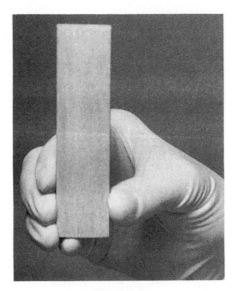

Fig. 25-6

2. Position the terminal shank of the bottom blade directly at 12:00.
3. Maintain a firm palm grasp of the entire instrument handle in the nondominant hand.
4. Counterbalance the opposite end of the instrument, with your index finger or thumb placed against the shank (Fig. 25-7).
5. Stabilize the entire arm by resting the elbow on the table top if seated, or stabilize the upper arm and elbow against your side and waist if standing.
6. Place the flat surface of the stone against the right lateral surface of the blade, with the top of the stone at the 12:00 position.
7. Tilt the top of the stone slightly toward 1:00 (Fig. 25-7).
8. Move the stone up and down against the right side of the blade to grind away metal from the right lateral surface.
9. Start the grinding process on the right lateral surface at the heel one-third of the blade (near the shank).
10. Gradually move the stone forward to grind the side at the middle one-third of the blade.

11. Advance the stone to grind metal away from the tip one-third of the blade.

Directions to Sharpen the Opposite Cutting Edge of the Same Blade

1. Maintain the same vertical palm grasp of the instrument. Turn the tip of the blade away from you.
2. Keep the terminal shank positioned at 12:00.
3. Place the stone against the right lateral surface. Tilt the top of the stone toward 1:00.
4. Repeat the grinding procedures start-

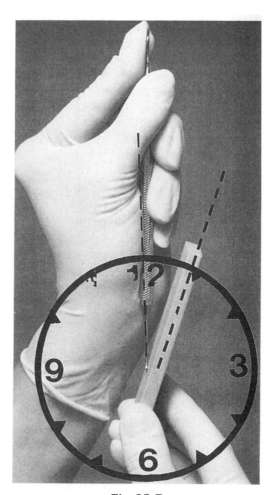

Fig. 25-7

ing at the heel one-third of the blade and advancing to the tip or toe one-third.

5. Focus only on the 12:00 position of the terminal shank and tilt the top of the stone toward 1:00.

DIRECTIONS TO ASSESS SHARPNESS OF THE SICKLE SCALER AND UNIVERSAL CURET WITH THE PLASTIC TEST STICK

1. Grasp the plastic test stick in your nondominant hand.
2. Hold the stick between your thumb and index finger approximately one-half inch from the end of the stick.
3. Position the top of the stick at 12:00 high noon (Fig. 25-8).
4. Hold the instrument in your dominant hand with a modified pen grasp, as you would for scaling.
5. To test each cutting edge, position the blade on the left side of the test stick with the tip (or toe) toward you or away from you as you did to grind the metal from the lateral surface. Slightly tilt the terminal shank toward 1:00.
6. Place your fulcrum on the side of the test stick directly opposite the cutting edge of the blade. Do not fulcrum on the top of the test stick.
7. Firmly press the cutting edge into the test stick. Make sure that the terminal shank is tilted slightly toward 1:00 so the blade is in the same position as used for scaling.
8. A sharp edge will bite into or grab the test stick so that the blade cannot shave or slide over the side of the stick.
9. If the cutting edge scales or shaves the plastic test stick, the edge is still dull or the terminal shank is not tilted slightly toward 1:00.
10. Assess your grinding progress frequently to avoid over-sharpening.

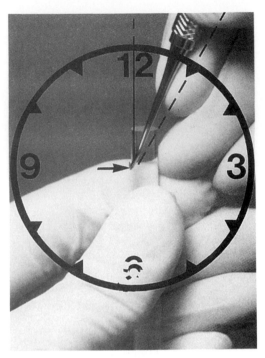

Fig. 25-8

DIRECTIONS FOR SHARPENING ALL GRACEY CURETS

1. Identify the design number of each Gracey blade by referring to the information on the handle of the instrument.
   a. For all odd-numbered Gracey blades, point the toe of the blade toward you.
   b. For all even-numbered Gracey blades, point the toe of the blade away from you.
2. Hold the instrument with a firm palm grasp in your nondominant hand, with the blade to be sharpened at the bottom and the toe pointed in the appropriate direction (see above).
3. Initially position the terminal shank of the instrument at 12:00. The lower cutting edge will be on the right side of the blade.
4. Tilt the terminal shank toward the 11:00 position to accommodate the "offset" angulation of the Gracey blade.
5. Position the stone against the right lat-

eral surface, with the top of the stone aimed at 12:00.

6. Tilt the top of the stone slightly toward, but a little less than, a 1:00 position (Fig. 25-9).

7. Grind the metal from the lateral (side) surface of the blade. Move the stone up and down with a rhythmic, fluid motion.

Important: Examine the cutting edge on a Gracey blade very closely (Fig. 25-10). Notice that the edge is straight as

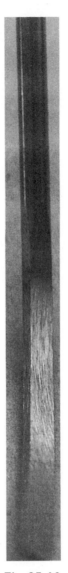

Fig. 25-10

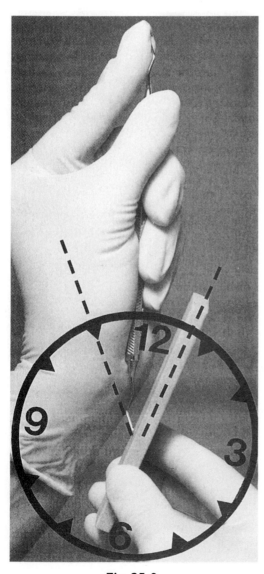

Fig. 25-9

it comes from the shank forward toward the toe. When viewed from the vantage point where the facial surface of the Gracey 13 blade can be seen slanting downward toward the right and the terminal shank is held at 12:00, the entire blade appears to be straight (Fig. 25-10). Compare this with the view seen while looking directly down on the facial surface with the terminal shank tilted toward 11:00 (Fig. 25-11). This perspective gives the illusion that the Gracey blade curves from the heel to

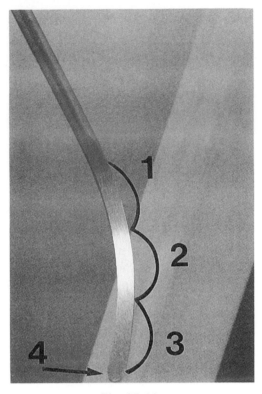

Fig. 25-11

8. Visually divide the blade into three equal segments. Grind away a consistent amount of metal from the lateral surfaces of each segment to preserve the original contours of the blade (Fig. 25-11).
9. Initiate the grinding process at the heel one-third of the blade.
10. Gradually advance the stone in the same plane to grind the middle one-third of the blade.
11. Advance the stone to contact the toe one-third of the blade.
12. Avoid the most common sharpening error of recontouring the toe one-third of a Gracey curet into a thin, pointed tip similar to that of a sickle scaler. Do not rotate the stone as you proceed to grind metal from the lateral surfaces. Remember the original design of the Gracey blade, as pictured in Figure 25-10.

the toe. The perceived curvature of the cutting edge is an optical illusion caused by the downward slant of the blade at a 60- to 70-degree angle to terminal shank.

Rounding the Toe of the Curet

1. To maintain the rounded shape of the curet toe, turn the toe to face your hand holding the stone.
2. Tilt the stone to a 2:00 position (Fig. 25-12).

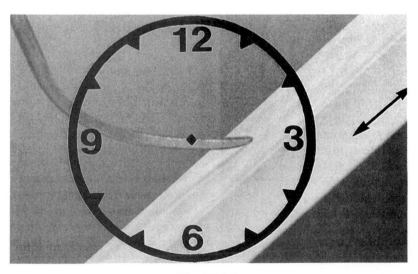

Fig. 25-12

3. Activate the stone in an up-and-down motion rotating around the toe (Fig. 25-11, section 4).
4. Do not apply heavy pressure.
5. Round the toe with approximately six to seven strokes.

DIRECTIONS TO ASSESS SHARPNESS FOR ALL GRACEY CURETS

1. Hold the plastic test stick at a 12:00 high-noon position in your nondominant hand.
2. Hold the Gracey curet in your dominant hand with a modified pen-grasp, as you would for scaling.
3. Place the cutting edge to be tested against the side of the test stick.

Note: The odd-numbered Gracey blades will be held with the toe pointed toward you. The even-numbered Gracey blades will be turned so the toe points away from you.

4. Position the fulcrum finger on the side of the test stick opposite the placement of the blade to be tested (Fig. 25-13). Do not position fulcrum on the top end of the test stick!
5. Hold the terminal shank exactly parallel to the test stick. Apply pressure against the instrument handle with the thumb, or pull the cutting edge into the stick toward the fulcrum. A sharp cutting edge will immediately "bite" into the plastic but should not shave the test stick.

DIRECTIONS TO REMOVE WIRE BURS BY "HONING" YOUR CURET BLADES

1. Wire edges or "burs" may result from grinding the metal away from the lateral surfaces of the blades. Minimize formation of these wire edges by finishing the grinding process on a downward stroke at each one-third segment of the blade.

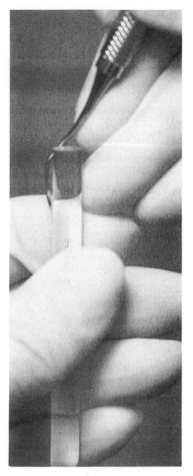

Fig. 25-13

2. The wire edges will form (or protrude upward) along the cutting edge on the facial surface of the blade (where you do not grind away the metal).
3. Use a conical or cylindrical stone to remove these wire edges by "honing" your curet blade.
4. For honing universal curets or curved sickles, hold the terminal shank at 12:00.
5. For honing Gracey curets, hold the toe of the blade toward you for visibility. If you are honing an odd-numbered Gracey blade, the terminal shank will be at 11:00 (Fig. 25-14). For even-numbered Gracey blades, hold the terminal shank at the 1:00 position with the toe pointed toward you.

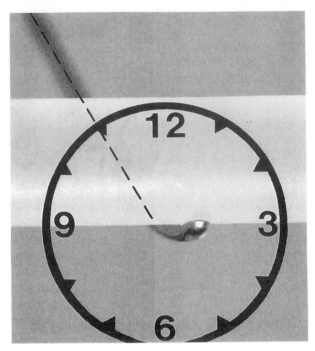

Fig. 25-14

6. Grasp the conical or cylindrical stone approximately one inch from the end for greater control and stability.
7. Place the stone flat across the facial surface of the blade in a 9:00 to 3:00 position.
8. Start at the heel one-third of the blade.
9. Roll the stone across the facial surface from the heel to the toe by rotating the wrist.
10. Carefully maintain the stone in a 9:00 to 3:00 position to avoid rolling over onto the cutting edge.
11. Repeat the process four to five times with light pressure.

SUMMARY

You will be able to sharpen any scaler or curet if you are familiar with the original design and contour of the blade. This simplified strategy will assist you in determining the correct placement of the stone to grind away metal. With the terminal shank held in the correct position (either 11:00 or 12:00), keep the stone against the lateral surface of the blade with the top tilted toward the 1:00 position. The purpose of this action is to position the stone against the blade so that (in traditional terms) an angle of approximately 110 degrees is formed with the facial surface.

SUGGESTED READINGS

Marquam BJ. Strategies to improve instrument sharpening. Dent Hyg 1988;62:334–338.
Pattison AM, Pattison GL. Periodontal instrumentation, 2nd ed. Norwalk, CT: Appleton & Lange, 1992.
Perry DA, Beemsterboer P, Carranza FA. Techniques and theory of periodontal instrumentation. Philadelphia: W.B. Saunders, 1990.
Sasse J. Cutting edges of curets: effects of repeated sterilization. Dent Hyg 1989;Jan:61.
Wilkins EM. Clinical practice of the dental hygienist, 7th ed. Baltimore: Williams & Wilkins, 1994.
Woodall I. Comprehensive dental hygiene care, 4th ed. St. Louis: C.V. Mosby, 1993.

Index

*Page numbers in *italics* denote figures; those followed by a *t* denote tables.

Aberrant frena (frenectomy), 158, *158*
Abscess
  acute periapical, 207
  gingival, 205–206
  periodontal, 206
Acatalasia, 23
Acetylpyridinium chloride, 128
Acquired pellicle, 14–15
Actinobacillus actinomycetemcomitans, 34
Acute gingivitis, 209, *210*
Acute inflammatory process in periodontal
    disease, 43
Acute necrotizing ulcerative gingivitis (ANUG),
    28, 31
Acute periapical abscess, 207
Adjunctive therapy for implant maintenance,
    204
After-five curets, 89
Age and wound healing, 105
Aging and periodontal disease, 22–23
Agranulocytes, 28
Agranulocytosis (malignant neutropenia), 26,
    212–213
AIDs-related periodontal diseases, 28–29
Allografts, 170
Alloplastic grafts, 171
Alpha-hemolytic (viridans) streptococci, 53
Alternate pathway, 46
Alveolar bone, 12
  supporting, 10
Alveolar fenestration, 12–13
Alveolar mucosa, 3–4
Alveolar process
  blood supply, *7,* 11
  bundle bone, 11
  contours, 11, *11, 12*
  dehiscence and fenestration, *12,* 12–13
  divisions, 9–10
  lability, 12
Anemia
  aplastic, 26
  sickle cell, 26
Anesthesia
  need for, in supragingival scaling, 92
  for periodontal surgery, 110–111
Antibiotics, (*See also* Antimicrobial agents)
  for at-risk patients, 53
  for periodontal surgery, 109–110
  systemic, 223
Antibodies, 49
Antibody-forming cells (AFCs), 47

Antigens, 49
Antimicrobial agents, 128–131, *129, 130,* (*See also*
    Antibiotics)
  applications for, 221–222
  controlled local delivery of, 222–223
  in mouthrinses, 203
  in plaque removal, 203
  in treating chronic adult periodontitis, 124–
    134
    indications, 125
    maintenance therapy, 134
    objectives, 125
    patient case analysis, 125–126, 127*t*
    patient education, 126–127
    personalized bacterial control, 131
    professional bacterial control, 127–128
    reevaluation, 131–134, 132*t*
Apically positioned flap, 149–151, *150*
Aplastic anemia, 26
Area-specific curet modifications, *89,* 89–90
Arkansas stone, 242
Armamentarium, 87
Articulators, 70
Asepsis and wound healing, 105
Attached gingiva, 1, 3
Attachment apparatus, 6, *7*
Attachment-retained overdenture (O-ring and ball
    abutments), 197–198
Autograft, 169–170

B cells, 47
B-1 cells, 47
B-2 cells, 47
Bacteremia, transient, 52–53, 83
Bacterial action, mechanisms of, 17–18
Bacterial analysis, 63
Bacterial control, 68
Bacterial factors in periodontal disease, 15–18
Bacterial plaque, 14, 18, 41, 75
  morphology of, 15–16
Bar overdenture, 196–197
Basophils, 42
Benign mucous membrane pemphigoid (cicatricial
    pemphigoid), 226, 227, *234*
Betadine, 129
Bifurcation, 66
Biologic width, *163,* 163–164
Bleeding
  control of, in periodontal surgery, 112–113
  and purulent exudation, 55

Blood supply for gingiva, 6
Bone, and wound healing
    bone replacement grafts, 104
    fate of bone autografts, 104
    guided tissue regeneration healing, 104–105
    infrabony defects, 103–104, *104*
Bone autografts, fate of, 104
Bone grafting
    advantages of, for implant placement, 189–190
    applications for, 190, *190, 191, 192*
Bone loss
    horizontal, 33
    vertical, 33
Bone replacement grafts, 104
    indications for, 168–169
    surgical procedures, 171–172
    types of, 169–171
Bradykinin, 42, 43
Brushing, 76–77
Bullous pemphigoid, 227

C5a, 43
Calculus, 15
    formation of, 20
Candidiasis, 28
Caries, 53
Catalase, 23
Cause in necrotizing ulcerative gingivitis, 208
Cavitron7, 93
Cellular components of inflammation, 42
Cellular elements of immune system, 47–48
Cementoenamal junction, 8–9, *9*
    relationship of, to bottom of pocket, 55
    relationship of gingival margin to, 55, *58*
Cementoid, 8
Cement-retained prosthesis, 195–196
Cementum
    cementoenamal junction, 8–9, *9*
    cervical projection of enamel, 9
    functions, 8
    palatogingival groove, 9, *10*
Ceramic stones, 241
Cervical projection of enamel, 9, *10*
Chediak-Higashi syndrome, 23
Chemical injury, 21
Chemokines, 42
Chemotactic factor, 46
Chisels, 88
Chlorhexidine, 130–131
Chlorhexidine digluconate, 129
Chondroitinase, 17
Chronic adult periodontitis, 34
Chronic desquamative gingivitis, 211–212
Chronic hepatitis and oral lichen planus, 226
Chronic idiopathic neutropenia, 23
Chronic inflammatory hyperplasia, 137
Chronic ulcerative stomatitis, 226, *233*
Circular group, 3, *4*
Classical pathway, 46
Clinically healthy gingiva, 4–5, *5*
Clot absorption, 97, *98*
Clotting factor deficiencies, 26
Collagenase, 17
Colony-stimulating factors (CSFs), 46, 49
Combination infrabony defect, 161

Combined periodontal trauma, 71
Comparison of full-thickness and partial-thickness
    flaps, 148
Complement, *44*
Composite grafts, 171
Contagion in necrotizing ulcerative gingivitis,
    207–208
Contiguous osseous autografts, 171
Coronally positioned flaps, 157, *157*
Cracked tooth syndrome, 54
Curets, 87, 88–89
Cyclic neutropenia, 23, 26
Cytokines, 49
    and other molecular components, 48–49
Cytotoxic agent, 17

Deep pocket retromolar area, *143,* 144
Dehiscence, 12
Delayed passive eruption, 137
Dental history, 53
Dental hygienist as member of dental implant
    team, 198
Dental implants, 188–199
    case types, 188
    classifications, 186
    fixed crown and bridge (cement-retained pros-
        thesis), 195–196
    indications, 186
    material, 186–188
    patient selection and considerations, 185–186
    placement, 190
    postoperative care, 194–195, *196, 197*
    presurgical checklist, 190–192
    prosthetic factors, determined before surgery,
        195
    prosthetics, 188
    restorative options, 195–198
    retainment, 188
    site preparation, 188–189, *189*
    surgical procedure, 192–194, *194, 195, 196*
    team for, 198–199
Dental laboratory technician as member of dental
    implant team, 199
Dentogingival junction, *5,* 6
Deposits survey, 62–63
Desquamative gingivitis, 31
Developmental defects, 67
Diabetes mellitus, 24–25
Diagnosis
    bacterial analysis, 63
    deposits survey, 62–63
    differential, in necrotizing ulcerative gingivitis,
        209–213, *210, 211, 212*
    general dental survey, 53–54
    health survey, 52
        dental history, 53
        medical history, 52–53
    limitations of techniques, 51
    in necrotizing ulcerative gingivitis, 208–209, *209*
    occlusal survey, 55, 57–61
    periodontal chart, 52
    periodontal survey, 54–55, *56*
    radiographic survey, 61–62, *62*
Differential diagnosis in necrotizing ulcerative gin-
    givitis, 209–213, *210, 211, 212*

Dilantin hyperplasia, 137
Disclosing agents, 76
Disease susceptibility and implant maintenance, 201–202
Distal wedge procedure, *143,* 144
Double-papillae flap, 154
Down's syndrome, 23
Drug-induced gingival enlargements, 28
Drugs, and periodontal disease, 27–28

E selectins, 43
Ehlers-Danlos phenomena, 24
Elastase, 46, 49
Emotional stress and periodontal disease, 23
Endocarditis, 52–53
Endocrine imbalances and periodontal disease, 24–26
Endotoxins, 17, 46
Epithelial cells, 16–17
Epithelium, 3
    junctional, 5–6
Erosive lichen planus, 225
Erythema multiforme, 186, 228–229, *237*
Erythrocytes, 17
Erythrosin, 76
Excessive occlusal force, 21
Exodontics, 20
Explorers, 87

Factitious disease, 20–21
Fenestration, alveolar, 12–13
Fibrinopeptides, 43
Fibroblasts, 48, 49
Files, 88
First-generation mouth rinses, 84
Fixed crown and bridge (cement-retained prosthesis), 195–196
Fixed-removable crown and bridge (screw-retained prosthesis), 196
Fixed-removable denture (screw-retained prosthesis), 198
Flap curettage/debridement, 181
Flaps, *101,* 101–102
    apically positioned, 149–151, *150*
    classification of, 145, *146,* 147–148, *148*
    comparison of full-thickness and partial-thickness, 148
    full-thickness (mucoperiosteal), 145, *146,* 147
    objectives of, 145
    palatal, 151
    partial-thickness (mucosal), 147–148, *148*
    replaced, 149, *149*
Fluorides, topical, 222
Food debris, 15
Food impaction, 21
Food particles, 17
Free gingival grafts, 102, 154–157, *155, 156*
Free osseous autografts, 169
Free soft tissue grafts, 152
Frenectomy, 158, *158*
Full-thickness flap, 145, *146,* 147
Furcation involvement, 66
    classifications, 175, *175, 176, 177*
    diagnosis, 174–175

philosophy, 174
prognosis, 175–177
pulpal-periodontal relationships, 177
therapy, 177–180, *179, 180*
Furcation plasty, 178

Gamma interferon (IFN-γ), 46
Gauze in plaque removal, 79–80
General dental survey, 53–54
Genetic disorders and periodontal disease, 23–24
Genetic factors, 18
Gingiva, 1, *2*
    attached, 1, 3
    blood, lymphatic, and nerve supply of, 6, *7*
    blood supply of, 6
    clinically healthy, 4–5, *5*
    excision of, 96–97, *97*
    keratinized, 1, *2*
    lymphatic drainage of, 6
    marginal (free), 1
Gingival abscess, 205–206
Gingival behavior, 162–164, *163, 164*
Gingival color, form, and consistency, 54–55
Gingival crevicular fluid, monitoring of, 203
Gingival fiber apparatus, 3, *4*
Gingival flap, 140
    contraindications, 141
    indications, 140–141
    objective, 141
    surgical procedure, *140, 141,* 141–142, *142, 143,* 144
Gingival groove, 1
Gingival group, 3, *4*
Gingival inflammatory hyperplasia, 25
Gingival margin, relationship of, to cementoenamal junction, 55, *58*
Gingival pocket, 32
Gingival recession, 152
Gingival sulcus, 1, 3
Gingivectomy, 96–97, *97,* 100
    contraindications, 137
    indications, 137
    technique, 137–140, *138, 139*
Gingivitis, 31
    desquamative, 31
    hormonal-influenced, 31
    medication-influenced, 31
    necrotizing ulcerative, 207–214
Gingivoplasty, 100, 178
    indications, 136
    technique, 136–137, *137*
Glow discharge treatment, 187
Glucoronidase, 49
Glycosuria, 24
Gracey curets, 89
    assessing sharpening for, 249, *249*
    directions for sharpening, 246–249
Gracey curvettes, 89–90
Granules, 45
Group function occlusion, 70
Guided tissue regeneration, 180, 181–182
Guided tissue regeneration healing, 104–105

Habits, 54
Hand instrumentation, technique for, 90–92, *91, 92*

Healing rate and wound healing, 105
Healing sockets, 170
Health survey
    dental history, 53
    medical history, 52–53
Hematologic disorders and periodontal disease, 26
Hemidesmosomes, 6
Hemisection, 180
Hereditary fibromatosis, 137
Histamine, 42, 43
History in necrotizing ulcerative gingivitis, 207
Hoes, 88
Home care aids for plaque removal, 203
Horizontal bone loss, 33
Hormonal-influenced gingivitis, 31
Host defenses and periodontal disease, 41–49
Human immunodeficiency virus (HIV), 28–29
Human leukocyte antigen (HLA), 18
Hyaluronidase, 17, 46, 49
Hydroxylapatite (HA), 186–187
Hyperglycemia, 24
Hyperparathyroidism, 24
Hypersensitivity, 214
    cause, 214
    treatment, 214–215
Hypersensitivity reactions, 28
Hypophosphatasia, 24

ICAMs, 49
IgA, 49
IgD, 49
IgE, 49
IgG, 49
IgM, 49
Immune response in periodontal disease, 49
Immune system, cellular elements of, 47–48
Immunoglobulins, 49
Immunology, 41, 47
    cellular elements of immune system, 47–48
    cytokines and other molecular components, 48–49
    immune response in periodontal disease, 49
    immunoglobulins (antibodies), 49
Implant maintenance, 201–204
    clinical measures
        adjunctive therapy, 204
        mobility/occlusion, 203
        monitoring of gingival crevicular fluid, 203
        patient's home care, 203
        probing, 202
        radiographs, 202–203
        therapist instrumentation, 203–204
        tissue health, 203
    peri-implant attachment apparatus and disease
        susceptibility, 201–202
        microbiology, 201–202
        reinfection, 201
Implant placement, advantages of bone grafting
    for, 189–190
Implant probing, 202
Incidence in necrotizing ulcerative gingivitis, 207
India oilstone, 242
Infectious mononucleosis, 213
Inflammation, 41
    acute process, in periodontal disease, 43

cellular components of, 42
molecular components of, 42–43
stages of, 41
Inflammatory response, *43*
Infrabony defects, 103–104, 160–161
Infrabony pockets, 32–33, 160
    etiology of, 33
Instrument sharpening, 239–250
    basic principles, 243–244
    characteristics of sharpening stones, 242–243
    design, 239, *240, 241*
    directions for, all sickle scalers and universal
        curets, 244–246
    directions for sharpening all Gracey curets,
        246–249
    directions to assess sharpness for all Gracey
        curets, 249, *249*
    directions to remove wire burs by honing your
        curet blades, 249–250, *250*
    directions to assess, of sickle scaler and univer-
        sal curet with plastic test stick, 246, *246*
    factors for consideration, 239
    methods to assess sharpness, *241,* 241–242,
        242
    simplified strategy for, 243
Instrumentation, 87
Interdental brushes and plaque removal, 203
Interdental cleansers, 80–81, *81, 82*
Interdental crater, 161, *161*
Interdental groove, 3
Interdental papilla, 3, *3*
Interferons, 48
Interleukin-1 (IL-1), 46, 48, 49
Interleukin-1 (IL-1) gene polymorphism, 23
Interleukin-2 (IL-2), 48, 49
Interleukin-4 (IL-4), 48
Interleukin-6 (IL-6), 46, 48, 49
Interleukin-8 (IL-8), 48, 49
Interleukin-10 (IL-10), 48
Interleukins, 48
Interproximal brush, 82
Interproximal plaque, removal of, 203
Intraoral donor sites, 169
Irrigation, 221

Jacquette Scaler, 88
Junctional epithelium, 5–6
Juvenile periodontitis, 34–35

Kaposi's sarcoma, 28
Keratinized gingiva, 1, *2*
Killer cells, 47
Kwashiorkor, 27

L selectins, 43
Lactoferrin, 45
Lamina propria, 3
Langer curets, 90, *90*
Laterally positioned flap, 152–154, *153, 154*
Leukemia, 26, 212, *212*
Leukocyte adhesion deficiency (LAD), 23
Leukocytes, 42

Leukotriene B2 (LTB2), 43
Leukotriene B4 (LTB4), 42, 43
Leukotriene D2 (LTD2), 43
Leukotriene D4 (LTD4), 42
Leukotrienes, 42, 48
Lichen planus, 225, 226, *231, 232*
Linear gingival erythema (LGE), 29
Lupus erythematosus, 187, 228, *236*
Lymphatic drainage of gingiva, 6
Lymphocytes, 42, 48, 49
Lymphotoxin (LT), 46, 48
Lysosomes, 45

Macrophages, 42, 48, 49
Magnetostrictive (ultrasonic), 93, *93*
Malocclusion, 64–65
Mandibular molars, osseous defects in, 174–175
Manual toothbrushes, 76
Marginal (free) gingiva, 1
Mast cells, 42
Materia alba, 15, 16*t*
Matrix metalloproteins (MMPs), 48–49
Matrix metalloprotineases, 46
Maxillary molars, osseous defects in, 174–175
Medical history, 52–53
Medication-influenced gingivitis, 31
Memory cells, 47
Metabolic disorders, nutritional deficiencies and, 26–27
Microbiology and implant maintenance, 201–202
Migration inhibitory factor (MIF), 48
Milled-bar overdenture, 198
Mini-five curets, 89
Minor tooth movement, 182–183
Mobility of implant fixture, 203
Mobility of teeth, 54, *54*
Modified Bass technique, 76
Molecular components of Inflammation, 42–43
Monocytes, 48
Mouth rinses, 83–84
Mucocutaneous diseases of periodontium, 225–238
    benign mucous membrane pemphigoid (cicatricial pemphigoid), 226, 227, *234*
    chronic ulcerative stomatitis, 226, *233*
    erythema multiforme, 228–229, *237*
    lichen planus, 225, 226, *231, 232*
    lupus erythematosus, 228, *236*
    pemphigus vulgaris, 227–228, *234, 235*
Mucogingival corrective surgery
    indications 2, 151
    objectives, 151
    techniques
        coronally positioned flaps, 157, *157*
        double-papillae flap, 154
        free gingival graft (free soft tissue autograft), 154–157, *155, 156*
        laterally positioned flap, 152–154, *153, 154*
        root coverage, 157
Mucogingival junction, *2, 3*
Mucoperiosteal flap, 145, *146,* 147
Mucous patch, 213
Multiple myeloma, 26
Myeloma, multiple, 26
Myeloperoxidase, 45

Nabors probe, 87
Natural killer (NK) cells, 48
Necrotizing ulcerative gingivitis (NUG), 29, 207–214
    cause, 208
    contagion, 207–208
    diagnosis, 208–209, *209*
    differential diagnosis, 209–213 *210, 211, 212*
    history, 207
    incidence, 207
    and smoking, 27–28
    treatment, 213–214
Necrotizing ulcerative gingivo-periodontitis, 35
Necrotizing ulcerative periodontitis (NUP), 29
Necrotizing ulcerative stomatitis (NUS), 29
Neoplasms, 21
Neutropenia, 26
Neutrophil chemotactic factor (NCF), 42, 43
Neutrophil chemotaxis, 43
Neutrophils, 42
Non-oxygen dependent phagocytosis in phagocytic system, 43
Nutrition and systemic disorders and wound healing, 105
Nutritional deficiencies and metabolic disorders, 26–27
    and periodontal disease, 26–27

Occlusal survey, 55, 57–61
Occlusal trauma, 71
    primary, 71, *72*
    secondary, 71, *72*
Occlusion
    analysis of, 57–58, *59*
    and implant maintenance, 204
    periodontal trauma from, 58, 60–61
    role of, in periodontal health and disease, 70–74, *72, 73*
Odontoplasty, 177
One-wall infrabony defect, 161
Oral hairy leukoplakia, 28
Oral hygiene instructions, 221
Oral irrigating devices, 82–83
O-ring and ball abutments, 197–198
Orthodontics, 20
Osseous coagulum, 169
Osseous defects, 160
    guidelines for treating, 183–184
    management of, 162–164, *163, 164,* 168–172
        bone replacement grafts, 168–172
        flap curettage/debridement, 181
        furcation involvement, 174–180, *175, 176, 177, 179, 180*
        guided tissue regeneration, 181–182
        minor tooth movement, 182–183
        selective extraction, 182, *182*
    structure of, 168
Osseous grafting materials, functions of, 168–169
Osseous resection, 164–166
    advantages of, 167
    contraindications for, 165
    disadvantages of, 167
    indications for, 165
    lingual approach to, 166
    modified, 166
    technique of, 165–166

Osseous surgery, 160
  classification, 160–161, *161, 162, 163*
  diagnosis, 160, *161*
  effect of bone removal, 166–167
  objectives, 161
Osteoconduction, 169
Osteogenesis, 169
Osteoplasty/ostectomy, 164–166
Oxygen-dependent phagocytosis, 45–46

P selectins, 43
Palatal flap, 151
Palatogingival groove, 9, *10,* 67
Papilla, interdental, 3, *3*
Papillon-Lefevre syndrome, 23
Partial-thickness (mucosal) flap, 147–148, *148*
Pathologic invasion of furcation areas, 55
Pedicle flap procedures, 152
Pellicle, acquired, 14–15
Pemphigoid, 186
  benign mucous membrane, 226, 227, *234*
Pemphigus, 187
Pemphigus vulgaris, 227–228, *234, 235*
Pericoronitis
  cause, 205
  signs and symptoms, 205
  treatment, 205
Peri-implant attachment apparatus and implant
    maintenance, 201–202
Peri-implant tissues, health of, 203
Periodontal abscess, 206
Periodontal chart, 52
Periodontal disease, linear versus burst theories
    of, 39
Periodontal diseases
  acute inflammatory process in, 43
  AIDs-related, 28–29
  bacterial factors in, 15–18
  critical pathway theory of, 39–40
  defined, 14
  etiology of, 14–21
  and host defenses, 41–49
  immune response in, 49
  local contributing factors and, 19–21
  pathogenesis of plaque-related, 35–40, *38, 39t*
    critical pathway theory of, 39–40
    disease progression, 37
    genetic factors in, 38
    histopathology, 36–37
    linear versus burst theories of activity, 39
    smoking and, 39
    spread of inflammation, 37–38, *38*
  risk factors and risk indicators in, 18
  systemic contributing factors, 22–30
    aging, 22–23
    AIDs-related, 28–29
    drugs and periodontium, 27–28
    emotional and psychosocial stress, 23
    endocrine imbalances, 24–26
    genetic disorders, 23–24
    hematologic disorders, 26
    infections, 29–30
    nutritional deficiencies and metabolic disor-
        ders, 26–27
  systemic factors and, 19

Periodontal emergencies, 205–216
  abscess formation, 205–207
  hypersensitivity, 214
  necrotizing ulcerative gingivitis, 207–214
  pericoronitis, 205
  primary, 215
  temporomandibular joint pain, 215–216
Periodontal examination instruments, 87
Periodontal health and disease, role of occlusion
    in, 70–74, *72, 73*
Periodontal infections and systemic diseases,
    29–30
Periodontal ligament
  blood supply of periodontal ligament, 8
  functions, 6
  nerve supply, 8
  width, 8
Periodontal maintenance therapy, 218–223
  effect of excellent program on total dental
      health, 223
  elements of program, *219,* 219–223, *222t*
  rationale for program, 218
  recall interval, 218–219
Periodontal pockets, reducing, 107
Periodontal probe, 87
Periodontal surgery, 64, 223
  considerations
    control of bleeding, 112–113
    dressing wound, 114, 117, 121
    instrumentation and flap design, *111,* 111–112,
        112
    surgical plan, 111
    suturing, 113–114, *115, 116, 117, 118, 119, 120*
    wound closure, 113, *113, 114*
  limitations of, 121, 123
  post-surgical considerations, 121, *122*
  presurgical considerations
    anesthesia, 110–111
    antibiotics, 109–110
    anxiety control, 108–109
    asepsis, 110
    contraindications for, 108
    emergencies, 110
    infection control/phase I therapy, 108, *109t*
    patient consent, 107–108
  reasons for, 107
  wound healing applied to, 105–106
Periodontal survey, 54–55, *56*
Periodontal trauma, from occlusion, 58, 60–61
Periodontal traumatism, 33
Periodontitis, 29
  causes of, 71
  chronic adult, 34
    role of antimicrobial agents in, 124–134, *127t,*
        129, 130, 132t
  classification of, 33–34, *35t*
  classification of pockets, 32–33
  genetic factors in, 38
  history of previous, 18
  juvenile, 34–35
  pathogens in, 202
  pocket formation, 31–32, *32*
  prepubertal, 34
  rapidly progressive, 35
  refractory, 35
  retrograde, 207

risk factors for, 18
risk indicators for, 18
and smoking, 39
smoking and, 18
Periodontium, 1–13
    alveolar process, 9–13
    cementum, 8–9
    and drugs, 27–28
    epithelium, 3–6
    gingiva, 1–3, *2*
    periodontal ligament, 6, 8
    repairing, 107
Periodontosis, 34–35
Phagocytes, *44,* 46
Phagocytic system
    destruction of host tissues, 46
    non-oxygen dependent phagocytosis in, 43
    oxygen-dependent phagocytosis, 45–46
    serum complement, 46–47
Phagocytosis, 43
    non-oxygen dependent, 43
Piezoelectric (ultrasonic), 93, *94*
Plaque
    bacterial, 14
    constituents of, 16–17
    microorganisms of, 16
    morphology of bacterial, 15–16
    subgingival, 16
Plaque control, 75–85
    aids for cleansing inaccessible areas, 81–82, *82*
    assessment of, 133
    brushing in, 76–77
    disclosing agents in, 76
    interdental cleansers in, 80–81, *81, 82*
    mouth rinses in, 83–84
    oral irrigating devices in, 82–83
    prebrushing mouthrinses in, 84
    proximal cleansing in, 77, *79,* 79–80
    teaching, 84–85
Plaque index, 62
Plaque removal, home care aids for, 204
Plaque-related periodontal disease, 36
    types of, 31–35
        chronic adult periodontitis, 34
        gingivitis, 31
        horizontal and vertical bone loss, 33–34
        juvenile periodontitis, 34–35
        periodontitis, 31–33
        prepubertal periodontitis, 34
        rapidly-progressive periodontitis, 35
        refractory periodontitis, 35
Plastic test stick, 240–241, *241*
Platelet activating factor (PAF), 42
Pocket, relationship of cementoenamal junction to
    bottom of, 55
Pocket (probing) depth, 55, *57*
Polishing, 95, 221
Polycythemia, 26
Polymorphonuclear neutrophils (PMNs), 17, 48, 64
    relationship of, to periodontal health and dis-
    ease, 45–46
Porphyromonas gingivalis, 202
Positioning, 53
Powered (mechanic) toothbrushes, 76–77, *77, 78*
Prebrushing mouthrinses, 84
Prepubertal periodontitis, 34

Prevotella intermedia, 202
Primary acute herpetic gingivostomatitis, 209–211,
    210
Primary occlusal trauma, 71, *72*
Primary periodontal traumatism
    definition, 215
    signs and symptoms, 215
    treatment, 215
Prognosis, 63–67
    of individual teeth, 65–67, *66, 67*
Promyelocytes, 42
Prophyjet7, 95
Proportional bone loss, 63
Prostaglandin E2 (PGE2), 42, 43
Prostaglandin-2, 46
Prostaglandins, 48
Proteases, 17
Protein deficiency, 27
Protozoa, 17
Protrusive excursion, 58
Proximal cleansing, 77, *79,* 79–80
Pruritus, 24
Pseudohypophosphatasia, 24
Pseudopockets, 31
Psychosocial stress and periodontal disease, 23
Pulpal status of teeth, 54
Pulpal-periodontal relationships, 177
Pyogenic granuloma, 25–26

Radiographic survey, 61–62, *62*
Radiographs in implant maintenance, 202–203
Rapidly progressive periodontitis, 35
Recurrent aphthous stomatitis (canker sores), 211,
    211
Refractory periodontitis, 35
Reinfection and implant maintenance, 201
Replaced flap, 148, *148*
Restorative dentist as member of dental implant
    team, 198
Restorative dentistry, 53–54
Retrograde periodontitis, 207
Rickets, 27
Root amputation, 178
Root concavities, 67
Root coverage, 157
Root detoxification, 86, 87, *102,* 102–103
Root planing, 68, 86, 87
Root preparation, 86
Root resection, 178
Round toothpicks, 80

Scalers, 87–88
    Jacquette, 88
    sickle, 88
    sonic, 92–95, *95*
    ultrasonic, 92–93
Scaling, 68, 86, 221
Scalloping, 163
Screw-retained prosthesis, 196, 198
Scurvy, 27
Secondary occlusal trauma, 71, *72*
Secondary syphilis, 214
Second-generation mouth rinses, 84
Selectins, 42–43, 49

Selective extraction, 182, *182*
Serotonin, 42, 43
Serum complement system, 46–47
Sex hormones, imbalances in, 25–26
Sharpening stones, characteristics of, 240–241
Sharpey's fibers, 11
Sickle cell anemia, 26
Sickle scaler, 88
Smoking
    and necrotizing ulcerative gingivitis, 27–28
    and periodontitis, 18, 39
Soft tissue
    classification based on positioning, 148–151, *149,*
        150
    healing of wounds in, 96–103, *97, 98, 99, 100, 101,*
        102
    management of, 145–151, *146, 148, 149, 150*
Soft tissue survey, 53
Sonic scaler, 92–95, *95*
Stannous fluoride, 129
Steam sterilization, 187
Stomatitis, chronic ulcerative, 226, *233*
Stomatognathic (gnathostomatic) system, 71
Subgingival area, tooth preparation in, 86
Subgingival deposit removal instruments, 88–89
Subgingival plaque, 16
Subperiosteal connective tissue grafts, 159–160
Sulcular (Bass) method of brushing, 76
Sulcus, 162
Superfloss, 79
Suprabony pocket, 32
Supragingival area, tooth preparation in, 86
Supragingival deposits removal instruments, 87–88
    scalers, 87–88
Surgery, periodontal, 64, 223
Surgical dentist as member of dental implant team,
    199
Systemic antibiotic therapy, 223
Systemic diseases, periodontal infections and, 29–30

T cells, 47, 48
T cytotoxic cells, 47
T helper cells, 47
T suppressor cells (Ts), 47
Tactile sensitivity, development of, 87
TAM, (*see* Tooth-accumulated materials (TAM))
Teeth
    extraction of, 68
    prognosis of individual, 65–67, *66, 67*
Temporomandibular joint pain dysfunction syn-
        drome, 215–216
    cause, 215–216
    symptoms, 216
    treatment, 216
Temporomandibular joints, 71
Tetracyclines, 129–130
Three-wall infrabony defect, 160–161
Thrombocytopenia, 26
Tooth accumulated materials (TAM), 14–15, 16*t*
Tooth mobility, effect of bone removal on, 166

Tooth morphology, 65
Tooth preparation, rationale for, 86
Toothbrush abrasion, 20
Toothbrushes
    manual, 76
    manual versus power, 77
    powered (mechanic), 76–77, *77, 78*
Tooth/tooth relationships, 58
Topical fluorides, 222
Transforming growth factor-β (TGF-β), 46, 48
Transient bacteremia, 52–53, 83
Transseptal group, 3, *5*
Treatment planning, 67–68
    bacterial control, 68
    maintenance, 69
    restorative, 69
    surgical therapy, 69
Tumor necrosis factor (TNF), 46, 48
Two-wall infrabony defect, 161

Ulcerative stomatitis, chronic, 226, *233*
Ultrasonic scalers, 92–93

Vertical bone loss, 33
Vertical releasing incisions, *150,* 150–151
Vitamin C deficiency, 27
Vitamin D, 27

Water irrigation systems and plaque removal,
    203
White blood cells, 17
Wound healing, 96–105
    age, 105
    applied to periodontal surgery, 105–106
    asepsis, 105
    healing rate, 105
    involving bone, 103
        fate of autografts, 104
        guided tissue regeneration healing, 104–105
        infrabony defects, 103–104
        replacement grafts, 104
    nutrition and systemic disorders, 105
    soft tissue
        excision of gingiva, 96–97
        flaps, *101,* 101–102
        free gingival grafts, 102
        new attachment, 99–100, *100*
        open, 100–101
        reattachment, 99, *99*
        root detoxification, *102,* 102–103
        simple incision, 97, *98, 99*

Xenografts, 170–171

Young Dental Manufacturing polishing instru-
    ments, 95